Biomarkers in Critical Care

Editor

MITCHELL M. LEVY

CRITICAL CARE CLINICS

www.criticalcare.theclinics.com

Consulting Editor
JOHN A. KELLUM

January 2020 • Volume 36 • Number 1

ELSEVIER

1600 John F. Kennedy Boulevard • Suite 1800 • Philadelphia, Pennsylvania, 19103-2899

http://www.theclinics.com

CRITICAL CARE CLINICS Volume 36, Number 1
January 2020 ISSN 0749-0704, ISBN-13: 978-0-323-68314-2

Editor: Colleen Dietzler
Developmental Editor: Casey Potter

Critical Care Clinics (ISSN: 0749-0704) is published quarterly by Elsevier Inc., 360 Park Avenue South, New York, NY 10010-1710. Months of issue are January, April, July, and October. Business and Editorial Offices: 1600 John F. Kennedy Blvd., Suite 1800, Philadelphia, PA 19103-2899. Customer Service Office: 6277 Sea Harbor Drive, Orlando, FL 32887-4800. Periodicals postage paid at New York, NY and additional mailing offices. Subscription prices are $250.00 per year for US individuals, $683.00 per year for US institutions, $100.00 per year for US students and residents, $285.00 per year for Canadian individuals, $856.00 per year for Canadian institutions, $318.00 per year for international individuals, $856.00 per year for international institutions, $100.00 per year for Canadian students/residents, and $150.00 per year for foreign students/residents. To receive student/resident rate, orders must be accompanied by name of affiliated institution, date of term, and the signature of program/residency coordinator on institution letterhead. Orders will be billed at individual rate until proof of status is received. Foreign air speed delivery is included in all *Clinics* subscription prices. All prices are subject to change without notice. POSTMASTER: Send address changes to *Critical Care Clinics*, Elsevier Periodicals Customer Service, 11830 Westline Industrial Drive, St. Louis, MO 63146. **Customer Service: 1-800-654-2452 (US). From outside of the US, call 1-314-447-8871. Fax: 1-314-447-8029. E-mail: journalscustomerservice-usa@elsevier.com (for print support) or journalsonlinesupport-usa@elsevier.com (for online support).**

Reprints. For copies of 100 or more of articles in this publication, please contact the Commercial Reprints Department, Elsevier Inc., 360 Park Avenue South, New York, NY 10010-1710. Tel.: 212-633-3874; Fax: 212-633-3820; E-mail: reprints@elsevier.com.

Critical Care Clinics is also published in Spanish by Editorial Inter-Medica, Junin 917, 1er A, 1113, Buenos Aires, Argentina.

Critical Care Clinics is covered in *MEDLINE/PubMed (Index Medicus), EMBASE/Excerpta Medica, Current Concepts/ Clinical Medicine, ISI/BIOMED, and Chemical Abstracts.*

Contributors

CONSULTING EDITOR

JOHN A. KELLUM, MD, MCCM
Professor, Critical Care Medicine, Medicine, Bioengineering and Clinical and Translational Science, Director, Center for Critical Care Nephrology, The CRISMA Center, Vice Chair for Research, Department of Critical Care Medicine, University of Pittsburgh School of Medicine, Pittsburgh, Pennsylvania, USA

EDITOR

MITCHELL M. LEVY, MD, MCCM
Professor of Medicine, Chief, Division of Pulmonary, Critical Care, and Sleep Medicine, The Warren Alpert Medical School of Brown University, Rhode Island Hospital, Providence, Rhode Island, USA

AUTHORS

ALFRED AYALA, PhD
Division of Surgical Research, Professor, Department of Surgery, Brown University, Rhode Island Hospital, Providence, Rhode Island, USA

JAN BAKKER, MD, PhD
Division of Pulmonary, Critical Care, and Sleep Medicine, New York University School of Medicine, Bellevue Hospital, Department Pulmonology and Critical Care, Columbia University Medical Center, New York, New York, USA; Department Intensive Care Adults, Erasmus MC University Medical Center, Rotterdam, Netherlands; Department of Intensive Care, Pontificia Universidad Católica de Chile, Santiago, Chile

DEBASREE BANERJEE, MD, MS
Division of Pulmonary, Critical Care, and Sleep Medicine, Assistant Professor, The Warren Alpert School of Medicine at Brown University, Division of Pulmonary, Critical Care, and Sleep Medicine, Rhode Island Hospital, Providence, Rhode Island, USA

ELISA BOGOSSIAN, MD
Fellow, Department of Intensive Care, Erasme University Hospital, Brussels, Belgium

CAROLYN S. CALFEE, MD, MAS
Professor, Departments of Medicine and Anesthesia, Cardiovascular Research Institute, University of California, San Francisco, San Francisco, California, USA

SUSAN R. CONWAY, MD
Division of Critical Care Medicine, Children's National Medical Center; Assistant Professor, Department of Pediatrics, George Washington University School of Medicine, Washington, DC, USA

SÉBASTIEN GIBOT, MD, PhD
CHRU Nancy, Hôpital Central, Service de Réanimation Médicale, Nancy, France;
INSERM UMRS-1116, Faculté de Médecine Nancy, Université de Lorraine, Vandoeuvre-les-Nancy, France

CHYNA C. GRAY, BA
Molecular Biology, Cell Biology and Biochemistry Department, Brown University, Rhode Island Hospital, Providence, Rhode Island, USA

BACHAR HAMADE, MD, MSc
Clinical Instructor, Department of Emergency Medicine, and Clinical Associate, Department of Surgery - Surgical Critical Care, American University of Beirut Medical Center, Beirut, Lebanon; Adjunct Faculty, Department of Critical Care Medicine, University of Pittsburgh Medical Center, Pittsburgh, Pennsylvania, USA

DAITHI S. HEFFERNAN, MD, FACS, AFRCSI
Divisions of Surgical Research and Trauma and Surgical Critical Care, Associate Professor, Department of Surgery, Brown University, Rhode Island Hospital, Providence, Rhode Island, USA

DAVID T. HUANG, MD, MPH
Professor, Departments of Critical Care Medicine and Emergency Medicine, The MACRO (Multidisciplinary Acute Care Research Organization) and CRISMA (Clinical Research, Investigation, and Systems Modeling of Acute illness) Centers, University of Pittsburgh, Pittsburgh, Pennsylvania, USA

GREGORY D. JAY, MD, PhD
Department of Emergency Medicine, Alpert Medical School, Brown University, Vice Chair for Research, Department of Emergency Medicine, Research Laboratory, Rhode Island Hospital, Providence, Rhode Island, USA

JOHN A. KELLUM, MD, MCCM
Professor, Critical Care Medicine, Medicine, Bioengineering and Clinical and Translational Science, Director, Center for Critical Care Nephrology, The CRISMA Center, Vice Chair for Research, Department of Critical Care Medicine, University of Pittsburgh School of Medicine, Pittsburgh, Pennsylvania, USA

GUNNAR LACHMANN, MD
Department of Anesthesiology and Operative Intensive Care Medicine (CCM, CVK), Charité – Universitätsmedizin Berlin, corporate member of Freie Universität Berlin, Humboldt-Universität zu Berlin, and Berlin Institute of Health, Berlin, Germany

JISOO LEE, MD
Division of Pulmonary, Critical Care, and Sleep Medicine, Fellow, The Warren Alpert School of Medicine at Brown University, Division of Pulmonary, Critical Care, and Sleep Medicine, Rhode Island Hospital, Providence, Rhode Island, USA

JÉRÉMIE LEMARIÉ, MD, PhD
CHRU Nancy, Hôpital Central, Service de Réanimation Médicale, Nancy, France;
INSERM UMRS-1116, Faculté de Médecine Nancy, Université de Lorraine, Vandoeuvre-les-Nancy, France

MITCHELL M. LEVY, MD, MCCM
Professor of Medicine, Chief, Division of Pulmonary, Critical Care, and Sleep Medicine, The Warren Alpert Medical School of Brown University, Rhode Island Hospital, Providence, Rhode Island, USA

MARCO MENOZZI, MD
Fellow, Department of Intensive Care, Erasme University Hospital, Brussels, Belgium

ABINAV K. MISRA, MD
Division of Pulmonary, Critical Care, and Sleep Medicine, Alpert Medical School of Brown University, Providence, Rhode Island, USA

SEAN F. MONAGHAN, MD, FACS
Divisions of Surgical Research and Trauma and Surgical Critical Care, Assistant Professor, Department of Surgery, Brown University, Rhode Island Hospital, Providence, Rhode Island, USA

VIKRAMJIT MUKHERJEE, MD
Division of Pulmonary, Critical Care, and Sleep Medicine, New York University School of Medicine, Bellevue Hospital, New York, New York, USA

CHRISTOPHER MULLIN, MD, MHS
Division of Pulmonary, Critical Care, and Sleep Medicine, Warren Alpert Medical School of Brown University, Providence, Rhode Island, USA

STEVEN M. OPAL, MD
Clinical Professor of Medicine, Infectious Disease Division, Alpert Medical School of Brown University, Ocean State Clinical Coordinating Center at Rhode Island Hospital, Providence, Rhode Island, USA

HOOMAN D. POOR, MD
Division of Pulmonary, Critical Care, and Sleep Medicine, Icahn School of Medicine at Mount Sinai Hospital, New York, New York, USA

RADU POSTELNICU, MD
Division of Pulmonary, Critical Care, and Sleep Medicine, New York University School of Medicine, Bellevue Hospital, New York, New York, USA

NATASHA M. PRADHAN, MBBS
Division of Pulmonary, Critical Care, and Sleep Medicine, Icahn School of Medicine at Mount Sinai Hospital, New York, New York, USA

KONRAD REINHART, MD
Department of Anesthesiology and Operative Intensive Care Medicine (CCM, CVK), Charité – Universitätsmedizin Berlin, corporate member of Freie Universität Berlin, Humboldt-Universität zu Berlin, and Berlin Institute of Health, Berlin, Germany; Jena University Hospital, BIH Visiting Professor/Stiftung Charité, Jena, Germany

HOLLY RICHENDRFER, PhD
Department of Emergency Medicine, Alpert Medical School, Brown University, Postdoctoral Fellow, Department of Emergency Medicine, Research Laboratory, Rhode Island Hospital, Providence, Rhode Island, USA

AARTIK SARMA, MD
Postdoctoral Fellow, Department of Medicine, University of California, San Francisco, San Francisco, California, USA

NATTACHAI SRISAWAT, MD, PhD
Division of Nephrology, Department of Medicine, Faculty of Medicine, Chulalongkorn University, and King Chulalongkorn Memorial Hospital, Bangkok, Thailand; Department of Critical Care Medicine, Center for Critical Care Nephrology, The CRISMA Center,

University of Pittsburgh School of Medicine, Pittsburgh, Pennsylvania, USA; Excellence Center for Critical Care Nephrology, King Chulalongkorn Memorial Hospital, Bangkok, Thailand; Critical Care Nephrology Research Unit, Chulalongkorn University, Bangkok, Thailand; Academic of Science, Royal Society of Thailand, Bangkok, Thailand; Tropical Medicine Cluster, Chulalongkorn University, Bangkok, Thailand

JEAN-LOUIS VINCENT, MD, PhD
Professor of Intensive Care Medicine, Université libre de Bruxelles, Consultant, Department of Intensive Care, Erasme University Hospital, Brussels, Belgium

MICHELLE E. WAKELEY, MD
Division of Surgical Research, Department of Surgery, Brown University, Rhode Island Hospital, Providence, Rhode Island, USA

NICHOLAS S. WARD, MD, FCCM
Division of Pulmonary, Critical Care, and Sleep Medicine, Alpert Medical School of Brown University, Providence, Rhode Island, USA

LORRAINE B. WARE, MD
Professor, Departments of Medicine, and Pathology, Microbiology, and Immunology, Vanderbilt University School of Medicine, Allergy, Pulmonary and Critical Care Medicine, Vanderbilt University Medical Center, Nashville, Tennessee, USA

XAVIER WITTEBOLE, MD
Assistant Professor, Critical Care Department, Cliniques Universitaires Saint-Luc, Brussels, Belgium

HECTOR R. WONG, MD
Division of Critical Care Medicine, Cincinnati Children's Hospital Medical Center, Cincinnati Children's Research Foundation; Professor, Department of Pediatrics, University of Cincinnati College of Medicine, Cincinnati, Ohio, USA

Contents

The History of Biomarkers: How Far Have We Come?   1

Gunnar Lachmann and Konrad Reinhart

> Sepsis is one of the oldest and most elusive syndromes in medicine that is still incompletely understood. Biomarkers may help to transform sepsis from a physiologic syndrome to a group of distinct biochemical disorders. This will help to differentiate between systemic inflammation of infectious and noninfectious origin and aid therapeutic decision making, hence improve the prognosis for patients, guide antimicrobial therapy, and foster the development of novel adjunctive sepsis therapies. To reach this goal requires increased systematic investigation that includes twenty-first century scientific approaches and technologies and appropriate clinical evaluation.

Biomarkers of Infection and Sepsis   11

Steven M. Opal and Xavier Wittebole

> The role of biomarkers for detection of sepsis has come a long way. Molecular biomarkers are taking front stage at present, but machine learning and other computational measures using bigdata sets are promising. Clinical research in sepsis is hampered by lack of specificity of the diagnosis; sepsis is a syndrome with no uniformly agreed definition. This lack of diagnostic precision means there is no gold standard for this diagnosis. The final conclusion is expert opinion, which is not bad but not perfect. Perhaps machine learning will displace expert opinion as the final and most accurate definition for sepsis.

Procalcitonin: Where Are We Now?   23

Bachar Hamade and David T. Huang

> Procalcitonin is a biomarker that is generally elevated in bacterial infections. This review describes a conceptual framework for biomarkers using lessons from the history of troponin, applies this framework to procalcitonin with a review of observational studies and randomized trials in and out of the intensive care unit, and concludes with clinical recommendations and thoughts on how to test a test.

Soluble Triggering Receptor Expressed on Myeloid Cells-1: Diagnosis or Prognosis?   41

Jérémie Lemarié and Sébastien Gibot

> The diagnosis of sepsis, and especially its differentiation from sterile inflammation, may be challenging. The triggering receptor expressed on myeloid cells-1 is an amplifier of the innate immune response. Its soluble form is detectable in various biological fluids and can be used as a

surrogate marker of triggering receptor expressed on myeloid cells-1 activation. In this article, we review the abundant literature evaluating the usefulness of soluble triggering receptor expressed on myeloid cells-1 for the diagnosis and the prognosis evaluation of sepsis or localized infections.

Proteoglycan 4 (or lubricin), a mucin-like glycoprotein, was originally classified as a lubricating substance within diarthrodial joints. More recently, lubricin has been found in other tissues and has been implicated in 2 inflammatory pathways within the cell, via the Toll-like receptors (TLRs) and CD44. Lubricin is an antagonist of TLR2 and TLR4, and appears to enter cells via the CD44 receptor. Because of lubricin's action on these receptors, downstream processes of inflammation are halted, thereby preventing release of cytokines (a hallmark of inflammation and sepsis) from the cell, indicating lubricin's role as a biomarker and possible therapeutic for sepsis.

Checkpoint regulators are a group of membrane-bound receptors or ligands expressed on immune cells to regulate the immune cell response to antigen presentation and other immune stimuli, such as cytokines, chemokines, and complement. In the context of profound immune activation, such as sepsis, the immune system can be rendered anergic by these receptors to prevent excessive inflammation and tissue damage. If this septic immunosuppression is prolonged, the host is unable to mount the appropriate immune response to a secondary insult or infection. This article describes the manner in which major regulators in the B7-CD28 family and their ligands mediate immunosuppression in sepsis.

Biomarker panels have the potential to advance the field of critical care medicine by stratifying patients according to prognosis and/or underlying pathophysiology. This article discusses the discovery and validation of biomarker panels, along with their translation to the clinical setting. The current literature on the use of biomarker panels in sepsis, acute respiratory distress syndrome, and acute kidney injury is reviewed.

Metabolomics is an emerging field of research interest in sepsis. Metabolomics provides new ways of exploring the diagnosis, mechanism, and prognosis of sepsis. Advancements in technologies have enabled significant improvements in identifying novel biomarkers associated with the disease progress of sepsis. The use of metabolomics in the critically ill may provide new approaches to enable precision medicine. Furthermore, the dynamic interactions of the host and its microbiome can lead to further progression of sepsis. Understanding these interactions and the changes in the host's genomics and the microbiome can provide novel preventive and therapeutic strategies against sepsis.

that are based on broad, clinically available criteria and include patients with heterogeneous biology. This heterogeneity is a barrier to developing and testing effective therapies for these syndromes. Biomarkers identify clinically distinct molecular phenotypes of ARDS and sepsis. These molecular phenotypes are associated with differences in mortality and predict response to several treatments in retrospective analyses of clinical trials. Biomarkers can be used for prognostic and predictive enrichment of clinical trials in critical illness to incorporate precision medicine in critical care.

It is now recognized that sepsis is not a uniformly proinflammatory state. There is a well-recognized counter anti-inflammatory response that occurs in many patients. The timing and magnitude of this response varies considerably and thus makes its identification and manipulation more difficult. Studies in animals and humans have now identified a small number of biologic responses that characterize this immunosuppressed state, such as lymphocyte death, HLA receptor downregulation, and monocyte exhaustion. Researchers are now trying to use these as markers of individual immunosuppression to predict outcomes and identify patients who would and would not benefit from new immune stimulatory therapies.

Numerous compounds have been tested as potential biomarkers for multiple possible applications within intensive care medicine but none is or will ever be sufficiently specific or sensitive for the heterogeneous syndromes of critical illness. New technology and access to huge patient databases are providing new biomarker options and the focus is shifting to combinations of several or multiple biomarkers rather than the single markers that research has concentrated on in the past. Biomarkers will increasingly be used as part of routine clinical practice in the future, complementing clinical examination and physician expertise to provide accurate disease diagnosis, prediction of complications, personalized treatment guidance, and prognosis.

CRITICAL CARE CLINICS

SERIES OF RELATED INTEREST

Emergency Medicine Clinics
Available at: https://www.emed.theclinics.com/

THE CLINICS ARE AVAILABLE ONLINE!
Access your subscription at:
www.theclinics.com

CRITICAL CARE CLINICS

Preface

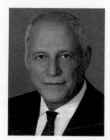

Mitchell M. Levy, MD, MCCM
Editor

Prompt diagnosis and early intervention are now recognized as an essential factor in survival of critical illness. This is certainly true for both sepsis and acute respiratory distress syndrome, the two most common disease states with which we are faced in critical care. We last edited an issue of *Critical Care Clinics* on "Biomarkers in the Critically Ill Patient" in 2011. It would be great if I were able to report that, over the past 9 to 10 years, we have made remarkable progress in the field and can now use biomarkers for early diagnosis, precision targeting for guiding the use of new therapeutic agents, inclusion criteria in large randomized controlled trials, or to determine specific risk profiles that facilitate clinical decision making in the emergency department and the medical wards. But clear and convincing studies, irrefutably establishing a single biomarker or biomarker panel for diagnosing sepsis, guiding sepsis therapeutics, or predicting morbidity and mortality are lacking.

A biomarker is a protein or specific molecule that can be objectively measured as an indicator of normal biological processes, pathogenic processes, or pharmacologic responses to a therapeutic intervention. The ideal biomarker would be highly sensitive and specific for a given disease state and have biologic plausibility. Biomarkers might be predictive or prognostic and be valuable in assessing the likelihood of patient outcomes or predicting response to therapeutic interventions. Ultimately, a widely utilized biomarker must have the capability of being easily measured and rapidly reported.

In this issue of *Critical Care Clinics*, a group of highly regarded experts in the field revisit the use of biomarkers in several areas and disease states in the critically ill. Without question, we are moving toward (albeit too slowly for many of us) the use of biomarkers for precision medicine and individualized therapy in critical care. This issue contains valuable articles that will guide the reader through a deeper understanding of the current and potential future role of biomarkers in various disease states commonly seen in the critically ill patient. There are helpful articles on rapid identification of infection as well as thorough reviews on procalcitonin, lactate, soluble TREM 1, and Lubricin, all potential markers or targets for therapeutic interventions. Biomarkers and right ventricular dysfunction are discussed along with the potential for using biomarkers for predicting renal dysfunction. There are also several articles in this issue

Crit Care Clin 36 (2020) xiii–xiv
https://doi.org/10.1016/j.ccc.2019.10.001
0749-0704/20/© 2019 Published by Elsevier Inc.

criticalcare.theclinics.com

in which the biomarkers that might identify the immunosuppressed phase of sepsis are discussed as well as the possible use of checkpoint inhibitors as therapeutic targets. Finally, there are important articles on the future of biomarkers as we move into the reality of precision medicine.

Overall, readers should find this issue both helpful and important in understanding the progress and potential for the use of biomarkers in critical care.

Mitchell M. Levy, MD, MCCM
Division of Pulmonary, Critical Care
and Sleep Medicine
The Warren Alpert Medical School of
Brown University
Rhode Island Hospital
593 Eddy Street
4th Floor Main Building
Providence, RI 02903, USA

E-mail address:
Mitchell_Levy@Brown.edu

The History of Biomarkers
How Far Have We Come?

Gunnar Lachmann, MD[a,b], Konrad Reinhart, MD[a,b,c],*

KEYWORDS

- Sepsis • Biomarker • History

KEY POINTS

- Despite a long history, diagnosis and therapy of sepsis remains challenging.
- The ideal sepsis biomarker still needs to be elucidated.
- Procalcitonin helps to guide antibiotic stewardship and other promising biomarkers are currently evaluated.
- Theranostics with biomarkers and omics approaches may help to foster precision medicine in sepsis.
- Identifying of more specific and sensitive sepsis biomarkers is crucial for the improvement of sepsis care and the development of novel therapeutic approaches.

THE HISTORY OF SEPSIS

The Greek physician Hippocrates (460–370 BC) first described "sepsis" as "when continuing fever is present, it is dangerous if the outer parts are cold, but the inner parts are burning hot"[1] (**Fig. 1**). The dilemma in the diagnosis and treatment of sepsis was then postulated by the Florentine philosopher Machiavelli (1469–1527): "As the physicians say of hectic fever, that in the beginning of the malady it is difficult to detect but easy to treat, but in the course of time, having been neither detected nor treated in the beginning, it becomes easy to detect but difficult to treat."[2] In 1904, Sir William Osler (1849–1919) was the first who pointed to the fundamental role of the host's immune response in sepsis: "Except on few occasions, the patient seems to die from the

Disclosure Statement: The authors declare no conflicts of interest.
[a] Department of Anesthesiology and Operative Intensive Care Medicine (CCM, CVK), Charité – Universitätsmedizin Berlin, corporate member of Freie Universität Berlin, Humboldt-Universität zu Berlin, and Berlin Institute of Health, Augustenburger Platz 1, D-13353 Berlin, Germany; [b] Berlin Institute of Health, Anna-Louisa-Karsch-Straße 2, D-10178 Berlin, Germany; [c] Jena University Hospital, Carl-Zeiss-Straße 12, D-07743 Jena, Germany
* Corresponding author. Department of Anesthesiology and Operative Intensive Care Medicine (CCM, CVK), Charité – Universitätsmedizin Berlin, corporate member of Freie Universität Berlin, Humboldt-Universität zu Berlin, and Berlin Institute of Health, Augustenburger Platz 1, D-13353 Berlin Germany.
E-mail address: Konrad.Reinhart@charite.de

Crit Care Clin 36 (2020) 1–10
https://doi.org/10.1016/j.ccc.2019.08.001
0749-0704/20/© 2019 Elsevier Inc. All rights reserved.

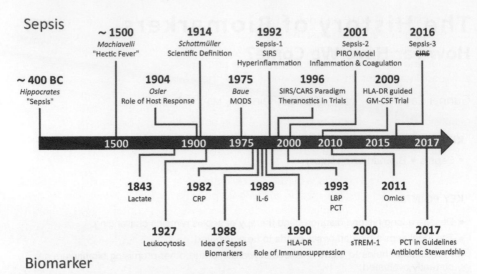

Fig. 1. History of sepsis and important biomarkers. CARS, compensatory anti-inflammatory response syndrome; GM-CSF, granulocyte-macrophage colony-stimulating factor; MODS, multiple-organ dysfunction syndrome.

body's response to infection rather than from it." A few years later in 1914, Hugo Schottmüller first defined sepsis in a scientific manner: "Sepsis is a state caused by microbial invasion from a local infectious source into the bloodstream which leads to signs of systemic illness in remote organs."[3] Before the development of intensive care therapy, patients with sepsis frequently succumbed due to irreversible shock within days to hours, before progressive multiple-organ failure, as known today, could develop. An important milestone was in 1975, when A. Baue described "Multiple, progressive or sequential systems failure. A syndrome of the 1970s," which was previously unknown in the pre–intensive care unit (ICU) era.[4]

According to the first sepsis consensus conference in 1992,[5] today termed "sepsis-1,"[5] sepsis was defined as a primarily proinflammatory systemic response syndrome (SIRS) due to an underlying or suspected infection. The presence of at least 2 of the 4 so-called SIRS criteria was mandatory for the definition of sepsis. Sepsis was graded into sepsis (at least SIRS criteria but no organ dysfunction), severe sepsis (sepsis plus at least 1 organ dysfunction), and septic shock (refractory shock despite adequate fluid resuscitation). Over the following years it was better understood that the proinflammatory SIRS from the very beginning is accompanied by an compensatory anti-inflammatory response.[6] In 2001, the sepsis-1 consensus definition was revised and acknowledged that a number of additional clinical signs and laboratory parameters may be present; in retrospect, this consensus was termed "sepsis-2."[7] Within sepsis-2, the PIRO conceptual framework (predisposition, pathogen, host response, and organ dysfunction) was introduced as a staging system for sepsis and critical illness, an analogy to the TNM system (tumor, metastasis, and lymph nodes) in oncology, which facilitated research and treatment of cancer by enabling practitioners to gauge the severity and prognosis of cancer.[8] Because the SIRS criteria are sensitive but lack specificity and, thus, sepsis may be present in 8% to 10% of cases without 2 SIRS criteria, a third sepsis consensus process was initiated by the American and the European societies of intensive care medicine: Society of Critical Care Medicine and European Society of Intensive Care Medicine. The results, called sepsis-3 definition, were published in 2016 and defined sepsis as a "Life-threatening organ dysfunction caused by a dysregulated host response to infection."[9] This definition no longer comprises the SIRS criteria as part of the sepsis definition but requires the presence of an infection-induced organ dysfunction sepsis and omits the term severe sepsis. An elevated lactate serum level became part of the definition of septic shock and is considered as an independent predictor of mortality. For 2 reasons, the sepsis-3 definition raised a lot of controversy, (1) because lactate has become part of the definition of septic shock, a laboratory parameter that is not easily available in low and middle income settings, and (2) the introduction of the quick sequential organ failure assessment score as a tool for the early detection of sepsis, which lacks sensitivity in comparison with the SIRS criteria or early warning scores like the National Early Warning Score.[10,11] Despite all efforts, a diagnostic gold standard for sepsis is still pending and the diagnosis remains on clinical judgment, positive blood cultures often taking several days, and nonspecific inflammatory biomarkers. Nowadays, sepsis and its long-term sequelae are seen as a "hidden public health disaster"[12] and the World Health Organization (WHO) recently acknowledged sepsis as a global health priority.[13] Overall, sepsis is the most common cause of death in hospitalized patients and the WHO recognizes most of the sepsis deaths are avoidable by better prevention, early recognition, and improved diagnosis and clinical management. Many patients with sepsis outside the ICU are frequently unrecognized due to incomplete documentation of infection-related organ dysfunctions.[14,15]

The understanding of sepsis pathophysiology has increased over the past decades, but is still incompletely understood.[16,17] Billions of dollars were invested for a therapeutic breakthrough to develop promising new sepsis diagnostics and therapies. However, until now no clinical interventional study has been able to show a modulation of the patients' immune response or an improved survival.[18] This failure must be attributed to a large degree to the lack of stratification systems targeting treatment toward those who are most likely to benefit.[19]

Biomarkers in Sepsis

Biomarkers have been defined as indicators of biological and pathogenic processes, or pharmacologic responses to a therapeutic intervention that defines what is normal while predicting or detecting what is abnormal.[20,21] Although microbial cultures take several days to obtain results and are nonspecific, biomarkers have been suggested to improve decision making for sepsis care by a rapid diagnosis of sepsis and initiation of therapy.[22]

The International Sepsis Forum in 2005 first systematically addressed the importance of biomarkers in sepsis research.[22] The ideal sepsis biomarker needs to be highly sensitive and specific for sepsis and reliably differentiate between infectious and noninfectious causes of inflammation, organ dysfunction, and shock. Furthermore, the biomarker should be present before the appearance of clinical sepsis signs, have prognostic value, and indicate the course of sepsis, as well as its severity. However, currently there is no ideal biomarker that fully fulfills all these requirements.

The idea of a sepsis biomarker came up in 1988, when Hoyt and colleagues[23] reported lymphocyte changes to be predictive of sepsis. Because of the complex sepsis pathophysiology that comprises a large number of molecular mechanisms, more than 180 markers over the past decades have been identified as potential biomarkers of sepsis, of which only 20% were examined in studies for diagnostic use in sepsis.[24] The most investigated biomarkers in sepsis are procalcitonin (PCT), C-reactive protein (CRP), interleukin (IL)-6, soluble triggering receptor expressed on myeloid cells 1 (sTREM-1), presepsin, and lipopolysaccharide binding protein (LBP).[25]

It was the German physician-chemist Johann Joseph Scherer (1814–1869) in 1843 who first described lactate in human blood as a pathologic finding in septic shock.[26] Centuries later, lactate emerged as a sepsis screening parameter with high specificity but low sensitivity.[27] As elevated lactate levels are positively correlated with sepsis mortality, they were included into the sepsis-3 definition for septic shock.[28]

In 1927, leukocytosis was first mentioned in a study of patients inter alia with sepsis.[29] Nowadays, leukocytosis is the commonly used laboratory parameter for prediction of bacterial infections and sepsis, although it has only a very low sensitivity and specificity.[30–32]

Discovered in 1930[33] and first described in the context of sepsis in 1982,[34] CRP constitutes the traditional marker of inflammation. It is besides leukocytes the most frequently used sepsis biomarker in clinical practice today but inferior to PCT in most sepsis studies.[25] The flaws of CRP are its delayed response and late peak after 36 to 50 hours.[35]

The IL-6 gene was isolated in 1986.[36] Three years later in 1989, IL-6 was studied in patients with sepsis.[37] Currently, IL-6 is less frequently used and also inferior to PCT.[25] However, the very fast response of IL-6 to infection is seen as a favorable feature of this biomarker.

CD64 on immune cells has been described since 1989,[38,39] whereas investigation of CD64 on neutrophils as a biomarker of sepsis started in 1999.[40] Currently, CD64 from neutrophils still needs to be elucidated in clinical routine, but first studies showed promising results with sensitivity and specificity of more than 80%, which would be superior to PCT.[25]

LBP was discovered in humans in 1990[41] and first studied in sepsis models in 1993.[42] During sepsis, LBP levels rise to median peak levels of 30 to 40 µg/mL within 24 hours.[43] Today it is known that LBP has only a low diagnostic accuracy for sepsis.[25]

In 1990, HLA-DR on monocytes was found as a marker of disease severity.[44] Today, HLA-DR on monocytes is a promising sepsis biomarker that allows monitoring of the immune status and recognition of immunosuppression, which may identify patients who might benefit from immune stimulatory treatment.

In 1993, Assicot and colleagues[45] were the first who described PCT as a potential biomarker for sepsis and infection. Currently, PCT is the most studied biomarker in sepsis and the only biomarker that is integrated into international ICU guidelines.[46] PCT shows a more convenient profile than CRP and cytokines because it increases within 4 to 12 hours after onset of infection.[47] Its sensitivity and specificity is in the range of 80%.[48] PCT is the first infection and sepsis biomarker whose use to guide antibiotic therapy was associated not only with a reduction of the duration of antimicrobial therapy but also with improved patient survival.[49] In a randomized controlled trial that comprised 1575 ICU patients with severe infections and sepsis, mortality at 28 days was 149 (20%) of 761 patients in the PCT-guided group and 196 (25%) of 785 patients in the standard-of-care group (between-group absolute difference 5.4%, 95% confidence interval 1.2–9.5, $P = .0122$).[49] A Cochrane meta-analysis on the impact of PCT-guided initiation or discontinuation of antibiotics found that the shorter time on antibiotics in this group was associated with a 1% lower mortality rate.[50]

In 2000, TREM-1 and its soluble form sTREM-1 were discovered.[51] Since then, several studies examined sTREM-1 levels as a biomarker for the diagnosis of sepsis suggesting sTREM-1 with modest diagnostic performance in differentiating sepsis from noninfectious SIRS, which is comparable to PCT.[52]

Presepsin, which is released from macrophages during sepsis, was found in 2004.[53] It is elevated before PCT and IL-6 and, therefore, seen as very early marker of sepsis.[54] However, results are inconsistent and need further investigation before being implemented as a routine sepsis marker.

Combinations of biomarkers reflecting various aspects of the host response have been proposed to overcome limitations of single biomolecules. A panel consisting of serum concentrations of sTREM-1 and PCT and the expression of the polymorpho-nuclear CD64 index in flow cytometry, called the "bioscore" was higher in patients with sepsis than in all others (P<.001 for the 3 markers).[55] These biomarkers were all inde-pendent predictors of infection, with the best receiver-operator characteristic curve being obtained for the PMN CD64 index, whereas the performance of the combination was better than that of each individual biomarker. This was also externally confirmed in a validation cohort.

The Role of Theranostic in the Evaluation of Novel Sepsis Therapies

The first theranostic approach in the evaluation of novel adjunctive sepsis therapies was derived from the RAMSES study in 2001. The results of this phase II trial suggested that a monoclonal antibody against tumor necrosis factor alpha (TNF-α) is more effective in patients with IL-6 blood concentrations of greater than 1000 pg/mL.[56] This hypothesis was tested in the follow-up phase III MONARCS trial for which patients with severe sepsis were prospectively stratified by IL-6 levels into low-risk and high-risk groups (IL-6 >1000 pg/mL) by an IL-6 bedside test.[57] However, the differences of the efficacy of this anti-TNF-α antibody in terms of mortality differences between the high and the low risk did not reach statistical difference. However, post-hoc analyses suggested that this antibody was highly effective in those patients with IL-6 levels over a cutoff of greater than 5000 pg/mL. In 1997, Docke and colleagues[58] reported the restoration of HLA-DR and sepsis recovery in 8 of 9 patients with low HLA-DR expression after interferon-γ application. In an investigator-initiated phase II trial, Meisel and col-leagues[59] in a small pilot study in 2009 also used a theranostic approach to investigate the impact of granulocyte-macrophage colony-stimulating factor (GM-CSF) in immune paralyzed patients for which HLA-DR testing was part of the inclusion criteria, and found decreased time of ventilation and a shortening of the ICU and hospital length of stay. Further studies that evaluate the efficacy of immune stimulation in which indicators of the immune status of patients are part of the inclusion criteria are in progress. The EUPHRATES trial used elevated blood endotoxin levels to compare conventional ther-apy alone among patients with septic shock and high endotoxin activity with removal of endotoxin by polymyxin B hemoperfusion in addition to conventional therapy but failed to show any survival benefit.[60]

The improved understanding of the interplay between coagulation and inflammation fostered the interest in coagulation parameters and tests like thrombocyte count, in-ternational normalized ratio (INR), antithrombin (AT) III, and protein C blood levels for the identification of patients who might benefit from therapies with recombinant AT III, activated protein C (APC), or recombinant tissue factor pathway inhibitor (rTFPI). However, the according trials with AT III[61] as well as with rTFPI,[62] albeit with promising results in phase II trials, were not effective in phase III trials. The PROWESS trial used APC treatment, which appeared to be promising in 2001 in patients with severe sepsis,[63] but was withdrawn in 2011 because of the lack of efficacy shown by the PROWESS-SHOCK trial.[12]

Recent advances in genetic and biochemical analyses now allow genotyping and biochemical characterization of large groups of patients via the "omics" technologies. In 2011, the upcoming technical progress and advances in bioinformatics led to ana-lyses of thousands of transcriptomics,[64] proteomics,[65] and metabolomics.[66] These new opportunities could lead to a paradigm shift in the approach to sepsis toward personalized treatments with interventions targeted toward specific pathophysiolog-ical mechanisms activated in the patient.

There is promise that omics-based molecular fingerprints may not only help to better understand the pathophysiology of sepsis but also to support clinical decision making in the near future.[67–69]

HOW FAR HAVE WE COME?

There is still a discrepancy between diagnosis and treatment of sepsis, which is elegantly characterized by C. Nathan: "It makes no sense to use twenty-first century technology to develop drugs targeted at specific infections whose diagnosis is delayed by nineteenth-century methods."[70] Importantly, the lack of reliable and safe biomarkers leads to diagnostic uncertainty possibly resulting in delays of lifesaving supportive and antiinfective therapies or overuse of antimicrobial agents.[71] No biomarker is currently available to discriminate reliably between infectious sepsis and noninfectious SIRS. Diagnosis and treatment initiation remains a clinical decision by the treating physicians based on the history of the patients, physiologic criteria, physical examination, laboratory values, symptoms of infection, and acute organ dysfunctions. However, first studies and meta-analyses suggest that the use of sepsis biomarkers may support the decision to initiate and to terminate antimicrobial therapy and even may contribute to improved patient relevant outcomes. Overall, the concept of personalized medicine appears to be promising also in the field of sepsis research, which has already been successfully established in other fields.[72] However, proof of the usefulness of sepsis biomarkers for identifying the most appropriate patient populations for the assessment of innovative adjunctive sepsis therapies is still missing. Nevertheless, there are a number of new single biomarkers and molecular fingerprints that are based on omics technologies that currently are under intense clinical evaluation.

An important issue in biomarker research is that to date there is no pathologic gold standard for sepsis. This makes the evaluation of the clinical utility of novel sepsis biomarkers more difficult. However, at the end of the day they will only become integrated into the diagnosis and clinical management of sepsis if they provide more information than conventional clinical judgment and laboratory parameters in terms of improved patient outcomes and cost-effectiveness. Likewise, their future role in the development of innovative adjunctive sepsis therapies will depend on the potential to enrich patient populations that might benefit most from such therapies, which are aimed at modifying the host response and related biochemical alterations or to augment the immune system in patients with immune suppression.

SUMMARY

Despite the undeniable progress of the understanding of the pathophysiology of sepsis over the past decades, we have not yet been able to identify a single sepsis biomarker that covers all diagnostic needs and this will probably also be the case for the future. However, there is progress especially in terms of support in the initiation and termination of antimicrobial therapy by the use of biomarkers and novel biomarkers. Moreover, molecular fingerprints will very likely help us to develop personalized medicine also in the field of sepsis and to foster the development of novel sepsis therapies.

ACKNOWLEDGEMENTS

Gunnar Lachmann is participant of the BIH Charité Clinician Scientist Program funded by the Charité – Universitätsmedizin Berlin and the Berlin Institute of Health (BIH).

REFERENCES

1. Gruithuisen VPF. Hippocrates des Zweyten. ächte medizinische Schriften, ins Deutsche übersetzt. Munich (Germany): Ignaz Josef Lentner; 1814.
2. Machiavelli N. The Prince, translated by WK Marriott. Adelaide (SA): eBooks@Adelaide, The University of Adelaide Library, University of Adelaide; 2002.
3. Schottmueller H. Wesen und Behandlung der Sepsis. Inn Med 1914;31:257–80.
4. Baue AE. Multiple, progressive, or sequential systems failure. A syndrome of the 1970s. Arch Surg 1975;110(7):779–81.
5. Bone RC, Balk RA, Cerra FB, et al. Definitions for sepsis and organ failure and guidelines for the use of innovative therapies in sepsis. The ACCP/SCCM consensus conference Committee. American College of Chest Physicians/Society of Critical Care Medicine. Chest 1992;101(6):1644–55.
6. Bone RC. Immunologic dissonance: a continuing evolution in our understanding of the systemic inflammatory response syndrome (SIRS) and the multiple organ dysfunction syndrome (MODS). Ann Intern Med 1996;125(8):680–7.
7. Levy MM, Fink MP, Marshall JC, et al. 2001 SCCM/ESICM/ACCP/ATS/SIS international sepsis definitions conference. Crit Care Med 2003;31(4):1250–6.
8. Marshall JC. The PIRO (predisposition, insult, response, organ dysfunction) model: toward a staging system for acute illness. Virulence 2014;5(1):27–35.
9. Singer M, Deutschman CS, Seymour CW, et al. The third international consensus definitions for sepsis and septic shock (Sepsis-3). JAMA 2016;315(8):801–10.
10. Machado FR, Assuncao MS, Cavalcanti AB, et al. Getting a consensus: advantages and disadvantages of Sepsis 3 in the context of middle-income settings. Rev Bras Ter Intensiva 2016;28(4):361–5.
11. Machado FR, Nsutebu E, AbDulaziz S, et al. Sepsis 3 from the perspective of clinicians and quality improvement initiatives. J Crit Care 2017;40:315–7.
12. Angus DC. Drotrecogin alfa (activated)...a sad final fizzle to a roller-coaster party. Crit Care 2012;16(1):107.
13. Reinhart K, Daniels R, Kissoon N, et al. Recognizing sepsis as a global health priority - a WHO resolution. N Engl J Med 2017;377(5):414–7.
14. Rohde JM, Odden AJ, Bonham C, et al. The epidemiology of acute organ system dysfunction from severe sepsis outside of the intensive care unit. J Hosp Med 2013;8(5):243–7.
15. Rhee C, Dantes R, Epstein L, et al. Incidence and trends of sepsis in US hospitals using clinical vs claims data, 2009-2014. JAMA 2017;318(13):1241–9.
16. Medzhitov R. Origin and physiological roles of inflammation. Nature 2008; 454(7203):428–35.
17. van der Poll T, Opal SM. Host-pathogen interactions in sepsis. Lancet Infect Dis 2008;8(1):32–43.
18. Christaki E, Anyfanti P, Opal SM. Immunomodulatory therapy for sepsis: an update. Expert Rev Anti Infect Ther 2011;9(11):1013–33.
19. Marshall JC. Why have clinical trials in sepsis failed? Trends Mol Med 2014;20(4): 195–203.
20. Dalton WS, Friend SI I. Cancer biomarkers–an invitation to the table. Science 2006;312(5777):1165–8.
21. Biomarkers Definitions Working G. Biomarkers and surrogate endpoints: preferred definitions and conceptual framework. Clin Pharmacol Ther 2001; 69(3):89–95.
22. Marshall JC, Reinhart K, International Sepsis F. Biomarkers of sepsis. Crit Care Med 2009;37(7):2290–8.

23. Hoyt DB, Ozkan AN, Ninnemann JL, et al. Trauma peptide induction of lymphocyte changes predictive of sepsis. J Surg Res 1988;45(4):342–8.
24. Pierrakos C, Vincent JL. Sepsis biomarkers: a review. Crit Care 2010;14(1):R15.
25. Liu Y, Hou JH, Li Q, et al. Biomarkers for diagnosis of sepsis in patients with systemic inflammatory response syndrome: a systematic review and meta-analysis. Springerplus 2016;5(1):2091.
26. Kompanje EJ, Jansen TC, van der Hoven B, et al. The first demonstration of lactic acid in human blood in shock by Johann Joseph Scherer (1814-1869) in January 1843. Intensive Care Med 2007;33(11):1967–71.
27. Singer AJ, Taylor M, Domingo A, et al. Diagnostic characteristics of a clinical screening tool in combination with measuring bedside lactate level in emergency department patients with suspected sepsis. Acad Emerg Med 2014;21(8):853–7.
28. Shankar-Hari M, Phillips GS, Levy ML, et al. Developing a new definition and assessing new clinical criteria for septic shock: for the third international consensus definitions for sepsis and septic shock (Sepsis-3). JAMA 2016;315(8):775–87.
29. Daland GA, Isaacs R. Cell respiration studies: II. A comparative study of the oxygen consumption of blood from normal individuals and patients with increased leucocyte counts (Sepsis; Chronic Myelogenous Leukemia). J Exp Med 1927; 46(1):53–63.
30. Mardi D, Fwity B, Lobmann R, et al. Mean cell volume of neutrophils and monocytes compared with C-reactive protein, interleukin-6 and white blood cell count for prediction of sepsis and nonsystemic bacterial infections. Int J Lab Hematol 2010;32(4):410–8.
31. Bogar L, Molnar Z, Kenyeres P, et al. Sedimentation characteristics of leucocytes can predict bacteraemia in critical care patients. J Clin Pathol 2006;59(5):523–5.
32. Muller B, Harbarth S, Stolz D, et al. Diagnostic and prognostic accuracy of clinical and laboratory parameters in community-acquired pneumonia. BMC Infect Dis 2007;7:10.
33. Tillett WS, Francis T. Serological reactions in pneumonia with a non-protein somatic fraction of pneumococcus. J Exp Med 1930;52(4):561–71.
34. Boyer KM. Diagnosis of neonatal sepsis. Mead Johnson Symp Perinat Dev Med 1982;(21):40–6.
35. Lelubre C, Anselin S, Zouaoui Boudjeltia K, et al. Interpretation of C-reactive protein concentrations in critically ill patients. Biomed Res Int 2013;2013:124021.
36. Hirano T, Yasukawa K, Harada H, et al. Complementary DNA for a novel human interleukin (BSF-2) that induces B lymphocytes to produce immunoglobulin. Nature 1986;324(6092):73–6.
37. Waage A, Brandtzaeg P, Halstensen A, et al. The complex pattern of cytokines in serum from patients with meningococcal septic shock. Association between interleukin 6, interleukin 1, and fatal outcome. J Exp Med 1989;169(1):333–8.
38. Unkeless JC. Function and heterogeneity of human Fc receptors for immunoglobulin G. J Clin Invest 1989;83(2):355–61.
39. Anselmino LM, Perussia B, Thomas LL. Human basophils selectively express the Fc gamma RII (CDw32) subtype of IgG receptor. J Allergy Clin Immunol 1989; 84(6 Pt 1):907–14.
40. Fjaertoft G, Hakansson L, Ewald U, et al. Neutrophils from term and preterm newborn infants express the high affinity Fcgamma-receptor I (CD64) during bacterial infections. Pediatr Res 1999;45(6):871–6.
41. Schumann RR, Leong SR, Flaggs GW, et al. Structure and function of lipopolysaccharide binding protein. Science 1990;249(4975):1429–31.

42. Geller DA, Kispert PH, Su GL, et al. Induction of hepatocyte lipopolysaccharide binding protein in models of sepsis and the acute-phase response. Arch Surg 1993;128(1):22–7 [discussion: 7–8].
43. Sakr Y, Burgett U, Nacul FE, et al. Lipopolysaccharide binding protein in a surgical intensive care unit: a marker of sepsis? Crit Care Med 2008;36(7):2014–22.
44. Hershman MJ, Cheadle WG, Wellhausen SR, et al. Monocyte HLA-DR antigen expression characterizes clinical outcome in the trauma patient. Br J Surg 1990;77(2):204–7.
45. Assicot M, Gendrel D, Carsin H, et al. High serum procalcitonin concentrations in patients with sepsis and infection. Lancet 1993;341(8844):515–8.
46. Rhodes A, Evans LE, Alhazzani W, et al. Surviving sepsis campaign: international guidelines for management of sepsis and septic shock: 2016. Intensive Care Med 2017;43(3):304–77.
47. Brunkhorst FM, Heinz U, Forycki ZF. Kinetics of procalcitonin in iatrogenic sepsis. Intensive Care Med 1998;24(8):888–9.
48. Wacker C, Prkno A, Brunkhorst FM, et al. Procalcitonin as a diagnostic marker for sepsis: a systematic review and meta-analysis. Lancet Infect Dis 2013;13(5): 426–35.
49. de Jong E, van Oers JA, Beishuizen A, et al. Efficacy and safety of procalcitonin guidance in reducing the duration of antibiotic treatment in critically ill patients: a randomised, controlled, open-label trial. Lancet Infect Dis 2016;16(7):819–27.
50. Schuetz P, Wirz Y, Sager R, et al. Procalcitonin to initiate or discontinue antibiotics in acute respiratory tract infections. Cochrane Database Syst Rev 2017;(10):CD007498.
51. Bouchon A, Dietrich J, Colonna M. Cutting edge: inflammatory responses can be triggered by TREM-1, a novel receptor expressed on neutrophils and monocytes. J Immunol 2000;164(10):4991–5.
52. Wu Y, Wang F, Fan X, et al. Accuracy of plasma sTREM-1 for sepsis diagnosis in systemic inflammatory patients: a systematic review and meta-analysis. Crit Care 2012;16(6):R229.
53. Yaegashi Y, Shirakawa K, Sato N, et al. Evaluation of a newly identified soluble CD14 subtype as a marker for sepsis. J Infect Chemother 2005;11(5):234–8.
54. Shozushima T, Takahashi G, Matsumoto N, et al. Usefulness of presepsin (sCD14-ST) measurements as a marker for the diagnosis and severity of sepsis that satisfied diagnostic criteria of systemic inflammatory response syndrome. J Infect Chemother 2011;17(6):764–9.
55. Gibot S, Bene MC, Noel R, et al. Combination biomarkers to diagnose sepsis in the critically ill patient. Am J Respir Crit Care Med 2012;186(1):65–71.
56. Reinhart K, Menges T, Gardlund B, et al. Randomized, placebo-controlled trial of the anti-tumor necrosis factor antibody fragment afelimomab in hyperinflammatory response during severe sepsis: the RAMSES Study. Crit Care Med 2001; 29(4):765–9.
57. Panacek EA, Marshall JC, Albertson TE, et al. Efficacy and safety of the monoclonal anti-tumor necrosis factor antibody F(ab')2 fragment afelimomab in patients with severe sepsis and elevated interleukin-6 levels. Crit Care Med 2004; 32(11):2173–02.
58. Docke WD, Randow F, Syrbe U, et al. Monocyte deactivation in septic patients: restoration by IFN-gamma treatment. Nat Med 1997;3(6):678–81.
59. Meisel C, Schefold JC, Pschowski R, et al. Granulocyte-macrophage colony-stimulating factor to reverse sepsis-associated immunosuppression: a double-

blind, randomized, placebo-controlled multicenter trial. Am J Respir Crit Care Med 2009;180(7):640–8.

60. Dellinger RP, Bagshaw SM, Antonelli M, et al. Effect of targeted polymyxin b hemoperfusion on 28-day mortality in patients with septic shock and elevated endotoxin level: the EUPHRATES randomized clinical trial. JAMA 2018;320(14): 1455–63.

61. Warren BL, Eid A, Singer P, et al. Caring for the critically ill patient. High-dose antithrombin III in severe sepsis: a randomized controlled trial. JAMA 2001;286(15): 1869–78.

62. Abraham E, Reinhart K, Opal S, et al. Efficacy and safety of tifacogin (recombinant tissue factor pathway inhibitor) in severe sepsis: a randomized controlled trial. JAMA 2003;290(2):238–47.

63. Bernard GR, Vincent JL, Laterre PF, et al. Efficacy and safety of recombinant human activated protein C for severe sepsis. N Engl J Med 2001;344(10):699–709.

64. Wong HR. Genetics and genomics in pediatric septic shock. Crit Care Med 2012; 40(5):1618–26.

65. Hartlova A, Krocova Z, Cerveny L, et al. A proteomic view of the host-pathogen interaction: the host perspective. Proteomics 2011;11(15):3212–20.

66. Serkova NJ, Standiford TJ, Stringer KA. The emerging field of quantitative blood metabolomics for biomarker discovery in critical illnesses. Am J Respir Crit Care Med 2011;184(6):647–55.

67. Atreya MR, Wong HR. Precision medicine in pediatric sepsis. Curr Opin Pediatr 2019;31(3):322–7.

68. Bauer M, Giamarellos-Bourboulis EJ, Kortgen A, et al. A transcriptomic biomarker to quantify systemic inflammation in sepsis - a prospective multicenter phase II diagnostic study. EBioMedicine 2016;6:114–25.

69. Miller RR 3rd, Lopansri BK, Burke JP, et al. Validation of a host response assay, SeptiCyte LAB, for discriminating sepsis from systemic inflammatory response syndrome in the ICU. Am J Respir Crit Care Med 2018;198(7):903–13.

70. Nathan C. Points of control in inflammation. Nature 2002;420(6917):846–52.

71. Kumar A, Roberts D, Wood KE, et al. Duration of hypotension before initiation of effective antimicrobial therapy is the critical determinant of survival in human septic shock. Crit Care Med 2006;34(6):1589–96.

72. Papadopoulos N, Kinzler KW, Vogelstein B. The role of companion diagnostics in the development and use of mutation-targeted cancer therapies. Nat Biotechnol 2006;24(8):985–95.

Biomarkers of Infection and Sepsis

Steven M. Opal, MD[a],*, Xavier Wittebole, MD[b]

KEYWORDS

- Rapid • Culture-independent • Microbial diagnostic techniques
- Host-derived biomarkers for early diagnosis of sepsis and septic shock
- Machine-learning systems to identify susceptible patients with sepsis
- Rapid genotypic and phenotypic methods to measure antimicrobial susceptibility patterns

KEY POINTS

- Promising molecular diagnostic techniques are under development, but not yet displaced the traditional rather insensitive, and slow microbial diagnostic measures in use today.
- Identifying a pathogen and determining its susceptibility to antimicrobial agents generally takes more than 24 hours, forcing clinicians to give empiric, broad-spectrum, antimicrobial agents to cover the likely pathogen(s).
- Clear evidence exists that correct administration of antimicrobial agents can be life-saving in patients with sepsis.
- Two major strategies are in development to assist treating physicians to make expeditious decisions on appropriate antibiotic choices that specifically targets the invading pathogens in the septic patient.
- This article reviews the current status of rapid molecular markers to optimally define which patients need urgent treatment.

INTRODUCTION

Intensive care unit (ICU) practitioners and emergency department clinicians are in urgent need of a major upgrade in their access to accurate and fast microbial diagnosis (**Table 1**). The diagnostic techniques for bloodstream infection available to most ICU clinicians today do not fundamentally differ from Robert Koch's laboratory methods circa 1887.[1,2] That was the year when 2 co-workers in Koch's laboratory, Fanny Hess and Richard Petri, first suggested using semisolid agar and 2 glass plates of slightly different size for isolation of bacteria in pure culture.

[a] Infectious Disease Division, Alpert Medical School of Brown University, Ocean State Clinical Coordinating Center at Rhode Island Hospital, 1 Virginia Avenue Suite 105, Providence, RI 02905, USA; [b] Critical Care Department, (Pr Laterre), Cliniques Universitaires Saint-Luc, Avenue Hippocrate 10, 1200 Brussels, Belgium
* Corresponding author.
E-mail address: Steven_Opal@brown.edu

Crit Care Clin 36 (2020) 11–22
https://doi.org/10.1016/j.ccc.2019.08.002
0749-0704/20/© 2019 Elsevier Inc. All rights reserved.

Table 1
Rapid detection methods and molecular biomarkers to improve the diagnosis of sepsis

Analytical Technique	Potential Uses	References
Microfluidics	Rapid antibiotic susceptibility method; neutrophil nuclear membrane deformability as an early diagnostic method	29,36–39
Proteomics and plasma protein biomarkers	Identify new patterns of plasma protein interactions and responses; predict outcomes and possibly direct new therapies by using plasma biomarkers	40–56
Genomics	Full genomic or exon-expressed SNPs as indicators for host susceptibility to infection and sepsis; rate of LPS removal in LDLRs by PCSK9 levels	53,57–59
Transcriptomics	Method to define DEGs to assess the acute and more chronic host–response to sepsis stimuli, determine the dominant host response from proinflammatory to immunosuppression to coagulopathic phenotypes	60–72
metabolomics	Measure metabolic perturbations in confined spaces such as pleural fluid or cerebrospinal fluid indicative of tissue stress, cell injury or immune–metabolic alterations for diagnosis and prognosis	73,74
Large data set machine learning	Identify pathophysiologic patterns of host response phenotypes and endotypes	75–79

Abbreviations: DEGs, differentially expressed genes; LDLR, low-density lipoprotein receptor; LPS, lipopolysaccharide; PCSK9, proprotein convertase subtilisin kexin type 9; SNP, single nucleotide polymorphism.

Most clinical microbiology laboratories still use the same basic method of single colony isolation before conducting antimicrobial susceptibility testing. The drug sensitivity results are usually not available for 24 to 72 hours. However, it should be noted that current treatment guidelines for treating sepsis promulgate initiation of effective antibiotics within 1 to 3 hours![3–5] Although clinicians at large medical centers might now have access to early microbial identification via innovations in mass spectrometry (MS) and nuclear magnetic resonance methods, rarely do they have antimicrobial susceptibility results at the critical moment of ordering the antibiotic treatment regimen. Antibiotic therapy is therefore empiric by nature and purposely given as broad-spectrum treatment to avoid missing the drug susceptibility profile of the causative pathogen.

Compelling but not uniformly accepted evidence exists in support of urgent administration of empiric antibiotics in patients with severe sepsis of septic shock.[5–9] Ideally, antibiotic intervention should be completed within 1 hour of initial diagnosis of sepsis or septic shock.[6–8] Living up to this 1-hour imperative is hampered by the fact that there is no single, rapid, and accurate diagnostic test for the syndrome of sepsis or septic shock. The diagnosis rests on a diagnosis of severe infection accompanied by a constellation of signs and symptoms, blood studies, and pathophysiologic findings clinically recognized as sepsis.[10]

Yet, choosing an effective, empiric, antimicrobial drug regimen, before knowing the sensitivity profile of the causative pathogen, is becoming a real challenge. Progressive emergence of antimicrobial resistance among bacterial and fungal pathogens is an omnipresent threat.[10–13] Widespread use of broad-spectrum antibiotics likely contributes to the spread of antibiotic resistance genes, further exacerbating the emergence of multidrug-resistant microbial pathogens and secondary fungal infections.[14,15] Antibiotic stewardship programs are focused on curbing excessive use of empiric antibiotics, placing the ICU clinician in a therapeutic conundrum.[15,16] To make matters worse, empiric antibiotics are often administered to patients before arriving in the hospital and before exhibiting progressive signs of sepsis, thereby precluding an accurate microbial diagnosis by standard culture methods.

What is needed now are a set of molecular tools that can provide (1) rapid diagnostic methods for invasive infection without the need for compulsory delays with laboratory cultivation, (2) the capacity for urgent determination of antimicrobial susceptibility results from the causative pathogen and (3), a new generation of biomarkers that can clearly distinguish between infection-mediated organ dysfunction and sepsis mimics with non–infection-mediated systemic inflammation. Progress is being made to advance the laboratory diagnosis of severe infection and early recognition of sepsis and septic shock.[16–18] We provide a brief review of the subject of biomarkers in sepsis and their status in clinical development. Hopefully, some of these innovations will soon be available as bedside tools for the diagnosis and treatment of the enigmatic syndrome called sepsis.

RAPID MICROBIAL DIAGNOSTIC METHODS

Advances in molecular diagnosis without the need for traditional, time-consuming culture methods is finally reaching the stage for actual clinical usage. This advance could revolutionize the clinical care and treatment decisions of critically ill, patients with sepsis. Knowing the molecular identity of the causative organism, and perhaps even the susceptibility data, in a few hours rather than 24 to 72 hours could allow the ICU physician to make more informed decisions on antibiotic choices.[16–23] Most of these rapid diagnostic methodologies are based on the polymerase chain reaction (PCR) to amplify the microbial DNA signal. This is followed by various analytical approaches to determine the genomic sequence identity by MS[16–23] or nuclear magnetic resonance.[14,24] The most common system currently used in clinical microbiology laboratory at present is matrix assisted laser desorption/ionization time of flight mass spectroscopy. Many studies report reduced mortality rates in comparative studies with traditional microbiologic diagnostic measurements.[16,19,21,22] Fast detection of specific pathogens such as *Staphylococcus aureus* versus coagulase-negative staphylococci by peptide–nucleic acid fluorescence in situ hybridization can inform the clinician with a rapid determination if the infection is a highly virulent or low virulence microorganism.[25–27] Linking rapid diagnostics results with antimicrobial stewardship programs with the hospital is particularly useful in realizing the maximum benefits of rapid microbial diagnostic testing[16,19,22]

Screening for the presence of antibiotic resistance genes is also certainly feasible as a part of rapid genomic testing, but there are hundreds of known antibiotic resistance genes and the list of new resistance genes continues to grow. Moreover, the resistance gene sequence might be present in the genomic DNA of the pathogen without being fully expressed.[16] Clinical correlation between genotype and phenotypic expression in vivo during infection needs further investigation.

The potential clinical usefulness of a rapid, non–culture-based microbial diagnosis was well-demonstrated in a recent large, multicenter, European observational trial. They simultaneously compared standard culture method s versus a PCR electrospray ionization mass spectroscopy–based diagnostic system in 616 bloodstream infections.[23] Routine blood cultures were positive in only 11% of patients with sepsis, whereas the PCR-based system from the same samples was positive for the pathogen in 37%. This large difference was attributed to the widespread use of empiric antibacterial therapy in these critical ill patients. Antibiotics limit the diagnostic validity of blood cultures but have little effect on the PCR-based samples with the ability to identify circulating bacterial DNA despite antibiotic exposure. If the PCR electrospray ionization mass spectroscopy data had been available to the investigators in real time, treatment would have been altered in up to 57% of these patients.

BIOMARKERS FOR RAPID DIAGNOSIS OF ANTIMICROBIAL SUSCEPTIBILITY TESTING

Another unmet medical need in managing critically ill patients with severe infection is the lack of ability to provide rapid and directed antibiotic therapy guided by specific, antimicrobial susceptibility testing.[21,22] In this era of progressive loss of antimicrobial activity from bacterial evolution of antibiotic resistance genes, rapid susceptibility testing is urgently needed but rarely available. There are exceptions of course. *Streptococcus pyogenes* (group A strep) remains uniformly susceptible to penicillin,[28] but for almost everything else direct antibiotic sensitivity testing to guide therapy is desirable if possible. Unfortunately, laboratory testing usually entails time-consuming incubation times to fully express and define the susceptibility pattern for each identified pathogen.

Progress is being made in the provision of novel methodologies to bring rapid susceptibility testing into clinical practice. Microfluidic systems with single cell imaging assays,[29] laser light scatter rapid imaging technologies,[30] and time-lapse microscopic imaging analyses[31] are only some of the antimicrobial sensitivity testing systems underway to fill the current void in rapid and clinically accessible susceptibility testing. These rapid diagnostic systems are best applied in normally sterile fluids like blood, cerebrospinal fluid, pleural fluid etc. and are not particularly useful at present for microbiologic diagnosis from tissues with an endogenous microbiome (sputum, urine, and gastrointestinal or genitourinary tract pathogens).[32–35]

BIOMARKERS FOR INFECTION VERSUS NONINFECTIOUS SYSTEMIC INFLAMMATION
Microfluidics

Advances in microfluidics and microchip assembly offer the potential to be a rapid diagnostic technique for distinguishing infection versus inflammation in the emergency department.[36] The internal flexibility and deformability of the nucleus found inside single cells of circulating neutrophils can be analytically measured within minutes in a microfluidics apparatus.[37] Activated neutrophils responding to systemic infection can be distinguished from resting neutrophils in the circulation by this technique. Deformability indices of thousands of neutrophils can be calculated over a few minutes. This technique could rapidly assess the state of neutrophil activation in a patient presenting acutely in the emergency department to aid in initial triage and management.[37–39]

Plasma Biomarkers, Proteomics, and Soluble Pattern Recognition Receptors

More than 100 proteins, soluble receptors, cytokines, and chemokines have proposed in the literature to serve as biomarkers to distinguish between infection and inflammation.[40,41] The most widely studied biomarkers as an indicator of sepsis are procalcitonin (PCT) and C-reactive protein (CRP). PCT is a prohormone synthesized and rapidly released by many cell types during period s of generalized inflammation. Plasma levels are usually highest during episodes of severe bacterial infection, but noninfectious injury such as major surgery, severe trauma, and some virus infections can also elevate PCT levels.[42–44] Serial measurement of PCT levels might prove to be useful in antibiotic stewardship programs to encourage clinicians to withdraw empiric antibiotics if PCT levels were never elevated or were low and drop precipitously. The clinical usefulness of applying PCT levels as a guide to discontinue antibiotics, if no objective evidence of bacterial infection is found, remains the subject of considerable debate.[40–44]

CRP is a hepatically synthesized, acute phase protein whose blood levels dramatically increase with tissue injury, infection, and acute severe inflammatory states.[45] The pentameric plasma protein functions as a soluble pattern recognition molecule that binds to C-polysaccharide of the pneumococcus. CRP also binds to dead or dying bacteria in the blood and promotes complement-mediated bacterial clearance. The binding site for CRP on bacteria and injured host cells is lysophosphatidal choline. The protein synthesis and secretion of CRP is IL-6 driven.[46] CRP levels in the blood can increase in sepsis and septic shock to greater than 10,000-fold greater resting levels. CRP has been used as a nonspecific but reliable measure of systemic inflammation of any type. CRP has been used by clinicians as a biomarker of inflammation for decades. It is highly sensitive for sepsis, but lacks specificity when compared with PCT.[47]

Several other protein biomarkers of recent interest include a neutrophil activation marker known as heparin-binding protein,[48,49] a mesenteric ischemia marker known as pancreatic stone protein,[50,51] and a detection assay for measuring circulating endothelial cells.[52] Elevated plasma levels of heparin-binding protein (>30 ng/mL) is an accurate indicator of neutrophil activation with evidence of neutrophil chemotaxis.[48] If left untended, progressive rise in heparin-binding protein levels portend endothelial damage, diffuse capillary leakage, sepsis, and shock. In a recent multicenter clinical trial, heparin-binding protein levels detected in the blood in 7 emergency departments compared favorably with other standard measures (CRP, blood lactate, and PCT) as a predictor of adverse outcomes.[49]

Another potentially promising biomarker is pancreatic stone protein. This protein is released during periods of splanchnic hypoperfusion and seems to be a good biomarker for mesenteric perfusion in patients with sepsis. Elevated levels can be readily detected with a rapid diagnostic assay, and pancreatic stone protein measurement might be able to outperform other biomarkers for sepsis like PCT and CRP.[50,51]

Another interesting detection assay in development for the prediction of sepsis is direct measurement of detached endothelial cells in the blood.[52] Sepsis-induced disruption of the endothelial barrier throughout the circulatory system is the hallmark pathophysiologic finding in septic shock.[53] A specific assay for endothelial cell damage might prove to be a useful tool to make an early diagnosis and management guide for novel sepsis therapeutics.

Measuring a biomarker that is the target of a new therapeutic intervention to prevent sepsis is a logical approach in using biomarkers. Measuring circulating endotoxin before starting an anti-endotoxin therapy[54] or measuring soluble triggering receptor expressed on myeloid cells before beginning a clinical trial targeting triggering receptor expressed on myeloid cells with a new experimental inhibitor.[55] Moreover, a holistic approach to proteomics where the entire plasma proteome is analyzed for critical interactions between signaling peptides in sepsis and septic shock could provide new insights on when and where to intervene.[56]

Genomics

Advances in DNA sequencing technologies now make it feasible to sequence the exon segments of the human genome and search for single nucleotide polymorphisms. Myriads of single nucleotide polymorphisms are already identified in the human genome that affect susceptibility to infection and alter the expression of the host response during sepsis.[53] We are just beginning to decipher the magnitude of interacting genomic elements induced by sepsis, and the computational biology, which will be essential to fully understanding the complexity of host susceptibility and resistance to infection.

At present we can only scratch the surface of the host–pathogen interactions that participate in the daily standoff between our genomes and an array of potential microbial pathogens.[53] Single nucleotide polymorphisms have already been identified in complement factors, immunoglobulin structure, intracellular signaling networks, and clearance capacity to eliminate lipopolysaccharides and other toxic biolipids.[57–59] Much basic research and applied science research is needed to bring advances in functional genomics to the bedside in support of sepsis management.

Transcriptomics

The major methodology now in use to analyze components of gene activation or inhibition of the host response in sepsis is with upregulation or downregulation of differentially expressed genes from a given specific baseline determination. Thousands of genes are differentially expressed in response to a powerful and pathologic pattern recognition molecule like bacterial endotoxin. Complicating matters further is that transcription gene profiles between individuals even with single site of infection (eg, pneumonia or blood stream infections) are markedly heterogeneous.[60] In response, investigators have endeavored to use unsupervised searches for common transcriptional clusters to detect recognizable and reproducible signatures of gene activation. This process requires a careful analysis for primary driver transcripts from different individuals with the same or similar acute disease process.[61–63]

Initial unsupervised clusters of transcripts are then linked in together from patients with similar disease features to determine recognizable, organ-specific, tissue-specific, and circulating blood transcript patterns. Meta-clustering and data pooling methods have improved the reproducibility of detection of common gene clusters associated with specific diseases. Research teams have now shown it is possible to distinguish infection-related systemic inflammatory states from noninfectious inflammatory states by analyzing differences in the transcription profiles.[64–67]

McHugh and colleagues[64] have been able to reduce the number of transcribed genes necessary to predict the presence or absence of infection in critically ill patients with only 4 targeted enzymes. The 4 gene products are *LAMP1* (lysosomal-associated membrane protein), *PLAG7* (phospholipase A2, group VII), *PLAC8* (placenta-specific gene 8), and *CEACAM 4* (carcinoembryonic antigen-related cell adhesion molecule 4). This work is of extreme importance in antibiotic stewardship practices in the ICU by avoiding the use of antibiotics if no infection is present.[67–69]

Efforts are underway to streamline this process and develop diagnostic tests by narrowing down the gene search to a small number of critical transcriptional determinants of infection versus noninfection. This promising approach is ongoing in many laboratories around the globe.[70,71] Although still in the developmental phase, these analyses are beginning to decipher patterns of host response genes that might help guide treatment strategies and improve patient selection in future experimental intervention trials. Sweeney and colleagues[71] have uncovered consistent patterns in transcriptome analysis that differentiate into 3 major clusters designated as inflammopathic, adaptive, and coagulopathic. Each of these groups are identifiable in numerous publicly available transcriptome databases and have significant outcomes. This work could begin to direct therapies in patients with sepsis with reduced heterogeneity in the patient population. Heterogeneity across different studies has stymied attempts to reproduce the results of interventional trials in sepsis. Hopefully, cluster analysis of transcriptomics-based classification will solve the problem of reproducibility of trial results by defining broadly relevant endotypes.[72]

Metabolomics

Another potentially rapid diagnostic methodology is the assessment of the metabolic state of tissues within the host by state-of-the-art ^{1}H nuclear magnetic resonance and gas chromatographic MS metabolomics.[73] Using principal components analysis for pattern recognition of unsupervised clustering behaviors of patient samples, it is possible to generate a 2-dimensional principal components analysis to rapidly recognize the presence of infection versus sterile inflammation and predict the risk of mortality in acutely ill patients. Both host-derived and pathogen-derived molecules can be measured by this technique and provide early distinction between bacterial and viral pathogens.[74]

Machine Learning Techniques and Early Sepsis Recognition Methods

A final novel biomarker strategy in development at present is instruction of ICU-focused machine-derived risk prediction and early recognition of sepsis.[75–79] Using large databases with thousands if not millions of physiologic and pathophysiologic data points from previous patients with sepsis, it is possible to train computers to recognize early patterns of sepsis development in real time. These pattern recognition elements can be improved on by adding more and more new data from ICU patients. Machine learning in the form of integrating input data points for early detection toward sepsis-specific patterns might serve as a monitoring assist device in ICU patients or ward patients who are developing sepsis. A number of groups are working on machine learning in the ICU and it is likely that this investigation will continue to evolve.

A recent study by Seymour and colleagues[75] in a machine learning in sepsis trial design is particularly intriguing. These investigators have used several large database assets from electronic medical records and focused on patients who developed sepsis. Unstructured clustering of patient physiologic elements repeatedly detected 4 specific patient phenotypes. Group 1 was the most common and were less ill with a lower need for vasopressors (33% of study population). Group 2 were older with lots of comorbid illnesses and acute kidney injury. Group 3 had more inflammatory markers and lung injury. Group 4 was least common (13%) with more septic shock and more liver dysfunction. Using statistics and machine learning, they then ran Monte Carlo simulations using different groupings of sepsis phenotypes at baseline against data available from several recent, phase 3 sepsis trials. Even though the clinical trial patients all met the standard sepsis definitions, changing the proportion of the 4 patient groups at baseline could alter the results. Some phenotype groups would drive outcomes toward harm and other phenotype ratios toward benefit. This information needs to be validated in future sepsis trials. If confirmed, this could serve as the basis for better patient phenotype selection into future trials. Most important, these patient phenotypes could be used to exclude patients at possible risk of harm.

SUMMARY

The role of biomarkers for the detection of sepsis has come a long way in the field of sepsis management and enrollment of patients into clinical trials. Molecular biomarkers are taking front stage at present but machine learning and other computational measures using big datasets is promising as well. Clinical research in sepsis is hampered but lack of specificity of the diagnosis itself as sepsis is a syndrome with no uniformly agreed definition.

One consequence of the lack of diagnostic precision in sepsis is who or what is the gold standard for the final diagnosis of sepsis. Currently the final conclusion is expert opinion, which is not bad but not perfect.[80,81] Perhaps machine learning (or some highly specific biomarker) will displace expert opinion as the final and most accurate definition for sepsis.

REFERENCES

1. Opal SM. The evolution of our understanding of the nature of infection and sepsis. Crit Care Clin 2009;25:637–63.
2. Artenstein A, Higgins T, Opal SM. Sepsis and scientific revolutions. Crit Care Med 2013;41(12):2770–2.
3. Pruinelli L, Westra BL, Yadav P, et al. Delay within the 3-hour Surviving Sepsis Campaign guideline on mortality for patients with severe sepsis and septic shock. Crit Care Med 2018;46:500–5.
4. Chen AX, Simpson SQ, Pallin DJ. Sepsis guidelines. N Engl J Med 2019;380(14): 1369–71.
5. Whiles BB, Deis AS, Simpson SQ. Increased time to initial antimicrobial administration is associated with progression to septic shock and in severe sepsis patients. Crit Care Med 2017;45:623–9.
6. Levy MM, Evans LE, Rhodes A. The surviving sepsis campaign bundle: 2018 update. Intensive Care Med 2018;44:925–8.
7. Seymour CW, Gesten F, Prescott, et al. Time to treatment and mortality during mandated emergency care of sepsis. N Engl J Med 2017;376:2235–44.
8. Kumar A, Roberts D, Wood KE, et al. Duration of hypotension before initiation of effective antimicrobial therapy is the critical determinant of survival in human septic shock. Crit Care Med 2006;34:1589–96.
9. Sterling SA, Miller WR, Pryor J, et al. The impact of timing of antibiotics on outcomes in severe sepsis and septic shock: a systematic review and meta-analysis. Crit Care Med 2015;43:1907–15.
10. Singer M, Deutschman CS, Seymour CW, et al. The third international definitions for sepsis and septic shock (Sepsis -3). JAMA 2016;315(8):801–10.
11. Pop-Vicas A, Opal SM. The clinical impact of multidrug resistant gram-negative bacilli in the management of septic shock. Virulence 2014;5(1):1–7.
12. Opal SM. Non-antibiotic treatments for pan-resistant bacterial pathogens. Crit Care 2016;20:397.
13. Opal SM, Pop-Vicas A. Molecular mechanisms of antibiotic resistance in bacteria. In: Bennett JE, Dolin R, Blaser M, editors. Principles and practice of infectious diseases. 9th edition. Elsevier Publishers: Philadelphia; 2019. p. 222–39.
14. Pfaller MA, Wolk DM, Lowery TJ. T2MR and T2 candida: novel technology for the rapid diagnosis of candidemia and invasive candidiasis. Future Microbiol 2016; 11:103–7.
15. Patel GP, Simon D, Scheetz M, et al. The effect of time to antifungal therapy on mortality in candidemia associated septic shock. Am J Ther 2009;16:508–11.

16. Beganovic M, McCreary EK, Mahoney MV, et al. Interplay between rapid diagnostic tests and antimicrobial stewardship programs among patients with bloodstream and other severe infections. J Appl Lab Med 2019;3(4):601–16.
17. Kerremans JJ, Verboom P, Stijnen T, et al. Rapid identification and antimicrobial susceptibility testing reduce antibiotic use and accelerate pathogen-directed antibiotic use. J Antimicrob Chemother 2008;61:428–35.
18. Timbrook TT, Morton JB, McConeghy KW, et al. The effect of molecular rapid diagnostic testing on clinical outcomes in bloodstream infections: a systematic review and meta-analysis. Clin Infect Dis 2017;64:15–23.
19. Cairns KA, Doyle JS, Trevillyan JM, et al. The impact of a multidisciplinary antimicrobial stewardship team on the timeliness of antimicrobial therapy in patients with positive blood cultures: a randomized controlled trial. J Antimicrob Chemother 2016;71:3276–83.
20. Banerjee R, Teng CB, Cunningham SA, et al. Randomized trial of rapid multiplex polymerase chain reaction-based blood culture identification and susceptibility testing. Clin Infect Dis 2015;61:1071–80.
21. Bookstaver PB, Nimmich EB, Smith TJ, et al. Cumulative effect of an antimicrobial stewardship and rapid diagnostic testing bundle on early streamlining of antimicrobial therapy in gram-negative bloodstream infections. Antimicrob Agents Chemother 2017;61 [pii:e00189-17].
22. Rivard KR, Athans V, Lam SW, et al. Impact of antimicrobial stewardship and rapid microarray testing on patients with gram-negative bacteremia. Eur J Clin Microbiol Infect Dis 2017;36:1879–87.
23. Vincent JL, Brealey D, Libert N, et al. Rapid diagnosis of infection in the critically ill, a multicenter study of molecular detection in bloodstream infections, pneumonia, and sterile site infections. Crit Care Med 2015;43(11):2283–91. https://doi.org/10.1097/CCM.001249.
24. Wilson NM, Alangaden G, Tibbetts RJ, et al. T2 magnetic resonance assay improves timely management of candidemia. JAMS 2017;1(1):12–8.
25. Forrest GN, Mankes K, Jabra-Rizk MA, et al. Peptide nucleic acid fluorescence in situ hybridization-based identification of Candida albicans and its impact on mortality and antifungal costs. J Clin Microbiol 2006;44:3381–3.
26. Forrest GN, Mehta S, Weekes E, et al. Impact of rapid in situ hybridization testing on coagulase-negative staphylococci positive blood cultures. J Antimicrob Chemother 2006;58:154–8.
27. Wenzler E, Wang F, Goff DA, et al. An automated, pharmacy-driven initiative improves quality of care for Staphylococcus aureus bacteremia. Clin Infect Dis 2017;65:194–200.
28. Horn DL, Zabriskie JB, Austrian R, et al. Why have group A Streptococci remained susceptible to penicillin? Clin Infect Dis 1998;26:1341–5.
29. Baltekin O, Boucharin A, Tano E, et al. Antibiotic susceptibility testing in less than 30 minutes using direct single-cell imaging. Proc Natl Acad Sci U S A 2017; 114(34):9170–5.
30. Choi J, Jeong HY, Lee GY, et al. Direct, rapid antimicrobial susceptibility test from positive blood cultures based on microscopic imaging analysis. Sci Rep 2017; 7(1148):1–26.
31. Hayden RT, Clinton LK, Hewitt C, et al. Rapid antimicrobial susceptibility testing using forward laser light scatter technology. J Clin Microbiol 2016;54(11):2701–6.
32. Mulpuru S, Aaron SD, Ronksley PE, et al. Hospital resource utilization and patient outcomes associated with respiratory viral testing in hospitalized patients. Emerg Infect Dis 2015;21:1366–71.

33. Potage CR, Cohen SH. State-of-the-art microbiologic testing for community-acquired meningitis and encephalitis. J Clin Microbiol 2016;54:1197–202.
34. Leber AL, Everhart K, Balada-Llasat JM, et al. Multicenter evaluation of Biofire Film Array meningitis/encephalitis panel for detection of bacteria, viruses and yeast in cerebrospinal fluid specimens. J Clin Microbiol 2016;54:2251–61.
35. Hanson KE, Couturier MR. Multiplexed molecular diagnostics for respiratory, gastrointestinal and central nervous infections. Clin Infect Dis 2016;63:1361–7.
36. Whitesides GM. The origins and the future of microfluidics. Nature 2006; 442(7101):368–73.
37. Crawford K, DeWitt A, Brierre S, et al. Rapid biophysical analysis of host immune cell variations associated with sepsis. Am J Respir Crit Care Med 2018;198(2): 280–2.
38. Khismatullin DB. The cytoskeleton and deformability of white blood cells. Curr Top Membr 2009;64:47–111.
39. Gossett DR, Tse HT, Lee SA, et al. Hydrodynamic stretching of single cells for large population mechanical phenotyping. Proc Natl Acad Sci U S A 2012; 109(20):7630–5.
40. Cho SY, Choi JH. Biomarkers for sepsis. Infect Chemother 2014;46(1):1–2.
41. Reinhart K, Meisner M. Biomarkers in the critically ill patient: procalcitonin. Crit Care Clin 2011;27:253–63.
42. Kopterides P, Siempos II, Tsangaris A, et al. Procalcitonin-guided algorithms of antibiotic therapy in the intensive care unit: a systematic review and meta-analysis of randomized controlled trials. Crit Care Med 2010;38:2229–41.
43. Anand D, Das S, Bhargava S, et al. Procalcitonin as a rapid diagnostic biomarker to differentiate between culture-negative bacterial sepsis and systemic inflammatory response syndrome: a prospective, observational, cohort study. J Crit Care 2015;30:218.e7-12.
44. Huang DT, Yealy DM, Filbin MR, et al. Procalcitonin–guided use of antibiotics for lower respiratory tract infection. N Engl J Med 2018;379:236–49.
45. Thompson D, Pepys MB, Wood SP. The physiological structure of human C-reactive protein and its complex with phosphocholine. Structure 1999;7(2):169–77.
46. Pepys MB, Hirschfield GM. C-reactive protein: a critical update. J Clin Invest 2003;111(12):1805–12.
47. Danesh J, Wheeler JG, Hirschfield GM, et al. C-reactive protein and other circulating markers of inflammation in the prediction of coronary heart disease. N Engl J Med 2004;350(14):1387–97.
48. Linder A, Arnold R, Boyd JH, et al. Heparin-binding protein measurement improves the prediction of severe infection with organ dysfunction in the emergency department. Crit Care Med 2015;43(11):2378–86.
49. Linder A, Akesson P, Inghammar M, et al. Elevated plasma levels of heparin-binding protein in intensive care unit patients with severe sepsis and septic shock. Crit Care 2012;16:R90.
50. Que YA, Delodder F, Guessous I, et al. Pancreatic stone protein as an early biomarker predicting mortality in a prospective cohort of patients with sepsis requiring ICU management. Crit Care 2012;16:R114.
51. García de Guadiana-Romualdo L, Berger M, Jiménez-Santos E, et al. Pancreatic stone protein and soluble CD25 for infection and sepsis in an emergency department. Eur J Clin Invest 2017;47(4):297–304.
52. Tapia P, Gatica S, Cortez-Rivera C, et al. Circulating endothelial cells from septic shock patients convert to fibroblasts are associated with the resuscitation fluid

dose and are biomarkers for survival prediction. Crit Care Med 2019. https://doi.org/10.1097/CCM 003778.

53. Hotchkiss RS, Moldawer LL, Opal SM, et al. Sepsis and septic shock. Nat Rev Dis Primers 2016;2:1–21.

54. Dellinger RP, Bagshaw SM, Antonelli M, et al. Effect of targeted polymyxin B hemoperfusion on 28-day mortality in patients with septic Shock and elevated endotoxin level. JAMA 2018;320(14):1455–63.

55. Gibot S, Cravoisy A, Levy B, et al. Soluble triggering receptor expressed on myeloid cells and the diagnosis of pneumonia. N Engl J Med 2004;350:451–8.

56. Oved K, Cohen A, Bioco O, et al. A novel host-proteome signature for distinguishing between acute bacterial and viral infections. PLoS One 2015;10:e0120012.

57. Walley KR, Francis GA, Opal SM, et al. The central role of proprotein convertase subtilisin/kexin type 9 in septic pathogen lipid transport and clearance. Am J Respir Crit Care Med 2015;192(11):1275–86.

58. Boyd JH, Fjell CD, Russel JA, et al. Increased plasma PCSK9 levels are associated with reduced endotoxin clearance and the development of acute organ failures during sepsis. J Innate Immun 2016. https://doi.org/10.1159/000442976.

59. Giamarellos-Bourboulis E, Opal SM. The role of genetics and antibodies in sepsis. Ann Transl Med 2016;4(17):328, 1-8.

60. Tsalik EL, Langley RJ, Dinwiddlie DL, et al. An integrated transcriptome and expressed variant analysis of sepsis survival and death. Genome Med 2014;6:111.

61. Maslove DM, Wong HR. Gene expression profiling in sepsis: timing, tissue and translational considerations. Trends Mol Med 2014;20:204–13.

62. Sweeney TE, Shidham A, Wong HR, et al. A comprehensive time-course-based multicohort analysis of sepsis and sterile inflammation reveals a robust diagnostic gene set. Sci Transl Med 2015;7:287ra271.

63. Geiss RK, Bumgarner RE, Birditt B, et al. Direct multiplexed measurement of gene expression with color-coded probe pairs. Nat Biotechnol 2008;26(3):317–25.

64. McHugh L, Seldon TA, Brandon RA, et al. A molecular host response assay to discriminate between acute bacterial infection and infection-negative systemic inflammation in critically ill patients; discovery and validation in independent cohorts. PLoS Med 2015;12:e1001916.

65. Miller RR, Lopansri BK, Burke JP, et al. Validation of a host response assay, SteriCycle LAB, for discriminating sepsis from systemic inflammatory syndrome in the ICU. Am J Respir Crit Care Med 2018;198(7):904–13.

66. Bauer M, Giamarellos-Bourboulis EJ, Kortgen A, et al. A transcriptomic biomarker to quantify systemic inflammation in sepsis-a prospective multicenter, phase II diagnostic study. EBioMedicine 2016;6:114–25.

67. Zimmerman JJ, Sullivan E, Yager TD, et al. Diagnostic accuracy of a host gene expression signature that discriminates clinical severe sepsis syndrome and infection-negative systemic inflammation among critically ill children. Crit Care Med 2017;45:e418–25.

68. Herberg JA, Kaforou M, Wright VJ, et al. Diagnostic test accuracy of a 2-transcript host RNA signature for discriminating bacterial from viral infection in febrile children. JAMA 2016;316:835–45.

69. Burham KL, Davenport EE, Radhakrishnan J, et al. Shared and distinct aspects of the sepsis transcriptomic response to fecal peritonitis and pneumonia. Am J Respir Crit Care Med 2017;196:328–9.

70. Davenport EE, Burnham KL, Radhakristnan J, et al. Genomic landscape and outcomes in sepsis: a prospective cohort study. Lancet Respir Med 2016;4:257–71.

71. Sweeney TE, Azad TD, Donato M, et al. Unsupervised analysis of transcriptomics in bacterial sepsis across multiple datasets reveals three robust clusters. Crit Care Med 2018;46(6):916–25.
72. Scicluna BP, van Vught LA, Zwiderman AH, et al. Classification of patients according to blood genomic endotype: a prospective cohort study. Lancet Respir Med 2017;5:816–26.
73. Coen M, O'Sullivan M, Bubb WA, et al. Proton nuclear magnetic resonance-based metabolomics for rapid diagnosis of meningitis and ventriculitis. Clin Infect Dis 2005;41(1):1582–90.
74. Banoei MM, Vogel HJ, Weljie AM, et al. Plasma metabolomics for the diagnosis and prognosis of H1N1 influenza pneumonia. Crit Care 2017;21:97.
75. Seymour CW, Kennedy JN, Wang S, et al. Novel clinical phenotypes in sepsis: derivation, validation, and potential treatment implications. JAMA 2019;321(20): 2003–17.
76. Shimabukuro DW, Barton CW, Feldman MD, et al. Effect of a machine-learning-based severe sepsis prediction algorithm on patient survival and hospital length of stay: a randomised clinical trial. BMJ Open Respir Res 2017;4:e000234.
77. Desautels T, Calvert J, Hoffman J, et al. Prediction of sepsis in the intensive care unit with minimal electronic medical record data: a machine learning approach. JMIR Med Inform 2016;4(3):e28.
78. Calvert J, Desautels T, Chettipally U, et al. High-performance detection and early prediction of septic shock for alcohol-use disorder patients. Ann Med Surg (Lond) 2016;8:50–5.
79. Rajkomar A, Dean J, Kohane I. Machine learning in medicine. N Engl J Med 2019; 380(14):1347–57.
80. Lopansri BK, Miller RR, Burke JP, et al. Physician agreement on the diagnosis of sepsis in the intensive care unit: estimation of concordance and analysis of underlying factors in a multicenter cohort. J Intensive Care 2019;7:13.
81. Klein Klouwenberg PM, Ong DS, Bos LD, et al. Interobserver agreement of the Centers for Disease Control and Prevention criteria for classifying infections in critically ill patients. Crit Care Med 2013;41:2373–8.

Procalcitonin
Where Are We Now?

Bachar Hamade, MD, MSc[a,b], David T. Huang, MD, MPH[c],*

KEYWORDS

- Sepsis • Respiratory tract infection • Procalcitonin • Antibiotics • Mortality

KEY POINTS

- Procalcitonin is a biomarker generally elevated in bacterial infections but not viral.
- Procalcitonin guidance may aid physicians in modestly decreasing antibiotic use in critically ill patients.
- However, impact in settings with low baseline antibiotic use may be muted, and the effect on antibiotic resistance is unclear.
- As with troponin and all tests, procalcitonin requires extensive observational and interventional studies to best determine its role.

History

Procalcitonin (PCT) is a protein that consists of 116 amino acids and is the peptide precursor of calcitonin. Calcitonin is initially biosynthesized as PCT, which, under normal conditions, is found in low levels in the circulation (≤ 0.1 ng/mL).[1,2]

PCT was first described as a marker of bacterial infection in 1993 when high concentrations of calcitonin-like immunoreactivity were detected in the blood of patients with extrathyroid diseases.[3] Using a monoclonal immunoradiometric assay for calcitonin precursors, investigators measured the serum concentrations of PCT

Disclosures: Dr D.T. Huang received funding from the National Institute of General Medical Sciences, National Institutes of Health (1R34GM102696-01, 1R01GM101197-01A1) and procalcitonin assays and laboratory training from Biomerieux for the ProACT randomized trial, and funding from ThermoFisher for an observational study of the microbiome in respiratory infection.
Dedication: Dedicated to Jia Liu.
a Department of Emergency Medicine, American University of Beirut Medical Center, 2nd Floor, Cairo Street, Beirut, Lebanon; b Department of Critical Care Medicine, University of Pittsburgh Medical Center, 3550 Terrace Street, Room 651, Scaife Hall, Pittsburgh, PA 15261, USA; c Departments of Critical Care Medicine and Emergency Medicine, The MACRO (Multidisciplinary Acute Care Research Organization) and CRISMA (Clinical Research, Investigation, and Systems Modeling of Acute illness) Centers, University of Pittsburgh, 3550 Terrace Street, Room 606B, Scaife Hall, Pittsburgh, PA 15261, USA
* Corresponding author.
E-mail address: huangdt@upmc.edu

Crit Care Clin 36 (2020) 23–40
https://doi.org/10.1016/j.ccc.2019.08.003
0749-0704/20/© 2019 Elsevier Inc. All rights reserved.
criticalcare.theclinics.com

in 79 children with bacterial and viral infections. They found serum PCT levels to be very high (6–53 ng/mL) in patients with severe invasive bacterial infections when compared with patients with mild local bacterial infections or viral infections (0.1–1.5 ng/mL); additionally, they noticed that the PCT levels decreased rapidly during antibiotic therapy and that calcitonin levels were normal in all patients irrespective of PCT levels. They concluded that PCT levels are increased during bacterial septic conditions and that serum concentrations are correlated with severity of microbial invasion.

A 1994 study also found PCT levels increase in response to bacterial infection, by injecting healthy volunteers with endotoxin and measuring serial PCT levels.[4] Levels were detectable at 4 hours, peaked at 6 hours, and maintained a plateau through 8 and 24 hours before they began to decrease, thus, exhibiting a half-life of 24 hours.[4,5] Several other studies also demonstrated superior diagnostic accuracy of PCT for sepsis compared with other markers, and additionally showed PCT itself is a mediator of the deleterious effects of systemic infection.[6,7]

Subsequently, PCT has received substantial interest as a potential marker of infection to assess the presence, clearance, and eradication of infection; predict mortality; and guide antibiotic management.

This review describes a conceptual framework for biomarkers using lessons from the history of troponin, applies this framework to PCT with a review of observational studies and randomized trials in and out of the intensive care unit (ICU), and concludes with clinical recommendations and thoughts on how to test a test.

LESSONS FROM TROPONIN

The evolution of PCT as a marker of sepsis is similar to the evolution of biomarkers of other disease processes. One biomarker used in everyday practice, and specifically in cardiac disease processes, is troponin. Here we discuss how troponin came to be the dominant cardiac injury marker.

Up until the early 1990s, creatine kinase muscle/brain (CKMB) was the biomarker of choice for diagnosing acute coronary syndromes (ACS) and cardiac ischemia. However, CKMB had both imperfect sensitivity to detect myocardial injury and imperfect specificity, with increased levels also noted in patients with skeletal muscle injury and renal failure.[8] Troponin is a contractile protein released into the circulation after loss of integrity of myocardial cell membranes and is undetectable in the serum of healthy people.[9] Several observational studies began to show the potential usefulness of troponin as a prognostic indicator in ACS. They showed that patients with unstable angina (ACS without biomarker elevation) who had negative values of CKMB but positive troponin values, had subsequently higher rates of myocardial infarction and cardiac events, as well as increased mortality.[9–11] Other observational studies also showed that patients with negative CKMB and positive troponin also exhibited worse echocardiographic findings and wall motion abnormalities,[12] and had worse cardiac pathology at autopsy.[13] Going beyond prognostication, other studies suggested that troponin could be of potential value in identifying patients that would benefit from specific treatments. For example, long-term anticoagulation was found to be associated with reduced infarction and death only in patients with positive troponin values,[14] and similar beneficial long-term outcomes were observed in patients with positive troponin placed on antiplatelet agents.[15] These observational studies were followed by interventional trials such as the randomized trial of 2220 patients by Morrow and colleagues[16] that demonstrated troponin identified ACS patients that would benefit from an early invasive strategy compared with a conservative strategy.

Currently, troponin is the gold standard cardiac biomarker, and critical care clinicians and investigators often wish we had a similar tool for sepsis. In the midst of our "troponin envy," we should recognize, however, that even troponin is not perfect. A recent editorial by a prominent troponin investigator noted that even now, "integration of troponin…-with clinical decision pathways…remains an area of active investigation" and that "what represents a significant change in troponin remains contentious."[17]

Nonetheless, there are several lessons to be learned from the history of troponin. Clinically, it is clear a thoughtful clinician is needed to decide when to order a test in the first place, and then how to interpret the test, to avoid, as has been stated for troponin, an "erosion of the importance of the clinical findings [and] the electrocardiogram."[18] Academically, it is clear many studies are needed, both observational and interventional, to fully understand the true clinical usefulness of a test, with a particular focus on understanding the discordance between the old and new tests. Ideally, a goal standard is available to help understand the discordance. In the case of troponin and CKMB, serial echocardiograms were used as a clinical gold standard for true myocardial infarction, "which kept [cardiology investigators] out of the logic loop of simply comparing 2 blood tests and trying to prove one is better by seeing who could shout louder."[19] Finally, and most important, any test needs to be tied to a treatment strategy to improve outcomes.

Overall, we should be clear and specific in what exactly we want a biomarker, or any test, to do. First, one could imagine a biomarker aiding in identification, both to detect occult cases early, as well as rule out. Second, a test that predicted the development of a condition could be useful, by prompting a clinician to order additional preventive measures. However, outcome prediction may of minimal use, as noted by another prominent troponin researcher who wrote that it is "easy to show prognosis…[yet] difficult to show prognostic value"[18] For example, whether or not your patient has a 30% mortality risk (based on routinely available data and your clinical judgment) or a 60% mortality risk (based on the additive value of a novel prognostic test), both scenarios represent a high risk, and you will likely offer maximal therapy in both scenarios. Third, the ideal test would also be able to guide treatment, with a subsequent improvement in outcomes.

Applying this framework to sepsis is challenging (**Table 1**). Sepsis is defined as life-threatening organ dysfunction owing to a dysregulated host response to infection.[20]

Table 1
Potential roles of a novel biomarker in sepsis, a clinical syndrome of infection and organ dysfunction

	Infection	Organ Dysfunction
Identify	Yes/No Etiology	No usefulness, as organ dysfunction defined clinically
Predict	Development—potential value in prompting increased preventive measures Outcomes—limited value unless huge change in predictive likelihood	
Guide treatment	Start, stop, or change antibiotics	Fluids—limited usefulness beyond existing hemodynamic monitoring technologies Organ support—can, and should, any novel test alter a clinician's judgment as to when to intubate, start vasopressors, start dialysis, etc?
Improve outcomes	The hardest bar to cross; troponin required multiple observational and interventional studies to determine clinical role	

The greatest challenge is that, unlike in ACS, there is no gold standard for infection or sepsis. The ideal biomarker would identify the presence or absence of infection, etiology, and some measure of antibiotic resistance and microbial burden. However, organ dysfunction is defined clinically via known guidelines such as Sepsis-3, thus, obviating any nonresearch role for a novel test in defining organ dysfunction.[21] With respect to guiding treatment, a biomarker could conceivably aid in deciding when to start, stop, or change antibiotics, but it is difficult to imagine a biomarker having incremental value in guiding fluid management beyond existing hemodynamic monitoring technologies, or aiding in deciding when to offer organ support beyond clinician judgment and routinely available data. For example, it would seem unlikely for a clinician to decide to intubate a patient based on a biomarker. Finally, improving outcomes is a high bar to cross, requiring multiple rigorous studies, as was done with troponin.

EVIDENCE: OBSERVATIONAL STUDIES
Identification

Several studies have examined the diagnostic usefulness of PCT both in and out of the ICU for multiple conditions (**Table 2**). Overall, most, but not all, studies have found PCT to have good performance characteristics for the identification of bacterial infection and sepsis.

A 2013 systematic review and meta-analysis by Wacker and colleagues[22] of PCT as a diagnostic marker of sepsis in critically ill patients included 30 observational ICU and

Table 2
Selected recent observational studies across a variety of conditions

Authors, Year	Type of Study	Sample Size (n)	PCT Cut-Off (ng/mL)	Identification
El-Solh et al,[36] 2011	Prospective observational	65	Multiple thresholds	Aspiration pneumonia
Maisel et al,[35] 2012	Prospective, international	1641	<0.25	Reduces pneumonia diagnosis uncertainty by 82%
Hattori et al,[23] 2014	Retrospective	1331	>0.9	+ Blood cultures
Laukemann et al,[24] 2015	Observational cohort	1083	>0.1	+ Blood cultures
Rast et al,[33] 2015	Observational quality control	48	>0.25	100% specificity for distinguishing erysipelas from deep venous thrombosis
Facy et al,[30] 2016	Prospective, multicenter observational	501	>0.25	Postoperative intra-abdominal infection
Rodriguez et al,[34] 2016	Prospective, multicenter, observational	972	<0.29	Excludes bacterial coinfection in influenza patients
Sharma et al,[26] 2016	Prospective	100	>7	Identifies cardiac surgery patients with infection
Dominguez-Comesana E et al,[29] 2017	Prospective observational	120	>0.45 on postoperative day 3	Postoperative intra-abdominal infection after colon surgery

non-ICU studies. The authors included articles that investigated PCT for the differentiation of sepsis from noninfectious inflammation, and had a well-defined reference standard for sepsis based on national medical society definitions. Pooled sensitivity and specificity were 0.77 (95% confidence interval [CI], 0.72–0.81) and 0.79 (95% CI, 0.74–0.81), respectively. The authors concluded PCT is a potentially helpful marker for identification of sepsis, when carefully interpreted within the context of the clinical presentation.

Two large emergency department (ED) studies demonstrated that PCT was a useful marker in excluding bacteremia and predicting severe bacteremia.[23,24] In the ICU, PCT and potentially change in PCT[25] were found to be a predictor of bacterial infection in the surgical population.[26,27] PCT was also able to predict anastomotic leaks[28] and infection after colorectal surgery[29,30] as well as mesenteric ischemia after cardiac surgery.[31] Other small outpatient and ED studies showed the diagnostic usefulness of PCT in identifying infection in patients with rheumatoid arthritis,[32] and differentiating erysipelas from deep vein thrombosis.[33] However, a study by Facy and colleagues[30] showed that C-reactive protein (CRP) outperformed PCT in detecting postoperative infections.

The diagnostic ability of PCT to indicate infection was also demonstrated in observational studies of respiratory diseases. In a large prospective, multicenter ICU study in patients with H1N1 influenza, a PCT of less than 0.29 ng/mL had a 94% negative predictive value for excluding bacterial coinfection, and outperformed CRP.[34] In the ED, the BACH study prospectively examined 1641 patients with a chief complaint of dyspnea and found PCT increased the accuracy of diagnosing pneumonia, particularly in cases with diagnostic uncertainty, such as in patients with concomitant acute heart failure.[35] In patients with acute heart failure, a PCT of greater than 0.21 ng/mL was associated with increased mortality if not treated with antibiotics. However, other observational studies have shown less impressive performance characteristics; for example, a study by El-Solh and colleagues[36] concluded that PCT had poor ability to differentiate aspiration pneumonia from pneumonitis.

Prediction

Several observational studies assessed the prognostic ability of PCT (**Table 3**). A 2015 systematic review and meta-analysis of PCT in predicting mortality in sepsis included 23 observational studies with 3944 patients. Studies had different PCT cut-offs, but all

Table 3
Selected observational studies of PCT predicting outcome

Authors, Year	Type of Study	Sample Size (n)	PCT Cut-Off (ng/mL)	Prediction
Bloos et al,[44] 2011	Multicenter observational	175	>0.6	Increased mortality in ventilator associated pneumonia
Jain et al,[42] 2014	Prospective observational	54	>7	Increased mortality
Sager et al,[45] 2017	Multinational prospective observational	6970	>0.5	Increased mortality
Schuetz et al,[46] 2017	Multicenter prospective observational	858	Delta-PCT >80% by day 4	Increased mortality

measured PCT serially. The authors found that elevated PCT and nonclearance of PCT were associated with increased mortality in septic patients with pooled relative risks of 2.60 (95% CI, 2.05–3.30) and 3.05 (95% CI, 2.35–3.95), respectively.[37] A small prospective study showed that a PCT of greater than 2.0 ng/mL was associated with ICU admission and 30-day mortality in patients with health care associated pneumonia,[38] and another study found similar associations and additionally showed a value of greater than 0.85 ng/mL predicted *Streptococcus pneumoniae* infection.[39] Other small prospective ICU studies showed elevated PCT levels at admission were associated with increased mortality in patients with sepsis,[40–42] infective endocarditis,[43] and community-acquired or ventilator-associated pneumonia.[44] The 2 largest studies were the TRIAGE[45] and MOSES[46] studies. TRIAGE was a multicenter prospective observational study of 6970 undifferentiated adult medical patients presenting to the EDs of 3 tertiary-care hospitals in Switzerland, France, and the United States. Irrespective of presenting diagnosis and independent of underlying infection, PCT was a strong and independent predictor of 30-day mortality, with an increased mortality as well as ICU admission and hospital readmission seen with higher PCT values. PCT also improved the prognostic accuracy of the quick sequential organ failure assessment score.[20] Similarly, the ED- and ICU-based MOSES study of 858 patients showed that, when the PCT did not decrease by more than 80% from baseline to day 4, the 28-day mortality doubled.

Guiding Treatment and Improving Outcomes

There have been several publications reporting either conceptual PCT guidance based on retrospective analysis of observational data, or actual implementation of a hospital protocol with PCT guidance. One single-center study assessed multiple clinical scores and biomarkers and concluded that the combination of a clinical score and PCT could potentially decrease unnecessary blood cultures with minimal false-negative rates.[24] Similarly, an observational Japanese study suggested that theoretic PCT guidance could safely decrease antibiotic duration in community-acquired pneumonia from 12.6 to 8.6 days,[47] and an observational Spanish study suggested PCT guidance might reduce antibiotic duration in secondary peritonitis.[48] Other studies have implemented a PCT guided protocol, and then used a before/after design to determine impact. A French study of 245 patients with an exacerbation of chronic obstructive pulmonary disease found a PCT protocol was associated with a decrease in antibiotic initiation, but not duration, with 60% physician compliance with the protocol.[49] Finally, some outcome prediction studies have suggested that like lactate clearance, PCT clearance could be used to identify treatment failure, and thus guide treatment.[50] However, not all studies concur, with some finding that PCT kinetics fail to predict treatment response, such as in perioperative abdominal infection with septic shock.[51]

Overall, although most of the observational literature of PCT suggest potential clinical usefulness, good performance characteristics alone are insufficient, with the central issue for PCT, or any biomarker or test, that it be tied to a treatment decision. For infection and sepsis, the lack of a gold standard is challenging, with the microbial etiology unknown for most cases of pneumonia, and even with septic shock, approximately 30% to 40% of such cases are culture negative.[52–54] To circumvent this issue, pioneering Swiss investigators developed a PCT treatment guideline, tested this guideline in a randomized trials, and thus used patient outcomes as the gold standard.[55] In the following section, we discuss the most recent systematic reviews and metanalysis of RCTs of adult patients admitted to ICUs with a diagnosis of sepsis, where antibiotic duration and mortality were compared between a PCT-guided intervention arm and a usual care arm (**Table 4**). We then individually cover the largest of these ICU trials, as well as the 2 largest ED trials.

EVIDENCE: RANDOMIZED, CONTROLLED TRIALS

A 2018 systematic review and meta-analysis examined 10 RCTs containing 3489 ICU patients to estimate the efficacy (antibiotic duration) and safety (mortality, ICU length of stay) of PCT guidance for suspected or confirmed sepsis.[56] Most trials used a cutoff of 0.5 ng/mL to recommend antibiotic cessation among patients with sepsis or when PCT levels had decreased by 80% to 90% from peak. Two trials were excluded from the efficacy analysis as their antibiotic metric differed from the other 8 (one of the excluded trials showed no antibiotic reduction, the other showed antibiotic reduction with PCT guidance); both were included in the safety analysis.[57,58] The review concluded PCT guidance reduced antibiotic duration by 1.49 days (7. days 35 vs 8.85 days), with no adverse impact on mortality or length of ICU stay.

Another 2018 meta-analysis had a slightly different methodology and focus. The authors used individual patient data from 4482 ICU patients with infection and sepsis from 11 randomized trials to primarily assess the impact of PCT guidance on mortality within 30 days.[59] None of the individual trials were powered for mortality, except for one trial that showed no significant difference.[60] This meta-analysis reported PCT guidance reduced mortality (21.1% vs 23.7%; adjusted odds ratio; 0.89; 95% CI, 0.8–0.99), and decrease antibiotic duration by 1.19 days (9.3 days vs 10.4 days), with no difference in length of ICU or hospital stay.

The most recent 2019 systematic review and meta-analysis focused on PCT-guided antibiotic discontinuation and mortality in ICU patients, and sought to resolve and understand the discrepant mortality findings of prior meta-analyses. The authors analyzed 16 RCTs with 5158 patients and found that PCT-guided antibiotic discontinuation was associated with decreased mortality (risk ratio, 0.89; 95% CI, 0.83–0.97) and antibiotic duration (mean difference of 1.31 days). However, the authors noted these findings represented low-certainty evidence with a high risk of bias, and that decreased mortality was not found in patients with sepsis, trials with high PCT-guidance algorithm adherence, and trials that used PCT-guidance algorithms without CRP.[61]

Overall, the systematic reviews found a decrease of 1.0 to 1.5 antibiotic days with the use of PCT-guided antibiotic therapy in ICU patients, with a null or small survival benefit, and no evidence of harm.

For greater detail, we next review the 4 largest individual RCTs done in critically ill patients of PCT antibiotic guidance, where the primary goal was antibiotic reduction.

Table 4
Selected systematic reviews and meta-analysis comparing PCT-guided antibiotic therapy versus control in patients with sepsis

Authors, Year	Number of Trials	Number of Patients	Outcome in PCT Group Compared With Control
lankova et al,[56] 2018	10	3489	No effect on mortality, 1.49 reduction in days on antibiotics
Wirz et al,[59] 2018	11	4482	Decreased mortality, 1.19 reduction in days on antibiotics
Pepper et al,[61] 2019	16	5158	Decreased mortality, 1.31 reduction in days on antibiotics, low certainty of evidence with a high risk of bias

- Bouadma and colleagues[62] (2010): ProRATA
  - Prospective, randomized, parallel-group, open-label trial in 7 ICUs in France
  - Dates of enrollment: June 2007 to May 2008
  - Population: Critically ill patients with suspected bacterial infection, who had not received antibiotics for more than 24 hours
  - N = 621 (PCT n = 307, control n = 314)

Enrolled patients were mostly medical (90%), and patients with neutropenia or infections where long-term antibiotic therapy is standard (eg, endocarditis) were excluded. PCT was assessed daily until antibiotic treatment was finished. Investigators were encouraged to discontinue antibiotics when PCT levels were less than 80% of peak, or less than 0.5 µg/L. This guidance was not followed in 219 episodes. Mortality met the noninferiority margin of 10%; however, the point estimates for mortality were higher in the PCT group versus the control group (30.0% vs 26.1% at 60 days, respectively). There was no difference in the proportion of patients with emerging multidrug-resistant bacteria from clinically obtained specimens (17.9% vs 16.6%).

- Shehabi and colleagues[63] (2014): ProGUARD
  - Multicenter, prospective, single-blind, randomized controlled trial in 11 ICUs in Australia
  - Dates of enrollment: March 2011 to December 2012
  - Population: Critically ill patients with suspected bacterial infection, receiving antibiotics, and with 2 or more systemic inflammatory response syndrome criteria
  - N = 394 (PCT n = 196, control n = 198)

PCT was measured at randomization and then daily until ICU discharge or up to 7 days, whichever came first. The PCT algorithm recommended antibiotic cessation for a PCT of less than 0.1 ng/mL, 0.1 to 0.25 ng/mL and infection deemed highly unlikely, or if PCT levels decreased by more than 90% from baseline. The primary outcome of median number of antibiotic days at day 28 did not differ between arms (9 days; interquartile range, 6–21 days) versus 11 days (interquartile range, 6–22 days), nor did the 90-day mortality (35% vs 31%). Compared with other ICU trials, this trial used a very low PCT cut-off to recommend antibiotic cessation. PCT was not measured after ICU discharge, however median ICU length of stay (6 days; interquartile range, 3–10 days) was shorter than the median number of antibiotic days. These 2 factors may have contributed to the lack of significant antibiotic reduction.

- Bloos and colleagues[60] (2016): SISPCT
  - Multicenter, placebo-controlled, randomized 2 × 2 factorial trial in 33 ICUs in Germany
  - Dates of enrollment: November 2009 to June 2013
  - Population: Adults admitted to the ICU with a diagnosis of severe sepsis or septic shock
  - N = 1089 (PCT n = 552, control n = 537)

This trial was the only RCT powered for mortality. Patients were randomized to PCT antibiotic guidance or usual care, as well as to intravenous sodium selenite or placebo. PCT was measured on days 0, 1, 4, 7, 10, and 14, and PCT guidance sought to both optimize antibiotic therapy and source control (if PCT had not decreased by ≥50% from baseline), as well as discontinue antibiotics (if on day 7 or later, PCT was ≤1 ng/mL, or ≥50% lower compared with the previous value). PCT guidance did not decrease mortality or antibiotic costs, but was associated with a 4.5% decrease in antibiotic exposure (823 days vs 862 days, antibiotic exposure per 1000 ICU days).

- de Jong and colleagues[64] (2016): SAPS
  o Multicenter randomized controlled trial in 15 ICUs in the Netherlands
  o Dates of enrollment: September 2009 to July 2013
  o Population: Critically ill patients receiving antibiotics with suspected or proven infection
  o N = 1546 (PCT n = 761, control n = 785)

The SAPS trial tested the potential superiority of PCT guidance for antibiotic exposure, and the potential noninferiority for mortality and recurrent infection. PCT was measured daily until ICU discharge or until 3 days after antibiotics were stopped, and the protocol recommended antibiotic discontinuation when PCT decreased by 80% or more from peak, or was 0.5 ng/mL or lower. There was a significant decrease in median number of antibiotic days in the PCT group (5 days) compared with the control group (7 days) with an absolute difference of 1.2 days (95% CI, 0.65–1.78; $P<.0001$).

The authors also reported an unexpected finding of a lower 28-day mortality (20% vs 25%), and postulated that PCT levels may have aided in consideration of alternative diagnoses when low, and optimization of infection management when persistently high. A meta-analysis by Pepper and colleagues[61] noted that, if 9 patients in the intervention arm changed from survived to died, the survival benefit would no longer have been statistically significant.

We summarize all ICU trials comparing PCT antibiotic guidance to usual care in **Table 5**. Overall, most, but not all, trials showed a modest reduction in antibiotic exposure, patients were predominantly medical, and PCT algorithm cut-offs varied widely between trials. Only 1 trial showed increased mortality.[65]

The 2 largest non–ICU-based trials of PCT antibiotic guidance are the ProHOSP[75] and ProACT[76] trials. Both enrolled adult ED patients with lower respiratory tract infection (LRTI).

- Schuetz and colleagues[75] (2009): ProHOSP
  o Multicenter, randomized, controlled trial in 6 EDs in Switzerland
  o Dates of enrollment: October 2006 to March 2008
  o Population: adult ED patients with LRTIs
  o N = 1359 (PCT n = 671, control n = 688)

Antibiotics were strongly discouraged for a PCT of less than 0.1 ng/mL, discouraged for a PCT of 0.25 ng/mL or less, encouraged for a PCT of greater than 0.25 ng/mL, and strongly encouraged for a PCT of greater than 0.5 ng/mL. PCT was measured in hospitalized patients after 6 to 24 hours, and on days 3, 5, and 7. PCT guidance was enforced by requiring the treating physician to follow Web-based instructions on the study website before registering and entering baseline data. Physicians could overrule PCT guideline recommendations only after consulting with the coordinating center, for critical illness, or for legionella infection. Overall adverse outcomes were similar between groups (15.4% PCT, 18.9% control); and met the a priori noninferiority margin of 7.5%. The mean antibiotic duration differed between groups (5.7 days PCT vs 8.7 days control). The authors concluded PCT guidance decrease antibiotic exposure without adverse effects in LRTI. The results of smaller but similar trials conducted between 2004 and 2016 were summarized in a 2018 meta-analysis of 4090 trials from 11 trials, and found PCT guidance in LRTI resulted in shorter mean antibiotic use (mean difference, −2.15 days) with no adverse effect on mortality or length of stay.[77] The ProACT trial was published in 2018, and not included in this meta-analysis.

Table 5
ICU RCTs comparing PCT-guided algorithm antibiotic administration with usual care

Authors, Year	Sample Size	PCT Algorithm for Antibiotic Cessation (ng/mL)	Mean Antibiotic Duration	Mortality
Nobre et al,[66] 2008	79	<0.25 or >90% change if initial level ≥1.0	12.3 (PCT), 13.5 (control)	21% (PCT), 20% (control)
Hochreiter et al,[67] 2009	110	<1.0; ≥65%–75% change from initial level and current level>1.0	5.9 (PCT), 7.9 (control)	26% (PCT), 26% (control)
Schroeder et al,[68] 2009	27	≤1.0; ≥65%–75% change from initial level	6.6 (PCT), 8.3 (control)	21% (PCT), 23% (control)
Stolz et al,[69] 2009	101	After 72 h <0.25; between 0.25 and 0.5 with a decrease ≥80% from day 0	27% reduction	16% (PCT), 24% (control)
Bouadma et al,[62] 2010	621	<0.5; >80% change from peak	10.3 (PCT), 13.3 (control)	21% (PCT), 20% (control)
Jensen et al,[70] 2011	1200	<1.0 for ≥3 d	6 (PCT), 4 (control) [median values]	31.5% (PCT), 32% (control)
Layios et al,[57] 2012	509	<0.5	NA	22% (PCT), 21% (control)
Qu et al,[71] 2012	71	<0.5 on day 3	10.89 (PCT), 16.06 (control)	Not mentioned
Annane et al,[72] 2013	62	<0.5	4.7 (PCT), 4.0 (control)	23% (PCT), 32% (control)
Deliberato et al,[73] 2013	81	<0.5; >90% change from peak	15.5 (PCT), 17.3 (control)	2% (PCT), 10% (control)
Oliviera et al,[74] 2013	94	Initial <1.0, day 4 <0.1; initial ≥1.0, day 5 decrease of ≥90%	7.0 (PCT), 6.0 (CRP)	32.7% (PCT), 33.3% (CRP)
Shehabi et al,[63] 2014	394	<0.1; <0.10–0.25 if infection unlikely; >90% change from baseline level	11.7 (PCT), 13.0 (control)	11% (PCT), 8% (control)
Najafi et al,[58] 2015	60	≤0.5	NA	17% (PCT), 13% (control)
Bloos et al,[60] 2016	1089	<1; >50% change from baseline	4.5% reduction	25.6% (PCT), 28.2% (control)
de Jong et al,[64] 2016	1545	≤0.5; >80% change from peak	5.7 (PCT), 7.3 (control)	20% (PCT), 25% (control)
Daubin et al,[65] 2018	302	<0.1	5.2 (PCT), 5.4 (control)	20% (PCT), 14% (control)

- Huang and colleagues[76] (2018): ProACT
  - Multicenter, randomized, controlled trial in 14 EDs in the United States
  - Dates of enrollment: November 2014 to May 2017
  - Population: adult ED patients with LRTIs
  - N = 1656 (PCT n = 826, control n = 830)

ProACT used the same PCT guidance cut-offs and serial measurements used in ProHOSP, and guidance was deployed using quality improvement principles, with extensive use of education, prompts, and feedback. Overall adverse outcomes were similar between the groups (11.7% vs 13.1%) and met the a priori noninferiority margin of 4.5%. However, there was no difference between groups in mean antibiotic days by day 30 (4.2 days PCT vs 4.3 days control). In patients with acute bronchitis, antibiotic prescription in the ED seems to be lower in the PCT group versus control group (17.3% vs 32.1%), even after adjustment for multiple comparisons. However, this finding was a secondary outcome of a subgroup. The authors concluded provision of a PCT guideline to ED and hospital clinicians did not decreased antibiotic use among patients with suspected LRTI. The authors speculated that potential reasons for the lack of difference included limited incremental information from PCT to guide decision making (because PCT was associated with antibiotic prescription in both groups, as well as clinical signs and symptoms), PCT-guided decisions to withhold antibiotics in the ED and hospital were overruled in the outpatient setting, lower control group antibiotic use compared with that in ProHOSP, and lower clinician adherence to PCT guidance than in ProHOSP. Notably, control group antibiotic use was lower than U. norms, with less than one-third of acute bronchitis patients in ProACT receiving antibiotics, versus approximately 70% in multiple large US studies.[78–80]

CURRENT USE

Between 2007 and 2015, PCT use in US ICUs increased from 0.0% to 11.7%, compared with CRP use, which only increased by 3% during that time. Currently, PCT is ordered in 1 of every 20 adult US patients in hospitals found in the Premier Healthcare Database.[81] A retrospective study of patients with sepsis in US ICUs registered in the Premier Healthcare Database found that 18% had PCT measured and 30% had serial PCT measurements.[82] Another retrospective study of 933,591 patients with sepsis showed an increase in PCT use compared with CRP, and that multiple PCT measurements were associated with more interventions such as ICU admission, and use of vasopressors and mechanical ventilation.[83]

National authorities and medical societies have reached varying conclusions about PCT guidance in LRTI and sepsis. The US Food and Drug Administration first approved PCT as an aid, in conjunction with other laboratory findings and clinical assessments, to predict which patients on their first day of ICU admission would progress to sepsis and septic shock. Subsequently, the US Food and Drug Administration also approved serial PCT as an aid to predict risk of 28-day mortality in critically ill patients with sepsis and septic shock. In 2017, the US Food and Drug Administration cleared the expanded use of PCT to help ED or hospital clinicians determine if antibiotics should be started or stopped in patients with LRTI, and stopped in patients with sepsis.[84] In 2016, the US Agency for Healthcare Research and Quality concluded PCT had moderate strength evidence for reducing antibiotic prescription in uncomplicated acute respiratory tract infections, with low strength evidence for safety.[85] In 2015, the United Kingdom National Institute for Health and Care Excellence concluded that there was insufficient evidence for use of PCT in sepsis,[86,87] and in 2016 the Infectious Diseases Society of America did not recommend PCT to guide antibiotic initiation in suspected hospital- or ventilator-associated pneumonia.[84] The current international 2016 Surviving Sepsis Campaign guidelines suggested that PCT could be used to support shortening antibiotic duration in patients with sepsis, and in patients who initially seemed to have sepsis but subsequently had limited clinical evidence of infection (weak recommendation, low quality of evidence).[88,89] The Infectious Diseases Society of America did not endorse these guidelines, stating that they failed to provide specific recommendations that providers can follow, and noting that their interpretation of the RCT literature is that PCT guidance for antibiotic duration is feasible and safe in critically ill patients with infections.[86]

Although disparate evidence and recommendations are common in medicine, what should hospitals and clinicians do today? We believe that in hospitals similar to those in ProACT—tertiary care academic centers with a relatively low baseline antibiotic use for LRTI—PCT guidance, even if deployed using extensive education, will have a minimal impact. It is possible that PCT guidance, combined with a robust antibiotic stewardship program, may have a greater impact. However, an antibiotic stewardship program alone might be sufficient in decreasing antibiotic use. It is also possible that PCT guidance in hospitals with more liberal use of antibiotics for LRTI may have a greater impact. However, simpler interventions such as basic education might also be impactful in such settings. For critically ill patients in the ICU and those with sepsis, we believe PCT should not be used for antibiotic initiation decisions, but could play a modest role in shortening antibiotic duration. However, the increased attention to antibiotic overuse and stewardship, and evidence-based movement toward shorter antibiotic courses, may limit incremental opportunity for PCT to further shorten duration. The most current meta-analyses in fact have only found a reduction of 1.0 to 1.5 antibiotic days from PCT guidance in the ICU. Although any decrease is laudable, the impact of a 1.0- to 1.5-day decrease in antibiotic duration on the ultimate target of antibiotic resistance is unclear. At the individual clinician level, we concur with the basic precepts of the Choosing Wisely Campaign, which urges thoughtful consideration of when to order tests and how to use their results. We recommend that should a physician choose to order PCT, that it be ordered in cases of clinical uncertainty so as to have the greatest chance of changing management, that the physician be prepared to follow the PCT guidance recommendation, and that above all traditional means of diagnosis and assessment should continue to be used, with PCT as only 1 part of clinical decision making.

HOW DO YOU TEST A TEST?

We should recognize that the story of PCT is not unique, and the generic question of how to prove a test is useful—or not—applies to all diagnostics in all fields. For example, it took decades to realize that the routine use of pulmonary artery catheters in the ICU was unnecessary,[90] and authorities still disagree on the optimal timing of mammograms for breast cancer screening,[91–93] as well as prostate-specific antigen testing for prostate cancer screening.[94] More recently, B-type natriuretic peptide–guided treatment was found to minimally change management in congestive heart failure and did not improve outcomes, in hospitals with expertise in heart failure and robust usual care.[95] Conversely, advanced testing has had positive impact in some areas, such as use of computed tomography scan screening to decrease lung cancer mortality, and use of a novel gene expression array to safely avoid chemotherapy use in breast cancer.[96,97] We believe that, as with troponin, not only PCT, but all tests, require extensive observational and interventional studies to best determine their role. Several currently enrolling trials of PCT guidance will aid in this determination (**Table 6**).

Title	ClinicalTrials. gov Identifier	Study Type	Aim
Table 6 **Ongoing PCT clinical trials**			
A Clinical Trial of Procalcitonin-guided Antimicrobial Therapy in Sepsis (PROGRESS)	NCT03333304	Randomized prospective open-label clinical trial	Can 1 PCT-guided rule of stop antimicrobials decrease the incidence of infections by *C difficile* and multidrug-resistant bacteria
Biomarker Guided Antibiotic Treatment in Community-Acquired Pneumonia (BIO-CAP)	NCT03146182	Randomized prospective parallel assignment open-label clinical trial	To determine the efficacy of CRP and PCT based guidelines vs standard of care in reducing duration of antibiotic exposure in hospitalized patients with community-acquired pneumonia
A Randomized Double-Blinded, Placebo-Controlled Trial of Antibiotic Therapy in Patients with Lower Respiratory Tract Infection (LRTI) and a Procalcitonin Level (TRAP-LRTI)	NCT03341273	Randomized double-blinded placebo controlled noninferiority multicenter clinical trial	Compare the efficacy of azithromycin vs placebo on day 5 in patients with suspect LRTI and PCT levels ≤0.25 ng/mL

REFERENCES

1. Muller B, White JC, Nylen ES, et al. Ubiquitous expression of the calcitonin-i gene in multiple tissues in response to sepsis. J Clin Endocrinol Metab 2001;86(1):396–404.
2. Wiedermann FJ, Kaneider N, Egger P, et al. Migration of human monocytes in response to procalcitonin. Crit Care Med 2002;30(5):1112–7.
3. Assicot M, Gendrel D, Carsin H, et al. High serum procalcitonin concentrations in patients with sepsis and infection. Lancet 1993;341(8844):515–8.
4. Dandona P, Nix D, Wilson MF, et al. Procalcitonin increase after endotoxin injection in normal subjects. J Clin Endocrinol Metab 1994;79(6):1605–8.
5. Brunkhorst FM, Heinz U, Forycki ZF. Kinetics of procalcitonin in iatrogenic sepsis. Intensive Care Med 1998;24(8):888–9.
6. Muller B, Becker KL, Schachinger H, et al. Calcitonin precursors are reliable markers of sepsis in a medical intensive care unit. Crit Care Med 2000;28(4):977–83.
7. Nylen ES, Whang KT, Snider RH Jr, et al. Mortality is increased by procalcitonin and decreased by an antiserum reactive to procalcitonin in experimental sepsis. Crit Care Med 1998;26(0).1001–6.
8. Adams JE 3rd, Bodor GS, Davila-Roman VG, et al. Cardiac troponin I. A marker with high specificity for cardiac injury. Circulation 1993;88(1):101–6.
9. Hamm CW, Ravkilde J, Gerhardt W, et al. The prognostic value of serum troponin T in unstable angina. N Engl J Med 1992;327(3):146–50.
10. Galvani M, Ottani F, Ferrini D, et al. Prognostic influence of elevated values of cardiac troponin I in patients with unstable angina. Circulation 1997;95(8):2053–9.

11. Stubbs P, Collinson P, Moseley D, et al. Prospective study of the role of cardiac troponin T in patients admitted with unstable angina. BMJ 1996;313(7052):262–4.

12. Adams JE 3rd, Sicard GA, Allen BT, et al. Diagnosis of perioperative myocardial infarction with measurement of cardiac troponin I. N Engl J Med 1994;330(10): 670–4.

13. Ooi DS, Isotalo PA, Veinot JP. Correlation of antemortem serum creatine kinase, creatine kinase-MB, troponin I, and troponin T with cardiac pathology. Clin Chem 2000;46(3):338–44.

14. Lindahl B, Venge P, Wallentin L. Troponin T identifies patients with unstable coronary artery disease who benefit from long-term antithrombotic protection. Fragmin in Unstable Coronary Artery Disease (FRISC) Study Group. J Am Coll Cardiol 1997;29(1):43–8.

15. Hamm CW, Heeschen C, Goldmann B, et al. Benefit of abciximab in patients with refractory unstable angina in relation to serum troponin T levels. c7E3 Fab Antiplatelet Therapy in Unstable Refractory Angina (CAPTURE) Study Investigators. N Engl J Med 1999;340(21):1623–9.

16. Morrow DA, Cannon CP, Rifai N, et al. Ability of minor elevations of troponins I and T to predict benefit from an early invasive strategy in patients with unstable angina and non-ST elevation myocardial infarction: results from a randomized trial. JAMA 2001;286(19):2405–12.

17. Collinson PO, Garrison L, Christenson RH. Cardiac biomarkers - a short biography. Clin Biochem 2015;48(4–5):197–200.

18. Jesse RL. On the relative value of an assay versus that of a test: a history of troponin for the diagnosis of myocardial infarction. J Am Coll Cardiol 2010; 55(19):2125–8.

19. Ladenson JH. Reflections on the evolution of cardiac biomarkers. Clin Chem 2012;58(1):21–4.

20. Seymour CW, Liu VX, Iwashyna TJ, et al. Assessment of clinical criteria for sepsis: for the third international consensus definitions for sepsis and septic shock (sepsis-3). JAMA 2016;315(8):762–74.

21. Singer M, Deutschman CS, Seymour CW, et al. The third international consensus definitions for sepsis and septic shock (sepsis-3). JAMA 2016;315(8):801–10.

22. Wacker C, Prkno A, Brunkhorst FM, et al. Procalcitonin as a diagnostic marker for sepsis: a systematic review and meta-analysis. Lancet Infect Dis 2013;13(5): 426–35.

23. Hattori T, Nishiyama H, Kato H, et al. Clinical value of procalcitonin for patients with suspected bloodstream infection. Am J Clin Pathol 2014;141(1):43–51.

24. Laukemann S, Kasper N, Kulkarni P, et al. Can we reduce negative blood cultures with clinical scores and blood markers? results from an observational cohort study. Medicine (Baltimore) 2015;94(49):e2264.

25. Trasy D, Tanczos K, Nemeth M, et al. Delta procalcitonin is a better indicator of infection than absolute procalcitonin values in critically ill patients: a prospective observational study. J Immunol Res 2016;2016:3530752.

26. Sharma P, Patel K, Baria K, et al. Procalcitonin level for prediction of postoperative infection in cardiac surgery. Asian Cardiovasc Thorac Ann 2016;24(4):344–9.

27. Jhan JY, Huang YT, Shih CH, et al. Procalcitonin levels to predict bacterial infection in surgical intensive care unit patients. Formos J Surg 2017;50:135–41.

28. Zielinska-Borkowska U, Dib N, Tarnowski W, et al. Monitoring of procalcitonin but not interleukin-6 is useful for the early prediction of anastomotic leakage after colorectal surgery. Clin Chem Lab Med 2017;55(7):1053–9.

29. Dominguez-Comesana E, Estevez-Fernandez SM, Lopez-Gomez V, et al. Procal-citonin and C-reactive protein as early markers of postoperative intra-abdominal infection in patients operated on colorectal cancer. Int J Colorectal Dis 2017; 32(12):1771–4.
30. Facy O, Paquette B, Orry D, et al. Diagnostic accuracy of inflammatory markers as early predictors of infection after elective colorectal surgery: results from the IMACORS study. Ann Surg 2016;263(5):961–6.
31. Klingele M, Bomberg H, Poppleton A, et al. Elevated procalcitonin in patients af-ter cardiac surgery: a hint to nonocclusive mesenteric ischemia. Ann Thorac Surg 2015;99(4):1306–12.
32. Tsujimoto K, Hata A, Fujita M, et al. Presepsin and procalcitonin as biomarkers of systemic bacterial infection in patients with rheumatoid arthritis. Int J Rheum Dis 2018;21(7):1406–13.
33. Rast AC, Knobel D, Faessler L, et al. Use of procalcitonin, C-reactive protein and white blood cell count to distinguish between lower limb erysipelas and deep vein thrombosis in the emergency department: a prospective observational study. J Dermatol 2015;42(8):778–85.
34. Rodriguez AH, Aviles-Jurado FX, Diaz E, et al. Procalcitonin (PCT) levels for ruling-out bacterial coinfection in ICU patients with influenza: a CHAID decision-tree analysis. J Infect 2016;72(2):143–51.
35. Maisel A, Neath SX, Landsberg J, et al. Use of procalcitonin for the diagnosis of pneumonia in patients presenting with a chief complaint of dyspnoea: results from the BACH (Biomarkers in Acute Heart Failure) trial. Eur J Heart Fail 2012; 14(3):278–86.
36. El-Solh AA, Vora H, Knight PR 3rd, et al. Diagnostic use of serum procalcitonin levels in pulmonary aspiration syndromes. Crit Care Med 2011;39(6):1251–6.
37. Liu D, Su L, Han G, et al. Prognostic value of procalcitonin in adult patients with sepsis: a systematic review and meta-analysis. PLoS One 2015;10(6):e0129450.
38. Hong DY, Park SO, Kim JW, et al. Serum procalcitonin: an independent predictor of clinical outcome in health care-associated pneumonia. Respiration 2016;92(4): 241–51.
39. Julian-Jimenez A, Timon Zapata J, Laserna Mendieta EJ, et al. Diagnostic and prognostic power of biomarkers to improve the management of community ac-quired pneumonia in the emergency department. Enferm Infecc Microbiol Clin 2014;32(4):225–35 [in Spanish].
40. Azevedo JR, Torres OJ, Czeczko NG, et al. Procalcitonin as a prognostic biomarker of severe sepsis and septic shock. Rev Col Bras Cir 2012;39(6): 456–61.
41. de Azevedo JR, Torres OJ, Beraldi RA, et al. Prognostic evaluation of severe sepsis and septic shock: procalcitonin clearance vs Delta Sequential Organ Fail-ure Assessment. J Crit Care 2015;30(1):219.e9-12.
42. Jain S, Sinha S, Sharma SK, et al. Procalcitonin as a prognostic marker for sepsis: a prospective observational study. BMC Res Notoo 2014,7.458.
43. Cornellssen CG, Frechen DA, Schreiner K, et al. Inflammatory parameters and prediction of prognosis in infective endocarditis. BMC Infect Dis 2013;13:272.
44. Bloos F, Marshall JC, Dellinger RP, et al. Multinational, observational study of pro-calcitonin in ICU patients with pneumonia requiring mechanical ventilation: a multicenter observational study. Crit Care 2011;15(2):R88.
45. Sager R, Wirz Y, Amin D, et al. Are admission procalcitonin levels universal mor-tality predictors across different medical emergency patient populations? Results

from the multi-national, prospective, observational TRIAGE study. Clin Chem Lab Med 2017;55(12):1873–80.

46. Schuetz P, Birkhahn R, Sherwin R, et al. Serial procalcitonin predicts mortality in severe sepsis patients: results from the multicenter procalcitonin MOnitoring SEpsis (MOSES) study. Crit Care Med 2017;45(5):781–9.

47. Ito A, Ishida T, Tokumasu H, et al. Impact of procalcitonin-guided therapy for hospitalized community-acquired pneumonia on reducing antibiotic consumption and costs in Japan. J Infect Chemother 2017;23(3):142–7.

48. Maseda E, Suarez-de-la-Rica A, Anillo V, et al. Procalcitonin-guided therapy may reduce length of antibiotic treatment in intensive care unit patients with secondary peritonitis: a multicenter retrospective study. J Crit Care 2015;30(3):537–42.

49. Picart J, Moiton MP, Gauzere BA, et al. Introduction of a PCT-based algorithm to guide antibiotic prescription in COPD exacerbation. Med Mal Infect 2016;46(8):429–35.

50. Shi Y, Xu YC, Rui X, et al. Procalcitonin kinetics and nosocomial pneumonia in older patients. Respir Care 2014;59(8):1258–66.

51. Jung B, Molinari N, Nasri M, et al. Procalcitonin biomarker kinetics fails to predict treatment response in perioperative abdominal infection with septic shock. Crit Care 2013;17(5):R255.

52. Phua J, Ngerng W, See K, et al. Characteristics and outcomes of culture-negative versus culture-positive severe sepsis. Crit Care 2013;17(5):R202.

53. de Prost N, Razazi K, Brun-Buisson C. Unrevealing culture-negative severe sepsis. Crit Care 2013;17(5):1001.

54. Gupta S, Sakhuja A, Kumar G, et al. Culture-negative severe sepsis: nationwide trends and outcomes. Chest 2016;150(6):1251–9.

55. Christ-Crain M, Muller B. Procalcitonin in bacterial infections–hype, hope, more or less? Swiss Med Wkly 2005;135(31–32):451–60.

56. Iankova I, Thompson-Leduc P, Kirson NY, et al. Efficacy and safety of procalcitonin guidance in patients with suspected or confirmed sepsis: a systematic review and meta-analysis. Crit Care Med 2018;46(5):691–8.

57. Layios N, Lambermont B, Canivet JL, et al. Procalcitonin usefulness for the initiation of antibiotic treatment in intensive care unit patients. Crit Care Med 2012;40(8):2304–9.

58. Najafi A, Khodadadian A, Sanatkar M, et al. The comparison of procalcitonin guidance administer antibiotics with empiric antibiotic therapy in critically ill patients admitted in intensive care unit. Acta Med Iran 2015;53(9):562–7.

59. Wirz Y, Meier MA, Bouadma L, et al. Effect of procalcitonin-guided antibiotic treatment on clinical outcomes in intensive care unit patients with infection and sepsis patients: a patient-level meta-analysis of randomized trials. Crit Care 2018;22(1):191.

60. Bloos F, Trips E, Nierhaus A, et al. Effect of sodium selenite administration and procalcitonin-guided therapy on mortality in patients with severe sepsis or septic shock: a randomized clinical trial. JAMA Intern Med 2016;176(9):1266–76.

61. Pepper D, Sun J, Rhee C, et al. Procalcitonin-guided antibiotic discontinuation and mortality in critically ill adults: a systematic review and meta-analysis. Chest 2019;155(6):1109–18.

62. Bouadma L, Luyt CE, Tubach F, et al. Use of procalcitonin to reduce patients' exposure to antibiotics in intensive care units (PRORATA trial): a multicentre randomised controlled trial. Lancet 2010;375(9713):463–74.

63. Shehabi Y, Sterba M, Garrett PM, et al. Procalcitonin algorithm in critically ill adults with undifferentiated infection or suspected sepsis. A randomized controlled trial. Am J Respir Crit Care Med 2014;190(10):1102–10.
64. de Jong E, van Oers JA, Beishuizen A, et al. Efficacy and safety of procalcitonin guidance in reducing the duration of antibiotic treatment in critically ill patients: a randomised, controlled, open-label trial. Lancet Infect Dis 2016;16(7):819–27.
65. Daubin C, Valette X, Thiolliere F, et al. Procalcitonin algorithm to guide initial antibiotic therapy in acute exacerbations of COPD admitted to the ICU: a randomized multicenter study. Intensive Care Med 2018;44(4):428–37.
66. Nobre V, Harbarth S, Graf JD, et al. Use of procalcitonin to shorten antibiotic treatment duration in septic patients: a randomized trial. Am J Respir Crit Care Med 2008;177(5):498–505.
67. Hochreiter M, Kohler T, Schweiger AM, et al. Procalcitonin to guide duration of antibiotic therapy in intensive care patients: a randomized prospective controlled trial. Crit Care 2009;13(3):R83.
68. Schroeder S, Hochreiter M, Koehler T, et al. Procalcitonin (PCT)-guided algorithm reduces length of antibiotic treatment in surgical intensive care patients with severe sepsis: results of a prospective randomized study. Langenbecks Arch Surg 2009;394(2):221–6.
69. Stolz D, Smyrnios N, Eggimann P, et al. Procalcitonin for reduced antibiotic exposure in ventilator-associated pneumonia: a randomised study. Eur Respir J 2009; 34(6):1364–75.
70. Jensen JU, Hein L, Lundgren B, et al. Procalcitonin-guided interventions against infections to increase early appropriate antibiotics and improve survival in the intensive care unit: a randomized trial. Crit Care Med 2011;39(9):2048–58.
71. Qu R, Ji Y, Ling Y, et al. Procalcitonin is a good tool to guide duration of antibiotic therapy in patients with severe acute pancreatitis. A randomized prospective single-center controlled trial. Saudi Med J 2012;33(4):382–7.
72. Annane D, Maxime V, Faller JP, et al. Procalcitonin levels to guide antibiotic therapy in adults with non-microbiologically proven apparent severe sepsis: a randomised controlled trial. BMJ Open 2013;3(2) [pii:e002186].
73. Deliberato RO, Marra AR, Sanches PR, et al. Clinical and economic impact of procalcitonin to shorten antimicrobial therapy in septic patients with proven bacterial infection in an intensive care setting. Diagn Microbiol Infect Dis 2013;76(3):266–71.
74. Oliveira CF, Botoni FA, Oliveira CR, et al. Procalcitonin versus C-reactive protein for guiding antibiotic therapy in sepsis: a randomized trial. Crit Care Med 2013; 41(10):2336–43.
75. Schuetz P, Christ-Crain M, Thomann R, et al. Effect of procalcitonin-based guidelines vs standard guidelines on antibiotic use in lower respiratory tract infections: the ProHOSP randomized controlled trial. JAMA 2009;302(10):1059–66.
76. Huang DT, Yealy DM, Filbin MR, et al. Procalcitonin-guided use of antibiotics for lower respiratory tract infection. N Engl J Med 2018;379(3):236–49.
77. Hey J, Thompson-Leduc P, Kirson NY, et al. Procalcitonin guidance in patients with lower respiratory tract infections: a systematic review and meta-analysis. Clin Chem Lab Med 2018;56(8):1200–9.
78. Barnett ML, Linder JA. Antibiotic prescribing for adults with acute bronchitis in the United States, 1996-2010. JAMA 2014;311(19):2020–2.
79. Gonzales R, Anderer T, McCulloch CE, et al. A cluster randomized trial of decision support strategies for reducing antibiotic use in acute bronchitis. JAMA Intern Med 2013;173(4):267–73.

80. Grigoryan L, Zoorob R, Shah J, et al. Antibiotic prescribing for uncomplicated acute bronchitis is highest in younger adults. Antibiotics (Basel) 2017;6(4) [pii:E22].
81. Sameer Kadri CR, Cao Z, Robinson SB, et al. The epidemiology of procalcitonin use in Unites States hospitals. Open Forum Infect Dis 2016;3:229.
82. Chu DC, Mehta AB, Walkey AJ. Practice patterns and outcomes associated with procalcitonin use in critically ill patients with sepsis. Clin Infect Dis 2017;64(11):1509–15.
83. Gluck E, Nguyen HB, Yalamanchili K, et al. Real-world use of procalcitonin and other biomarkers among sepsis hospitalizations in the United States: a retrospective, observational study. PLoS One 2018;13(10):e0205924.
84. Discussion and recommendations for the application of procalcitonin to the evaluation and management of suspected lower respiratory tract infections and sepsis. Gaithersburg, Maryland: FDA Executive Summary. November 10, 2016.
85. McDonagh M, Peterson K, Winthrop K, et al, AHRQ. Interventions to improve antibiotic prescribing for uncomplicated acute respiratory tract infections. North Bethesda (MD): Agency for Healthcare Research and Quality; 2016. 15(16)-EHC033-3-EF.
86. NICE. Procalcitonin testing for diagnosing and monitoring sepsis (ADVIA Centaur BRAHMS PCT assay, BRAHMS PCT Sensitive Kryptor assay, Elecsys BRAHMS PCT assay, LIAISON BRAHMS PCT assay and VIDAS BRAHMS PCT assay). Diagnostics guidance. October 7, 2015. Available at: nice.org.uk/guidance/dg18.
87. Kalil AC, Metersky ML, Klompas M, et al. Management of adults with hospital-acquired and ventilator-associated pneumonia: 2016 clinical practice guidelines by the infectious diseases Society of America and the American Thoracic Society. Clin Infect Dis 2016;63(5):e61–111.
88. Rhodes A, Evans LE, Alhazzani W, et al. Surviving sepsis Campaign: international guidelines for management of sepsis and septic shock: 2016. Crit Care Med 2017;45(3):486–552.
89. Force IST. Infectious Diseases Society of America (IDSA) POSITION STATEMENT: why IDSA did not endorse the surviving sepsis Campaign guidelines. Clin Infect Dis 2018;66(10):1631–5.
90. Chatterjee K. The Swan-Ganz catheters: past, present, and future. A viewpoint. Circulation 2009;119(1):147–52.
91. Monticciolo DL, Newell MS, Hendrick RE, et al. Breast cancer screening for average-risk women: recommendations from the ACR commission on breast imaging. J Am Coll Radiol 2017;14(9):1137–43.
92. Oeffinger KC, Fontham ET, Etzioni R, et al. Breast cancer screening for women at average risk: 2015 guideline update from the American Cancer Society. JAMA 2015;314(15):1599–614.
93. Siu AL, U.S. Preventive Services Task Force. Screening for breast cancer: U.S. preventive services task force recommendation statement. Ann Intern Med 2016;164(4):279–96.
94. Kim EH, Andriole GL. Prostate-specific antigen-based screening: controversy and guidelines. BMC Med 2015;13:61.
95. Felker GM, Anstrom KJ, Adams KF, et al. Effect of natriuretic peptide-guided therapy on hospitalization or cardiovascular mortality in high-risk patients with heart failure and reduced ejection fraction: a randomized clinical trial. JAMA 2017;318(8):713–20.
96. National Lung Screening Trial Research Team, Aberle DR, Adams AM, Berg CD, et al. Reduced lung-cancer mortality with low-dose computed tomographic screening. N Engl J Med 2011;365(5):395–409.
97. Sparano JA, Gray RJ, Makower DF, et al. Adjuvant chemotherapy guided by a 21-gene expression assay in breast cancer. N Engl J Med 2018;379(2):111–21.

Soluble Triggering Receptor Expressed on Myeloid Cells-1: Diagnosis or Prognosis?

Jérémie Lemarié, MD, PhD[a,b], Sébastien Gibot, MD, PhD[a,b,*]

KEYWORDS

- Sepsis • Diagnosis • Prognosis • Biomarker • sTREM-1

KEY POINTS

- Soluble triggering receptor expressed on myeloid cells-1 concentration can be used as a surrogate marker of triggering receptor expressed on myeloid cells-1 activation (a receptor that amplifies the innate immune response).
- Plasma soluble triggering receptor expressed on myeloid cells-1 has a moderate diagnostic performance in differentiating sepsis from sterile inflammatory response.
- Determination of soluble triggering receptor expressed on myeloid cells-1 concentrations at the site of the presumed infection is more useful in clinical practice.
- Soluble triggering receptor expressed on myeloid cells-1 concentrations have a moderate prognostic significance in assessing the mortality of infection in adult patients.

INTRODUCTION

Sepsis-related mortality and morbidity are major health care problems worldwide.[1] Clinical and laboratory signs of systemic inflammation are neither sensitive nor specific enough for the diagnosis of sepsis and can often be misleading. Patients with major trauma, burns, pancreatitis, acute autoimmune disorders, and many other conditions may present the same clinical signs as infected patients. There is no gold standard for diagnosing sepsis because nearly one-half of infected patients remain without microbial documentation. Moreover, microbiological results are not immediately available. While waiting, clinicians may administer unneeded antibiotics. However, the empirical use of broad-spectrum antibiotics in patients without infection is potentially harmful, facilitating colonization and superinfection with multidrug-resistant bacteria. Thus, there is an unsatisfied need for laboratory tools allowing

[a] CHRU Nancy, Hôpital Central, Service de Réanimation Médicale, 29 avenue de LAttre de Tassigny, 54000 Nancy, France; [b] INSERM UMRS-1116, Faculté de Médecine Nancy, Université de Lorraine, 9 avenue de la forêt de Haye, 54500 Vandoeuvre-les-Nancy, France
* Corresponding author.
E-mail address: s.gibot@chru-nancy.fr

Crit Care Clin 36 (2020) 41–54
https://doi.org/10.1016/j.ccc.2019.08.004
criticalcare.theclinics.com
0749-0704/20/© 2019 Elsevier Inc. All rights reserved.

distinguishing between sterile inflammation and sepsis. Among the markers of sepsis currently in use, procalcitonin (PCT) has been suggested to be the most promising one. However, its use as a diagnostic and staging tool has been questioned (discussed in Bachar Hamade and David T. Huang's article, "Procalcitonin: Where Are We Now?," in the issue).[2]

A biomarker has been defined as "a characteristic that is, objectively measured and evaluated as an indicator of normal biological processes, pathogenic processes, or pharmacologic responses to a therapeutic intervention."[3] In this article, we review the usefulness of a recently discovered biomarker, the soluble form of the triggering receptor expressed on myeloid cells-1 (sTREM-1) as a diagnostic and prognostic tool for sepsis.

THE TRIGGERING RECEPTOR EXPRESSED ON MYELOID CELLS-1

The TREM family encompasses several isoforms that share low sequence homology with each other and have only 1 immunoglobulin-like domain. The 5 identified *trem* genes are clustered on human chromosome 6 (and mouse chromosome 17). All TREMs associate with the adaptor DNA activating protein 12 (DAP12, also called KARAP) for signaling.[4] Engagement of TREMs triggers a signaling pathway leading to intracellular calcium mobilization, actin cytoskeleton rearrangement and activation of transcriptional factors such as nuclear factor κB. This eventually results in the production of metalloproteases, proinflammatory cytokines, and chemokines along with rapid neutrophil degranulation and oxidative burst.[5,6]

Among the TREM family, TREM-1 has been the subject of intense research. As suggested by its name, TREM-1 was first identified on both human and murine myeloid cells, especially neutrophils, mature monocytes and macrophages. Its expression at the cell surface of these effector cells is dramatically increased in skin, biological fluids and tissues infected by gram-positive or gram-negative bacteria as well as by fungi.[7] The activation of TREM-1 by its still unknown ligand in the presence of Toll-like receptor 2 (TLR2) or TLR4 ligands amplifies the production of proinflammatory cytokines. In addition, activation of these TLRs upregulates TREM-1 expression.[5] Thus, TREM-1 and TLRs cooperate to produce an inflammatory response. The role of TREM-1 as an amplifier of the inflammatory response has been confirmed in a mouse model of septic shock in which blocking signaling through TREM-1 partially protected animals from death.[7,8]

SOLUBLE TRIGGERING RECEPTOR EXPRESSED ON MYELOID CELLS-1

Besides its membrane-anchored form, a soluble form of TREM-1 (sTREM-1) is released and can be measured in several body fluids. Whether sTREM-1 originates from a splice variant isoform lacking the transmembrane domain or whether it is generated by proteolytic cleavage of membrane-bound TREM-1 is still a matter of debate and both mechanisms are likely to occur.[9,10] Soluble TREM-1 acts as a decoy receptor by sequestering the unknown TREM-1 ligand, hence, dampening cell-surface TREM-1 activation.[8] Because the sTREM-1 concentration can be used as a surrogate marker of TREM-1 activation, it has set the stage for the evaluation of sTREM-1 as a biomarker for diagnosing and prognosticating sepsis. We have previously reviewed this topic in 2011 and 2015.[11,12] This article is an update that includes the most recent evidence regarding the role of sTREM-1 as a diagnostic biomarker of systemic sepsis, as a diagnostic tool for localized infections, and as a prognostic biomarker of infection.

SOLUBLE TRIGGERING RECEPTOR EXPRESSED ON MYELOID CELLS-1 AS A DIAGNOSTIC BIOMARKER OF INFECTION

Considering the a priori specific involvement of TREM-1 during infectious processes, the usefulness of sTREM-1 in diagnosing sepsis has been the focus of many studies during the last 15 years.

Soluble Triggering Receptor Expressed on Myeloid Cells-1 and the Diagnosis of Systemic Sepsis

Many studies aimed to distinguish between sepsis and sterile inflammation (systemic inflammatory response syndrome) in various populations of patients. Main publications on the use of sTREM-1 as a diagnostic biomarker of sepsis in adult patients are summarized in **Table 1**. In their initial publication on 76 consecutive medical intensive care unit (ICU) patients, Gibot and colleagues[13] determined that plasma concentrations of C-reactive protein (CRP), PCT and sTREM-1 were higher in infected patients than in those with noninfectious inflammation. Soluble TREM-1 performed better than other markers in diagnosing infection. The same encouraging results were reported by Wang and Chen[14] (in a cohort of 56 ICU patients) and by Su and colleagues[15] (in 144 ICU patients). These results were not confirmed in 2 subsequent studies by Barati and colleagues[16] and Latour-Perez and colleagues,[17] involving a total of 246 critically ill patients. In these studies, sTREM-1 was inferior to CRP and PCT. In the emergency room, plasma sTREM-1 alone was also disappointing with an area under the receiver operating characteristic curve (AUC) at 0.61.[18] The most recent meta-analysis on sTREM-1 as a diagnostic biomarker of sepsis in adult patients was published by Wu and colleagues[19] in 2012. Its conclusion was that plasma sTREM-1 had a moderate diagnostic performance in differentiating sepsis from sterile inflammatory response and was not sufficient for sepsis diagnosis, especially when the pretest probability of systemic inflammatory response syndrome was high. Considering the low quality of the studies published from 2012 onwards (lack of external validation cohort and/or no assessment of the reclassification power of the biomarker), the conclusion of an updated meta-analysis is likely to remain disappointing.

The diagnostic accuracy of sTREM-1 in neonatal and pediatric sepsis has also been evaluated. As in adult patients, similar discrepancies were seen between studies. The first study in this field found that sTREM-1 was superior to CRP or immature to total neutrophil ratio in diagnosing severe bacterial infections in 44 neonates.[29] In contrast, Sarafidis and colleagues[30] reported that sTREM-1 performed lower than IL-6 in a neonatal ICU. Since then, a total of 9 studies have been combined in a meta-analysis by Pontrelli and colleagues[31] in 2016, whose conclusions were that "available data were insufficient to support a role for sTREM in the diagnosis and follow-up of pediatric sepsis."

Therefore, the measurement of plasma sTREM-1 concentrations does not seem to fulfill the unmet need for a diagnostic biomarker of sepsis. Indeed, it now seems that many inflammatory conditions may be responsible for an elevation of plasma sTREM-1 concentrations (discussed elsewhere in this article). Nevertheless, determination of plasma sTREM-1 concentrations in combination with other markers could help to overcome some of the limitations of its standalone measurement.[20,22]

Soluble Triggering Receptor Expressed on Myeloid Cells-1 and Localized Infections

Since 2004, with the publication by Gibot and colleagues[32] in the setting of pneumonia, many studies have dealt with the local measurement of sTREM-1 concentrations during a variety of localized infections.

Table 1
Soluble TREM-1 and systemic sepsis in adult patients

	Country	Setting	Patients	Assay Method	Cut-Off (pg/mL)	Sensitivity/specificity (%)	AUC
Gibot et al,[13] 2004	France	Medical ICU	76 consecutive patients with clinically suspected infection	ELISA (Dako, Glostrup, Denmark)	60	96/89	0.97
Kofoed et al,[20] 2007	Denmark	Medical ED	151 patients with suspected community-acquired infections	Luminex multiplex assay (Luminex corp, Austin, TX)	3500	82/40	0.61
Rivera-Chavez & Minei,[21] 2009	USA	Surgical ICU	108 patients with suspected infection	ELISA (R&D Systems, Minneapolis, MN)	230	98/91	0.97
Barati et al,[16] 2010	Iran	Medical and surgical ICUs	132 patients	ELISA (R&D Systems, Minneapolis, MN)	725	70/60	0.65
Latour-Perez et al,[17] 2010	Spain	General ICUs	114 patients	ELISA (R&D Systems, Minneapolis, MN)	463	49/79	0.62
Gamez-Diaz et al,[18] 2011	Colombia	ED	631 patients with suspected infection, fever, delirium, or acute hypotension of unexplained origin within 24 h of ED presentation	ELISA (R&D Systems, Minneapolis, MN)	135	60/59	0.61
Wang & Chen,[14] 2011	China	General ICU	56 patients with SIRS (32 with sepsis) and 25 controls without SIRS	ELISA (R&D Systems, Minneapolis, MN)	135	94/85	0.94
Gibot et al,[22] 2012	France	2 medical ICUs	300 consecutive patients (inceptive cohort) + 79 patients (validation cohort)	ELISA (R&D Systems, Minneapolis, MN)	755	53/86	0.73

Study	Country	Setting	Population	Assay			
Su et al,[15] 2012	China	General ICUs	144 patients	ELISA (R&D Systems, Minneapolis, MN)	109	83/81	0.87
Li et al,[23] 2013	China	Surgical ICU	52 patients with clinically suspected infection	ELISA (R&D Systems, Minneapolis, MN)	74	79/79	0.82
Su et al,[24] 2013	China	General ICUs	130 patients	ELISA (R&D Systems, Minneapolis, MN)	64	91/90	0.98
Halim et al,[25] 2015	Turkey	Hospitalized patients (53% ICU)	74 patients	ELISA (R&D Systems, Minneapolis, MN)	200	82/73	0.83
Aksaray et al,[26] 2016	Turkey	General ICU	90 patients	ELISA 9MyBioSource, Inc., San Diego, CA, USA)	133	71/73	0.78
Brenner et al,[27] 2017	Germany	Surgical ICU	60 septic shock, 30 postoperative control, 30 healthy volunteers (post hoc analysis of the RAMMSES trial[28])	ELISA (R&D Systems, Minneapolis, MN)	30	98/90	0.96

Abbreviations: ED, emergency department; ICU, intensive care unit; SIRS, systemic inflammatory response syndrome.

Pleuropulmonary Infections

Pleuropulmonary infections constitute the core of research on sTREM-1 diagnostic performance. The first study was published in 2004 by Richeldi and colleagues.[33] It showed an increased expression of TREM-1 at the surface of alveolar neutrophils and macrophages determined by flow cytometry during bacterial pneumonia as compared with levels found in patients with noninfectious interstitial lung diseases. Gibot and colleagues[32] investigated alveolar sTREM-1 as a marker of infectious pneumonia in 148 consecutive patients under mechanical ventilation. In this study, alveolar sTREM-1 concentrations were highly predictive of lung infection and performed better than any other clinical or biological findings in both community-acquired pneumonia (CAP) and ventilator-associated pneumonia (VAP), with a diagnostic odds ratio of 41.5. Several other studies then confirmed these preliminary results. Huh and colleagues[34] found that sTREM-1 concentrations were useful during bacterial or fungal pneumonias, whereas sTREM-1 concentrations remained low in case of viral infection. The study by Determann and colleagues[35] focusing on VAP added kinetics data. Alveolar sTREM-1 concentrations increased a few days before the clinical diagnosis of VAP, and the investigators concluded that the combination of more than 200 pg/mL of alveolar sTREM-1 with an increase of more than 100 pg/mL as compared with the value obtain 2 days earlier was highly predictive of the diagnosis of VAP. El Solh and colleagues[36] showed that alveolar sTREM-1 allowed for the discrimination between aspiration pneumonia and pneumonitis. Ramirez and colleagues[37] found that alveolar sTREM-1 concentration had the capacity to discriminate between a pulmonary and an extrapulmonary infection in the context of acute respiratory failure. Besides alveolar concentrations, sTREM-1 levels from blood samples to diagnose CAP are clearly not useful. Müller and colleagues[38] first addressed this question in 2007. In a cohort of 302 consecutive patients from the emergency department, they could not find any difference in sTREM-1 levels between patients with mild and severe CAP. In a cohort of 433 hospitalized children, Esposito and colleagues[39] found that plasma sTREM-1 had a poor ability to differentiate bacterial from viral CAP, as well as to identify severe cases. Several other studies, although confirming the increase of alveolar sTREM-1 concentrations during lung infections, reported a lower discriminative value. During VAP, alveolar sTREM-1 performed lower than the usual clinical pulmonary infection score. In a population of 23 patients clinically suspected of having VAP, Horonenko and colleagues[40] reported a very low specificity of sTREM-1 concentration from bronchoalveolar lavage samples, with a much lower informative value than sTREM-1 concentrations from exhaled ventilator condensates or than clinical pulmonary infection score. Recently, Li and colleagues[41] reported high sensitivity and specificity for sTREM-1 from bronchoalveolar lavage and exhaled ventilator condensates to diagnose VAP in children after cardiac surgery but there was a major overlap in the distribution of sTREM-1 levels from VAP and non-VAP patients, thus limiting its clinical usefulness. In the same way, Oudhuis and colleagues[42] found a significant difference between sTREM-1 concentrations from alveolar samples but an area under the receiving operating characteristic curve at 0.58 only. Finally, some studies revealed no predictive value for the diagnosis of VAP from alveolar samples.[43,44]

There is much less controversy over the diagnosis of pleural effusions. Seven different studies were pooled into a meta-analysis by Summah and colleagues[45] (733 patients). They found that pleural sTREM-1 was useful to distinguish between infectious (empyema, parapneumonia) and noninfectious pleural effusions (congestive heart failure, cancer).

Meningitis

Identifying the bacterial cause of meningitis can also be challenging, especially when patients have already received antibiotics. Three different studies showed that the increase in sTREM-1 concentrations in the cerebrospinal fluid was able to discriminate between infectious and viral meningitis, with cut-off values ranging from 20 to 25 pg/mL. Of note, sTREM-1 concentrations were similar during pneumococcal and meningococcal infections, and concentration was normal in a culture-proven tuberculous meningitis.[46–48]

Urinary Sepsis

Only 1 study investigated sTREM-1 concentrations in urine for the diagnosis of lower urinary tract infections, and the results were inconclusive.[49] It is worth noting that one study found an interesting role for urinary sTREM-1 as a marker of sepsis-associated acute kidney injury.[50]

Abdominal Sepsis

Determann and colleagues[51] showed in a cohort of 83 patients operated for secondary peritonitis that the peritoneal concentration of sTREM-1 progressively decreased in patients with a good outcome but remained persistently elevated and even increased during residual sepsis and tertiary peritonitis. Lu and colleagues[52] investigated the diagnosis value of sTREM-1 concentration in peripancreatic necrotic tissue to differentiate between infected necrosis from sterile in 30 patients with suspected secondary infection of necrotic tissue. They reported an interesting AUC of 0.972 and sensitivity and specificity of 94.4% and 91.7% respectively for a cut-off of 285.6 pg/mL. Ascitic fluid sTREM-1 was also evaluated in the setting of spontaneous bacterial peritonitis in patients with cirrhosis.[53] At 1595 pg/mL, the sensitivity and specificity of the test were 96% and 99% with an AUC of 0.98.

Periodontitis

Finally, elevated sTREM-1 concentrations were also reported from gingival crevicular fluid from patients with periodontitis.[54–56] As reported by Jiyong and colleagues[57] in their meta-analysis, nearly all of these studies suggest that the determination of sTREM-1 concentrations at the site of the presumed infection may be useful in clinical practice. Nevertheless, more research is required before implementing this assay into practical diagnostic algorithms. These positive results should now be translated into interventional studies, with the demonstration that measurement of sTREM-1 concentrations can safely guide and reduce the use of antibiotics.

SOLUBLE TRIGGERING RECEPTOR EXPRESSED ON MYELOID CELLS-1 AS A PROGNOSTIC MARKER OF INFECTION

The early recognition of patients with sepsis with the highest risk of death is of paramount importance because the outcome relies on the adequacy and timeliness of key therapeutic interventions, such as antibiotics and fluids administration. Beyond the use of sTREM-1 as a diagnostic biomarker, the determination of its concentration may also be helpful to prognosticate the outcome of a septic patient. Gibot and colleagues[58] sequentially measured plasma sTREM-1 concentrations in 63 consecutive patients with sepsis. The baseline plasma sTREM-1 concentration was higher in survivors and was found to be an independent factor associated with good outcome. The patterns of evolution were also different according to the outcome, with a progressive decrease in sTREM-1 concentrations in survivors, whereas concentrations remained high in nonsurvivors. Two different studies from Giamarellos-Bourboulis and colleagues[59] and Wu and colleagues[60] confirmed the prognostic value of sTREM-1 in VAP. Tejera and colleagues[61] investigated serum levels of sTREM-1 in a cohort of 226 patients with CAP and reported significantly lower values in survivors than in nonsurvivors.[61] In a mixed population of 52 patients with sepsis, one-half of them suffering from lower respiratory tract infection, Zhang and colleagues[62] demonstrated that serum sTREM-1 concentrations reflected the severity of sepsis more accurately than those of CRP and PCT and were more sensitive for dynamic evaluations of sepsis prognosis. Su and colleagues[63] shared the same conclusions. In the setting of chemotherapy-associated febrile neutropenia, a retrospective study from Kwofie and colleagues[64] reported that sTREM-1 levels were potentially useful to predict the clinical course of these patients. Nevertheless, some studies led to a different conclusion. This topic was recently reviewed in a meta-analysis by Su and colleagues.[65] They concluded that sTREM-1 concentrations had a moderate prognostic significance in assessing the mortality of infection in adult patients. Therefore, sTREM-1 alone was insufficient to predict mortality. The most recent high-quality study in this field was published by Charles and colleagues[66] in 2016. In a cohort of 190 patients with sepsis in the ICU, they compared sTREM-1, PCT, and leukocyte surface expression of CD64 with clinical severity scores. Although sTREM-1 was found to be the best prognostic biomarker among those tested, the Simplified Acute Physiology Score severity score II outperformed sTREM-1 regarding the prediction of ICU survival.

LIMITATIONS FOR THE USE OF SOLUBLE TRIGGERING RECEPTOR EXPRESSED ON MYELOID CELLS-1 AS A BIOMARKER OF SEPSIS

Recent evidence suggests that sTREM-1 concentrations increase in biological fluids even in the absence of infection. TREM-1 expression depends on the activation of several TLRs or NOD-like receptors, and it has become clear that many danger-associated molecular patterns that activate these receptors may be produced during sterile inflammation.

Moreover, TREM-1 expression was first found on cell of the myeloid lineage. However, TREM-1 has now been shown to be expressed on nonimmune cells. For instance, TREM-1 is expressed and inducible in endothelial cells and plays a direct role in vascular inflammation and dysfunction.[67] In an experimental model of septic shock, mice with a conditional knockdown of Trem-1 in endothelial cells had markedly decreased sTREM-1 concentrations compared with wild-type mice with normal expression of TREM-1 by the endothelium. Thus, endothelial cells are probably a major source of sTREM-1 during inflammation. TREM-1 is also constitutively expressed in platelet α-granules and mobilized at the membrane upon platelet activation to promote platelet aggregation.[68]

Therefore, it is not surprising that many studies have shown high sTREM-1 concentrations in a myriad of noninfectious inflammatory conditions, such as inflammatory bowel diseases,[69,70] pancreatitis,[71] lung cancer,[72] systemic lupus erythematosus,[73] vasculitis,[74] rheumatoid arthritis,[75] subarachnoid hemorrhage,[76] and cystic fibrosis.[77] There is also mounting evidence that TREM-1 activation is a critical mediator of the inflammatory response that occurs during cardiovascular diseases such as atherosclerosis and healing after myocardial infarction.[78,79] For instance, in a French cohort of more than 1000 patients admitted for acute myocardial infarction, a high sTREM-1 concentration at the time of presentation was associated with a higher risk of death after 2 years of follow-up, even after adjustment for several cardiovascular risk factors.[79]

THERAPEUTIC MODULATION OF THE TRIGGERING RECEPTOR EXPRESSED ON MYELOID CELLS-1 PATHWAY

A relevant biomarker should be of physiologic relevance. The therapeutic modulation of the TREM-1 pathway has been the subject of many experimental studies. Because the synthesis of TREM-1 antagonist peptides, numerous studies aimed to assess the effects of the modulation of the inflammatory response during various pathologic conditions. After successful interventions during experimental septic shock using small and large animal models,[80,81] one of these inhibitory peptide, nangibotide, has cleared the first safety hurdle in a phase I clinical trial[82] and shown promising results in a phase IIa clinical trial.[83]

SUMMARY

TREM-1 is an amplifier of the innate immune response. Initially thought to be expressed only on myeloid cells and involved mainly during bacterial infections, intense research has shown that TREM-1 is also expressed on nonimmune cells and is a critical player during various noninfectious inflammatory conditions. A soluble form of TREM-1 is present in many biological fluids and can be used as a surrogate marker of TREM-1 activation. sTREM-1 displays a moderate diagnostic performance in differentiating sepsis from sterile inflammatory response as well as a moderate prognostic significance in assessing the mortality of infection in adult patients. Local sTREM-1 concentration at the site of the presumed infection is more clinically useful. However, its role to guide antibiotic strategy is yet to be evaluated.

REFERENCES

1. Fleischmann C, Scherag A, Adhikari NKJ, et al. Assessment of global incidence and mortality of hospital-treated sepsis. Current estimates and limitations. Am J Respir Crit Care Med 2016;193(3):259–72.
2. Andriolo BN, Andriolo RB, Salomão R, et al. Effectiveness and safety of procalcitonin evaluation for reducing mortality in adults with sepsis, severe sepsis or septic shock. Cochrane Database Syst Rev 2017;(1):CD010959.
3. Biomarkers Definitions Working Group. Biomarkers and surrogate endpoints: preferred definitions and conceptual framework. Clin Pharmacol Ther 2001; 69(3):89–95.
4. Ford JW, McVicar DW. TREM and TREM-like receptors in inflammation and disease. Curr Opin Immunol 2009;21(1):38–46.
5. Bleharski JR, Kiessler V, Buonsanti C, et al. A role for triggering receptor expressed on myeloid cells-1 in host defense during the early-induced and adaptive phases of the immune response. J Immunol 2003;170(7):3812.
6. Bouchon A, Dietrich J, Colonna M. Cutting edge: inflammatory responses can be triggered by TREM-1, a novel receptor expressed on neutrophils and monocytes. J Immunol 2000;164(10):4991–5.
7. Bouchon A, Facchetti F, Weigand MA, et al. TREM-1 amplifies inflammation and is a crucial mediator of septic shock. Nature 2001;410(6832):1103–7.
8. Gibot S, Kolopp-Sarda M-N, Béné M-C, et al. A soluble form of the triggering receptor expressed on myeloid cells-1 modulates the inflammatory response in murine sepsis. J Exp Med 2004;200(11):1419–26.
9. Baruah S, Keck K, Vrenios M, et al. Identification of a novel splice variant isoform of TREM-1 in human neutrophil granules. J Immunol 2015;195(12):5725–31.

10. Gómez-Piña V, Soares-Schanoski A, Rodríguez-Rojas A, et al. Metalloproteinases shed TREM-1 ectodomain from lipopolysaccharide-stimulated human monocytes. J Immunol 2007;179(6):4065–73.
11. Barraud D, Gibot S. Triggering receptor expressed on myeloid cell 1. Crit Care Clin 2011;27(2):265–79.
12. Lemarié J, Barraud D, Gibot S. Host response biomarkers in sepsis: overview on sTREM-1 detection. Methods Mol Biol 2015;1237:225–39.
13. Gibot S, Kolopp-Sarda M-N, Béné MC, et al. Plasma level of a triggering receptor expressed on myeloid cells-1: its diagnostic accuracy in patients with suspected sepsis. Ann Intern Med 2004;141(1):9–15.
14. Wang H, Chen B. Diagnostic role of soluble triggering receptor expressed on myeloid cell-1 in patients with sepsis. World J Emerg Med 2011;2:190–4.
15. Su L, Han B, Liu C, et al. Value of soluble TREM-1, procalcitonin, and C-reactive protein serum levels as biomarkers for detecting bacteremia among sepsis patients with new fever in intensive care units: a prospective cohort study. BMC Infect Dis 2012;12(1):157.
16. Barati M, Bashar FR, Shahrami R, et al. Soluble triggering receptor expressed on myeloid cells 1 and the diagnosis of sepsis. J Crit Care 2010;25(2):362.e1-6.
17. Latour-Pérez J, Alcalá-López A, García-García M-A, et al. Diagnostic accuracy of sTREM-1 to identify infection in critically ill patients with systemic inflammatory response syndrome. Clin Biochem 2010;43(9):720–4.
18. Gámez-Díaz LY, Enriquez LE, Matute JD, et al. Diagnostic accuracy of HMGB-1, sTREM-1, and CD64 as markers of sepsis in patients recently admitted to the emergency department. Acad Emerg Med 2011;18(8):807–15.
19. Wu Y, Wang F, Fan X, et al. Accuracy of plasma sTREM-1 for sepsis diagnosis in systemic inflammatory patients: a systematic review and meta-analysis. Crit Care 2012;16(6):R229.
20. Kofoed K, Andersen O, Kronborg G, et al. Use of plasma C-reactive protein, procalcitonin, neutrophils, macrophage migration inhibitory factor, soluble urokinase-type plasminogen activator receptor, and soluble triggering receptor expressed on myeloid cells-1 in combination to diagnose infections: a prospective study. Crit Care 2007;11(2):R38.
21. Rivera-Chavez FA, Minei JP. Soluble triggering receptor expressed on myeloid cells-1 is an early marker of infection in the surgical intensive care unit. Surg Infect 2009;10(5):435–9.
22. Gibot S, Béné MC, Noel R, et al. Combination biomarkers to diagnose sepsis in the critically ill patient. Am J Respir Crit Care Med 2012;186(1):65–71.
23. Li L, Zhu Z, Chen J, et al. Diagnostic value of soluble triggering receptor expressed on myeloid cells-1 in critically-ill, postoperative patients with suspected sepsis. Am J Med Sci 2013;345(3):178–84.
24. Su L, Feng L, Song Q, et al. Diagnostic value of dynamics serum sCD163, sTREM-1, PCT, and CRP in differentiating sepsis, severity assessment, and prognostic prediction. Mediators Inflamm 2013;2013:969875.
25. Halim B, Özlem T, Melek Ç, et al. Diagnostic and prognostic value of procalcitonin and sTREM-1 levels in sepsis. Turk J Med Sci 2015;45(3):578–86.
26. Aksaray S, Alagoz P, Inan A, et al. Diagnostic value of sTREM-1 and procalcitonin levels in the early diagnosis of sepsis. North Clin Istanb 2016;3(3):175–82.
27. Brenner T, Uhle F, Fleming T, et al. Soluble TREM-1 as a diagnostic and prognostic biomarker in patients with septic shock: an observational clinical study. Biomarkers 2017;22(1):63–9.

28. Brenner T, Fleming T, Uhle F, et al. Methylglyoxal as a new biomarker in patients with septic shock: an observational clinical study. Crit Care 2014;18(6):683.

29. Chen H-L, Hung C-H, Tseng H-I, et al. Soluble form of triggering receptor expressed on myeloid cells-1 (sTREM-1) as a diagnostic marker of serious bacterial infection in febrile infants less than three months of age. Jpn J Infect Dis 2008; 61(1):31–5.

30. Sarafidis K, Soubasi-Griva V, Piretzi K, et al. Diagnostic utility of elevated serum soluble triggering receptor expressed on myeloid cells (sTREM)-1 in infected neonates. Intensive Care Med 2010;36(5):864–8.

31. Pontrelli G, De Crescenzo F, Buzzetti R, et al. Diagnostic value of soluble triggering receptor expressed on myeloid cells in paediatric sepsis: a systematic review. Ital J Pediatr 2016;42. https://doi.org/10.1186/s13052-016-0242-y.

32. Gibot S, Cravoisy A, Levy B, et al. Soluble triggering receptor expressed on myeloid cells and the diagnosis of pneumonia. N Engl J Med 2004;350(5):451–8.

33. Richeldi L, Mariani M, Losi M, et al. Triggering receptor expressed on myeloid cells: role in the diagnosis of lung infections. Eur Respir J 2004;24(2):247–50.

34. Huh J, Lim C-M, Koh Y, et al. Diagnostic utility of the soluble triggering receptor expressed on myeloid cells-1 in bronchoalveolar lavage fluid from patients with bilateral lung infiltrates. Crit Care 2008;12(1):R6.

35. Determann RM, Millo JL, Gibot S, et al. Serial changes in soluble triggering receptor expressed on myeloid cells in the lung during development of ventilator-associated pneumonia. Intensive Care Med 2005;31(11):1495–500.

36. El Solh AA, Akinnusi ME, Peter M, et al. Triggering receptors expressed on myeloid cells in pulmonary aspiration syndromes. Intensive Care Med 2008; 34(6):1012–9.

37. Ramirez P, Kot P, Marti V, et al. Diagnostic implications of soluble triggering receptor expressed on myeloid cells-1 in patients with acute respiratory distress syndrome and abdominal diseases: a preliminary observational study. Crit Care 2011;15(1):1–8.

38. Müller B, Gencay MM, Gibot S, et al. Circulating levels of soluble triggering receptor expressed on myeloid cells (sTREM)-1 in community-acquired pneumonia. Crit Care Med 2007;35(3):990–1.

39. Esposito S, Di Gangi M, Cardinale F, et al. Sensitivity and specificity of soluble triggering receptor expressed on myeloid cells-1, midregional proatrial natriuretic peptide and midregional proadrenomedullin for distinguishing etiology and to assess severity in community-acquired pneumonia. PLoS One 2016;11(11). https://doi.org/10.1371/journal.pone.0163262.

40. Horonenko G, Hoyt JC, Robbins RA, et al. Soluble triggering receptor expressed on myeloid cell-1 is increased in patients with ventilator-associated pneumonia: a preliminary report. Chest J 2007;132(1):58–63.

41. Li C, Zhu L, Gong X, et al. Soluble triggering receptor expressed on myeloid cells-1 as a useful biomarker for diagnosing ventilator-associated pneumonia after congenital cardiac surgery in children. Exp Ther Med 2019;17(1):147–52.

42. Oudhuis GJ, Beuving J, Bergmans D, et al. Soluble Triggering Receptor Expressed on Myeloid cells-1 in bronchoalveolar lavage fluid is not predictive for ventilator-associated pneumonia. Intensive Care Med 2009;35(7):1265–70.

43. Anand NJ, Zuick S, Klesney-Tait J, et al. Diagnostic implications of soluble triggering receptor expressed on myeloid cells-1 in BAL fluid of patients with pulmonary infiltrates in the ICU. Chest J 2009;135(3):641–7.

44. Palazzo SJ, Simpson TA, Simmons JM, et al. Soluble triggering receptor expressed on myeloid cells-1 (sTREM-1) as a diagnostic marker of ventilator-associated pneumonia. Respir Care 2012;57(12):2052–8.
45. Summah H, Tao L-L, Zhu Y-G, et al. Pleural fluid soluble triggering receptor expressed on myeloid cells-1 as a marker of bacterial infection: a meta-analysis. BMC Infect Dis 2011;11(1):280.
46. Determann RM, Weisfelt M, de Gans J, et al. Soluble triggering receptor expressed on myeloid cells 1: a biomarker for bacterial meningitis. Intensive Care Med 2006;32(8):1243–7.
47. Bishara J, Hadari N, Shalita-Chesner M, et al. Soluble triggering receptor expressed on myeloid cells-1 for distinguishing bacterial from aseptic meningitis in adults. Eur J Clin Microbiol Infect Dis 2007;26(9):647–50.
48. Guanghui G, Qiaoya J, Zhenhua S. Value of soluble triggering receptor expressed on myeloid cells-1 in the diagnosis of bacterial meningitis. Int J Lab Med 2011;9:952–4.
49. Determann RM, Schultz MJ, Geerlings SE. Soluble triggering receptor expressed on myeloid cells-1 is not a sufficient biological marker for infection of the urinary tract. J Infect 2007;54(6):e249–50.
50. Su L, Feng L, Zhang J, et al. Diagnostic value of urine sTREM-1 for sepsis and relevant acute kidney injuries: a prospective study. Crit Care 2011;15(5):R250.
51. Determann RM, Olivier van Till JW, van Ruler O, et al. sTREM-1 is a potential useful biomarker for exclusion of ongoing infection in patients with secondary peritonitis. Cytokine 2009;46(1):36–42.
52. Lu Z, Liu Y, Dong Y, et al. Soluble triggering receptor expressed on myeloid cells in severe acute pancreatitis: a biological marker of infected necrosis. Intensive Care Med 2012;38(1):69–75.
53. Ichou L, Carbonell N, Rautou PE, et al. Ascitic fluid TREM-1 for the diagnosis of spontaneous bacterial peritonitis. Gut 2016;65(3):536–8.
54. Belibasakis GN, Öztürk V-Ö, Emingil G, et al. Soluble triggering receptor expressed on myeloid cells 1 (sTREM-1) in gingival crevicular fluid: association with clinical and microbiologic parameters. J Periodontol 2014;85(1):204–10.
55. Bostanci N, Öztürk VÖ, Emingil G, et al. Elevated oral and systemic levels of soluble triggering receptor expressed on myeloid cells-1 (sTREM-1) in periodontitis. J Dent Res 2013;92(2):161–5.
56. Bisson C, Massin F, Lefevre PA, et al. Increased gingival crevicular fluid levels of soluble triggering receptor expressed on myeloid cells (sTREM) -1 in severe periodontitis. J Clin Periodontol 2012;39(12):1141–8.
57. Jiyong J, Tiancha H, Wei C, et al. Diagnostic value of the soluble triggering receptor expressed on myeloid cells-1 in bacterial infection: a meta-analysis. Intensive Care Med 2009;35(4):587–95.
58. Gibot S, Cravoisy A, Kolopp-Sarda M-N, et al. Time-course of sTREM (soluble triggering receptor expressed on myeloid cells)-1, procalcitonin, and C-reactive protein plasma concentrations during sepsis. Crit Care Med 2005;33(4):792–6.
59. Giamarellos-Bourboulis EJ, Zakynthinos S, Baziaka F, et al. Soluble triggering receptor expressed on myeloid cells 1 as an anti-inflammatory mediator in sepsis. Intensive Care Med 2006;32(2):237–43.
60. Wu C-L, Lu Y-T, Kung Y-C, et al. Prognostic value of dynamic soluble triggering receptor expressed on myeloid cells in bronchoalveolar lavage fluid of patients with ventilator-associated pneumonia. Respirology 2011;16(3):487–94.
61. Tejera A, Santolaria F, Diez M-L, et al. Prognosis of community acquired pneumonia (CAP): value of triggering receptor expressed on myeloid cells-1 (TREM-

1) and other mediators of the inflammatory response. Cytokine 2007;38(3): 117–23.

62. Zhang J, She D, Feng D, et al. Dynamic changes of serum soluble triggering receptor expressed on myeloid cells-1 (sTREM-1) reflect sepsis severity and can predict prognosis: a prospective study. BMC Infect Dis 2011;11(1):53.

63. Su L, Liu C, Li C, et al. Dynamic changes in serum soluble triggering receptor expressed on myeloid cells-1 (sTREM-1) and its gene polymorphisms are associated with sepsis prognosis. Inflammation 2012;35(6):1833–43.

64. Kwofie L, Rapoport BL, Fickl H, et al. Evaluation of circulating soluble triggering receptor expressed on myeloid cells-1 (sTREM-1) to predict risk profile, response to antimicrobial therapy, and development of complications in patients with chemotherapy-associated febrile neutropenia: a pilot study. Ann Hematol 2012; 91(4):605–11.

65. Su L, Liu D, Chai W, et al. Role of sTREM-1 in predicting mortality of infection: a systematic review and meta-analysis. BMJ Open 2016;6(5). https://doi.org/10. 1136/bmjopen-2015-010314.

66. Charles PE, Noel R, Massin F, et al. Significance of soluble triggering receptor expressed on myeloid cells-1 elevation in patients admitted to the intensive care unit with sepsis. BMC Infect Dis 2016;16. https://doi.org/10.1186/s12879-016-1893-4.

67. Jolly L, Carrasco K, Derive M, et al. Targeted endothelial gene deletion of Triggering Receptor Expressed on Myeloid cells-1 protects mice during septic shock. Cardiovasc Res 2018. https://doi.org/10.1093/cvr/cvy018.

68. Jolly L, Lemarie J, Carrasco K, et al. Triggering Receptor Expressed on Myeloid cells-1: a new player in platelet aggregation. Thromb Haemost 2017;117. https://doi.org/10.1160/TH17-03-0156.

69. Jung YS, Park JJ, Kim SW, et al. Correlation between soluble triggering receptor expressed on myeloid cells-1 (sTREM-1) expression and endoscopic activity in inflammatory bowel diseases. Dig Liver Dis 2012;44(11):897–903.

70. Tzivras M, Koussoulas V, Giamarellos-Bourboulis EJ, et al. Role of soluble triggering receptor expressed on myeloid cells in inflammatory bowel disease. World J Gastroenterol 2006;12(21):3416.

71. Yasuda T, Takeyama Y, Ueda T, et al. Increased levels of soluble triggering receptor expressed on myeloid cells-1 in patients with acute pancreatitis. Crit Care Med 2008;36(7):2048–53.

72. Kuemmel A, Alflen A, Schmidt LH, et al. Soluble triggering receptor expressed on myeloid cells 1 in lung cancer. Sci Rep 2018;8. https://doi.org/10.1038/s41598-018-28971-0.

73. Molad Y, Pokroy-Shapira E, Kaptzan T, et al. Serum soluble triggering receptor on myeloid cells-1 (sTREM-1) is elevated in systemic lupus erythematosus but does not distinguish between lupus alone and concurrent infection. Inflammation 2013; 36(6):1519–24.

74. Daikeler T, Regenass S, Tyndall A, et al. Increased serum levels of soluble triggering receptor expressed on myeloid cells-1 in antineutrophil cytoplasmic antibody-associated vasculitis. Ann Rheum Dis 2008;67(5):723–4.

75. Molad Y, Ofer-Shiber S, Pokroy-Shapira E, et al. Soluble triggering receptor expressed on myeloid cells-1 is a biomarker of anti-CCP-positive, early rheumatoid arthritis. Eur J Clin Invest 2015;45(6):557–64.

76. Sun X-G, Ma Q, Jing G, et al. Early elevated levels of soluble triggering receptor expressed on myeloid cells-1 in subarachnoid hemorrhage patients. Neurol Sci 2017;38(5):873–7.

77. Forrester DL, Barr HL, Fogarty A, et al. sTREM-1 is elevated in cystic fibrosis and correlates with proteases. Pediatr Pulmonol 2017;52(4):467–71.
78. Joffre J, Potteaux S, Zeboudj L, et al. Genetic and pharmacological inhibition of TREM-1 limits the development of experimental atherosclerosis. J Am Coll Cardiol 2016;68(25):2776–93.
79. Boufenzer A, Lemarie J, Simon T, et al. TREM-1 mediates inflammatory injury and cardiac remodeling following myocardial infarction. Circ Res 2015. https://doi.org/10.1161/CIRCRESAHA.116.305628.
80. Gibot S, Alauzet C, Massin F, et al. Modulation of the triggering receptor expressed on myeloid cells–1 pathway during pneumonia in rats. J Infect Dis 2006;194(7):975–83.
81. Derive M, Boufenzer A, Bouazza Y, et al. Effects of a TREM-like transcript 1-derived peptide during hypodynamic septic shock in pigs. Shock 2013;39(2):176–82.
82. Cuvier V, Lorch U, Witte S, et al. A first-in-man safety and pharmacokinetics study of nangibotide, a new modulator of innate immune response through TREM-1 receptor inhibition. Br J Clin Pharmacol 2018;84(10):2270–9.
83. Francois B, Wittebole X, Ferrer R, et al. Safety and pharmacodynamic activity of a novel TREM-1 pathway inhibitory peptide in septic shock patients phase IIa clinical trial results. Intensive Care Med Exp 2018;6:196.

Lubricin as a Therapeutic and Potential Biomarker in Sepsis

Holly Richendrfer, PhD[a,b], Gregory D. Jay, MD, PhD[a,b,*]

KEYWORDS

- Lubricin • PRG4 • Toll-like receptors • CD44 • Inflammasome • NF-κB
- Inflammation

KEY POINTS

- Lubricin is a lubricant and has a cellular protective effect as it prevents cellular death and decreases cellular inflammation.
- Lubricin is an antagonist of Toll-like receptors (TLRs) TLR2 and TLR4 and gains entry into the cell via CD44 to block inflammatory processes indicating a therapeutic role.
- Lubricin is down-regulated by several cytokines, indicating it could serve as an inflammatory and sepsis biomarker.

INTRODUCTION

Lubricin—Original Discoveries

Lubricin (also known as proteoglycan 4 [PRG4]), expressed by the *PRG4* gene, is a mucin-like 224-kDa glycoprotein known for its lubricating properties and was originally found within the synovial fluid of diarthrodial joints in bovine and human samples and secreted by synovial fibroblasts.[1–7] Lubricin contains many O-linked glycosylations located in a central post-translationally modified mucin domain. The length of the mucin-like repeats in its structure varies across species but is generally proportional to the size of the animal.[4,6] Lubricin also can be expressed with several different isoforms in the N-terminus and each isoform may have different functions.[8] Like other mucins and mucin-like substances, lubricin prevents the attachment of cells to surfaces, which enables its activity as a boundary lubricant by reducing friction.[9]

Funding source: NIH R01AR067748.
H. Richendrfer has no conflicts of interest. G. Jay has ownership and financial interest in the formation of recombinant human lubricin production (Lubris, LLC).
[a] Department of Emergency Medicine, Alpert Medical School, Brown University, 222 Richmond Street, Providence, RI 02903, USA, [b] Department of Emergency Medicine, Research Laboratory, Rhode Island Hospital, 1 Hoppin Street, CORO West, Room 4.303, Providence, RI 02903, USA
* Corresponding author. Department of Emergency Medicine, Alpert Medical School, Brown University, 222 Richmond Street, Providence, RI 02903.
E-mail address: gregory_jay_md@brown.edu

Friction and Apoptosis

The ability of lubricin to exert its lubricating effects and decrease friction is dependent on its concentration, indicated by an increase in joint friction with decreased lubricin concentrations.[4] Optimal concentrations of lubricin were found to be between 200 μg/mL and 260 μg/mL for proper lubricating activity and reduced friction coefficients in noncartilage surfaces.[7]

Patients born with a rare genetic mutation in the *PRG4* gene display camptodactyly-arthropathy-coxa vara-pericarditis (CACP) syndrome, which is characterized by increased joint friction, apoptosis, and cellular morphologic changes that eventually lead to joint failure.[10-12] Lubricin null mice (*Prg4* $^{-/-}$) (the orthologous genetic model of CACP syndrome in humans) were bred in order to study joint mechanics and to examine histologic abnormalities. *Prg4* gene trap ($^{GT/GT}$) mice have increased friction and activated caspase-3 staining in their chondrocytes, which is reversed after the *Prg4* gene is turned back on through Cre-mediated recombination.[13] The coefficient of friction and amount of activated caspase-3 staining in lubricin null mice given purified human synoviocyte lubricin was significantly lower than in mice that were lubricin null littermates receiving only sham injections.[14] Moreover, lubricin null mice had higher levels of $ONOO^-$ in femoral head cartilage and synoviocytes compared with controls.[14] Additionally, there was increased gene expression of the cytokines interleukin (IL)-1β and tumor necrosis factor (TNF)-α, and caspases-3, -6, and -7 in the cartilage of lubricin null mice compared with controls, indicating the anti-inflammatory role of lubricin in preventing apoptosis that is activated through the intrinsic pathway.[14]

Other studies reveal that lubricin has a cellular protective effect, because knee joints from lubricin null mice had increased numbers of apoptotic cells, which was measured via anti–caspase-3 and terminal deoxynucleotidyl transferase-mediated dUTP nick end labeling (TUNEL).[15] In rats with anterior cruciate ligament transection (ACLT), expression levels of lubricin and deposition of lubricin on cartilage surfaces were significantly decreased when assessed at 3 weeks and 5 weeks post-transection.[16] At 3 weeks, exercised rats with ACLT had expression levels of lubricin that were even lower than rats that had undergone ACLT only, indicating increased damage in the joint.[16] Moreover, the rats with ACLT plus exercise also showed an increase in activated caspase-3 staining of chondrocytes in comparison with ACLT-only rats, which was further increased at 5 weeks.[16] Treatment of ACLT rats with intra-articular purified human lubricin significantly lowered activated caspase-3 staining of chondrocytes compared with those with no lubricin.[16]

Osteoarthritis (OA) is a common age-related degenerative disease of the joints that consists of cartilage degeneration, inflammation, and bone remodeling, characterized by pain, joint stiffness, and swelling.[17] The causes of OA are still not well understood but are thought to stem from genetic and orthopedic abnormalities, gender, metabolic diseases, environmental factors such as sports injuries, and obesity.[17] There is still an unmet need for treatment of patients with OA, but several reports point to lubricin not only as a factor in the progression of the disease process but also as a potential effective therapy for its treatment.[11,18,19]

OA in humans presents with down-regulated *PRG4* in lateral femoral condyle cartilage, which may be location and isoform dependent.[20] In a sheep model of OA, lubricin immunostaining was decreased in cartilage, which also corresponded with down-regulated messenger RNA (mRNA) levels of lubricin in comparison to sham-treated animals.[19] Moreover, lubricin was shown to prevent OA in a mouse model using intra-articular injected adenoviral vectors conjugated to antibodies designed to overexpress *PRG4*.[21,22] It seems that one of the mechanisms of cellular protection is via lubricin inhibition of cellular pathways that led to catabolism of cartilage.[21]

Rheumatoid arthritis (RA) is a type of arthritis that has autoimmune and inflammatory components.[23] The symptoms of RA are similar to those of OA; however, the causes and comorbidities are different.[23,24] Autoimmunity leads to joint destruction and swelling in addition to inflammation of the synovium.[23,24] Lubricin concentrations in synovial fluid from both OA and RA patients is significantly lower than that of controls.[25] Moreover, synovial fluid from patients with RA failed to lubricate rabbit knee joints after induced injury, indicating that there is a loss of lubricin that occurs within the RA disease process similar to that of OA.[26]

These findings indicate the significant role that lubricin has in mitigating joint friction and in preventing chondrocyte cell death in normal and disease states. These studies also suggest that lubricin should be considered as an intra-articular therapeutic and potential biomarker in patients that sustain joint-related injuries or in patients with CACP, OA, and RA in order to provide a protective effect on the joint.[27]

MORE RECENT DISCOVERIES

Although lubricin was originally found in cartilage and synovial fluid and secreted by the synovial fibroblasts, it has since been found in other tissues, such as lung, heart, liver, eye, uterus, cervix, prostate, bladder, and bone, indicating that it has a multifunctional role that is not limited solely to joints and friction reduction.[5,6,28] Therefore, due to lubricin's ubiquitous nature, there have been numerous reports of lubricin as a potential therapeutic in several nontribologic disorders (discussed later).[29]

Extra-articular Nontribologic Functions of Lubricin: Bowel and Bladder Permeability

Interstitial cystitis-bladder pain syndrome (IC-BPS) is a common disorder characterized by painful and increased frequency of urination from disruption of epithelial cells in the bladder. Irritable bowel syndrome (IBS) is a common disorder of the large intestine, involving pain, cramping, bloating, gas, diarrhea, and/or constipation and has a high comorbidity with IC-BPS, indicating cross-talk of the disorders.[30] Currently, patients with either IBS or IC-BPS have few treatment options.[30,31] In rats, treatment with protamine sulfate (PS) induced bladder and subsequently colon permeability, which mimic IC-BPS and IBS in humans.[32] When rats that were exposed to PS and later treated with lubricin, there was a reduction of the PS-induced permeability in both the bladder and the colon.[29] Therefore, lubricin could have potential as a therapeutic for patients with IC-BPS or IBS.

Patients who undergo abdominal surgery have a high chance of developing intra-abdominal lesions, with up to 20% requiring treatment despite newer less invasive surgical techniques.[33,34] There currently are no proved methods to completely prevent the formation of intra-abdominal lesions, resulting in a clinical need for improved therapies.[35] Intra-abdominal adhesions were created in rats via both cecal abrasion and cecal enterotomy, with only the cecal abrasions leading to significant lesion formation.[35] In rats with cecal abrasions, recombinant human lubricin (rhPRG4) treatment applied directly after surgery prevented both inflammation and fibrosis of the lesioned areas, indicating a potential role for lubricin as a postoperative treatment in patients who undergo abdominal surgeries.[35]

Clinical Uses for Lubricin: Dry eye (xerophthalmia) and dry mouth (xerostomia) diseases

Dry eye (xerophthalmia) is a condition in which there are not enough tears produced in order to lubricate the ocular surface leading to discomfort, light sensitivity, burning sensations, inflammation, and potential eye damage.[36,37] There are several other conditions that lead to dry eye, including the use of contact lenses, dry eye disease, Sjögren syndrome (SS), Stevens-Johnson syndrome, vitamin deficiencies, RA, and refractive surgery.[37] The current treatments for dry eye include hyaluronic acid (HA), polyvinyl alcohol, povidone, hydroxypropyl guar, and cellulose derivatives, and treatment depends on the cause of dry eye.[36] Dry eye typically has an inflammatory component and, if it is severe enough, may need anti-inflammatory or immunosuppressant treatments.[36]

Dry mouth (xerostomia) is the feeling of oral dryness and most often occurs in older adult women.[38] The most common complaints with xerostomia are difficulty talking, chewing, and swallowing in addition to altered taste.[38] Some of the most common causes of xerostomia include cancer treatment, various medications, and SS.[38]

Sjögren syndrome is an autoimmune disease that mainly results in both dry eye and dry mouth but can affect other organ systems.[39] Women are more effected by SS than men and it most often occurs in later years.[39] The causes of SS, however, are not well known because it seems there are many contributing factors.[39] Due to the lubricating and anti-inflammatory properties of lubricin, several studies have suggested lubricin as a therapeutic for both dry eye and dry mouth. It has been documented that lubricin deficiency in the eye has a negative impact on corneal functioning.[28] In lubricin null mice, there was a significant increase in fluorescein staining and inflammation compared with wild-type animals, signifying that substantial corneal damage occurs without lubricin present.[28]

HA is commonly used in patients with dry eye and it is commercially available. Recently, a clinical trial indicated that lubricin is an excellent lubricating factor in patients with moderate dry eye disease and is more effective than HA at treating dry eye.[40] Moreover, a deficiency of lubricin, as seen in lubricin null mice, led to increased corneal fluorescein staining, illustrating the need for lubricin to reduce friction by acting as a natural lubricant in the space between the cornea and eyelid.[28] Recently, cathepsin S was found to be increased in the tears of patients with SS.[41] Cathepsin S was found to decrease ocular lubrication via degradation of lubricin in human tears.[42] Therefore, it seems that one of the mechanisms of dry eye in SS patients occurs via a reduction of lubricin at the ocular surface.[42]

These results, discussed previously, suggest that lubricin would be a better treatment of dry eye than current treatments, such as HA. Commercialization efforts currently are under way for production of lubricin intended for dry eye and dry mouth by Lubris, LLC (Framingham, MA).

Anti-inflammatory Actions of Lubricin: Toll-like Receptor 4, CD44, Nuclear Factor kB, and NOD-like Receptor Pyrin Domain Containing 3

Recently, lubricin has been studied to determine if it serves as a ligand for various receptors that are involved in cellular inflammatory cascades. Several studies indicate that lubricin binds to the integrin CD44 and some members of the Toll-like receptor (TLR) family, which suggests a role for lubricin in regulating inflammatory cascades.[43,44] Moreover, as detailed later, lubricin reduces nuclear factor (NF) kappa-light-chain-enhancer of activated B cells (NF-κB) nuclear translocation and

NOD-like receptor pyrin domain containing 3 (NLRP3) inflammasome activation, leading to decreases in the production of proinflammatory cytokines.

CD44 is a glycoprotein transmembrane cell surface receptor that is well known for binding to HA and internalizing it via receptor-mediated endocytosis and is highly involved in inflammatory cascades.[45–48] CD44 signaling seems to have function in both proinflammatory and anti-inflammatory pathways, because studies show contradictory reports about its function depending on ligand binding, cell type, and type of infection. For example, in CD44 knockout mice, renal dysfunction and inflammation were delayed after lipopolysaccharide (LPS) treatment.[49] On the contrary, CD44-deficient mice with *Escherichia coli* infections had increased lung inflammation and proinflammatory cytokine release.[50,51] Therefore, ligand binding to CD44 may elicit both proinflammatory and anti-inflammatory cascades, depending on cell type and other factors The ability of lubricin to disrupt the HA and CD44 interaction has also been observed in breast cancer cells.[52]

Besides HA, lubricin was found to be one of CD44's ligands. Using direct enzyme-linked immunosorbent assay (ELISA), rhPRG4 was found to bind to recombinant CD44 receptors with a higher affinity than CD44's known ligand, HA and was concentration dependent.[44] HA blocked the binding of rhPRG4 to CD44, however, in a concentration-dependent manner.[44] Removal of the mucin domain's sialic acid and O-glycosylations of rhPRG4 resulted in an even greater affinity of rhPRG4 to CD44. In the same study, RA fibroblast-like synoviocytes (RA-FLS) proliferation was induced via IL-1β and TNF-α, which was suppressed with rhPRG4.[44] IM7, an antibody directed against CD44, blocked the suppressive effects of rhPRG4, further verifying that CD44 is one of lubricin's receptors.[44]

The TLRs are a large 11-member family of receptors that are associated with host defense mechanisms for innate immunity.[53,54] The TLR family of receptors is responsible for the detection of pathogen-associated molecular patterns from bacteria, fungi, and viruses and are considered 1 family of the pathogen-recognition receptors.[53] On recognition of said pathogens, a cascade of immune events occurs in the host, including cytokine release and transcriptional factor activation.[53] Therefore, antagonists of the TLRs have been utilized as a means to reverse immune cascades in order to treat various immune-related disorders.[55,56]

Both rhPRG4 and native human lubricin (nhPRG4) bind to TLR2 and TLR4, and binding is concentration dependent, which was verified via ELISA and via a TLR2/TLR4 HEK-293 reporter cell line.[43] Moreover, nhPRG4 was effectively able to block TLR2 and TLR4 activation when the agonists Pam3CSK4 and LPS were used.[43] TLR2 and TLR4 activation can also be stimulated via human synovial fluid samples from patients with OA and RA, which are effectively blocked with both rhPRG4 and nhPRG4.[43] OA and RA synovial fluid have naturally depleted levels of lubricin, which coincides with increased TLR2 and TLR4 activation.[43] Therefore, lubricin seems to be an effective antagonist of both TLR2 and TLR4, thus blocking downstream inflammatory cellular responses.

Activation of inflammatory pathways including ligand binding of both the TLRs and CD44 stimulates NF-κB translocation into the nucleus, which triggers a cascade of inflammatory related events.[44,57] NF-κB is a family of transcription factors and are well known for being activated during innate and acquired immune responses and subsequently stimulate the release of chemokines, cytokines, antiapoptotic proteins, and stress-response proteins.[57,58] Moreover, these same chemokines, cytokines, and proteins also can trigger NF-κB translocation in a reciprocal fashion.[57] More recent findings indicate, however, that the role of NF-κB is tissue specific and is implicated in the production of both inflammatory and anti-inflammatory genes spurring characterization of the canonical and alternative NF-κB signaling pathways.[57] These results indicate that the function of NF-κB is difficult to elucidate and that activation of NF-κB stimulates release of both proinflammatory and anti-inflammatory factors, which would increase or decrease apoptosis depending on cellular dynamics.

Recent reports indicate that lubricin can prevent NF-κB translocation. For example, treatment of RA-FLS with TNF-α induces NF-κB translocation into the nucleus, which can be blocked with both rhPRG4 or MG132 (a known inhibitor of NF-κB translocation).[44] Moreover, blockade of NF-κB translocation from rhPRG4 was significantly reduced with the IM7 antibody.[44] Similarly, in THP-1 macrophages treated with monosodium urate (MSU) crystals, NF-κB translocation was significantly increased, which was reversed by lubricin treatment.[59]

The NLRP3 inflammasome is another facilitator of inflammatory cascades within the cell.[59–61] NLRP3 can be stimulated by a variety of factors within the cell, such as NF-κB translocation and, when primed, initiates pro–caspase-1 activity, creating the inflammasome that promotes the cleavage of pro–IL-1β and pro–IL-18 into their mature forms to further drive the inflammatory response.[59–61] Lubricin inhibited both the inflammasome and pro–caspase-1 activation in macrophages that were induced into an inflammatory state via MSU crystals, which typically are deposited in joints in patients with gout.[59]

Proinflammatory cytokines and growth factors also play a role in regulating the production and release of lubricin.[62,63] The cytokines TNF-α and IL-1 decrease both lubricin mRNA and protein expression from both articular chondrocytes and synoviocytes whereas the growth factor TGF-β increased lubricin mRNA expression.[62,63] Lubricin also has been shown to regulate the release of various cytokines and chemokines.[59] For example, MSU-treated THP-1 macrophages induced significant increases in the cytokines IL-1β and TNF-α, and the chemokines IL-8 and monocyte chemoattractant protein-1, all of which were significantly reduced with treatment of rhPRG4.[59]

Due to these findings, a role for lubricin as an anti-inflammatory biologic has emerged and indicates that lubricin may serve as a biomarker of inflammatory processes and inflammation. In fact, lubricin is upregulated in the liver in a mouse sepsis model, indicating its potential as a sepsis biomarker[64] lubricin's antagonism of TLR receptors and interaction with the CD44 integrin indicate that it may be an important treatment option in a variety of disorders with an immunologic basis (**Fig. 1**). Therefore, further studies of rhPRG4 and its interaction in immune pathways have more recently been performed, as discussed below.

Potential Therapeutic Role of Lubricin in Sepsis: Sepsis background

Sepsis is a major health concern due to its high mortality rate and ineffective current treatments. Sepsis was previously technically defined as a syndrome resulting from systemic inflammatory response syndrome, which stems from bacterial and viral infections, creating a cascade of inflammatory responses within the host, also known as the cytokine storm. Newer reports have proposed, however, that certain terminology be removed in order for clinicians to more accurately diagnosis sepsis and initiate treatment.[65] There also are cases in which sepsis can occur from noninfectious conditions, such as pancreatitis, burns, and tissue injury.[66] In the absence of adequate intervention or treatment, the inflammatory cascades and cytokine storm usually lead to septic shock, organ failure, and death.[66]

Because sepsis is a highly multifactorial syndrome, it is difficult to treat, and most treatments that have been tested in clinical trials were ineffective.[66] Another reason

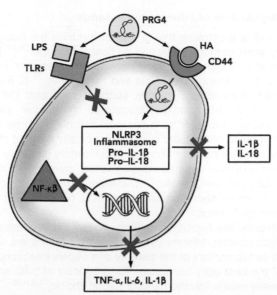

Fig. 1. Proposed mechanism of action of lubricin in inflammatory cascades. Various ligands bind to both the TLRs and CD44, namely, LPS and HA. Activation of these receptors activate internal cellular pathways involved in inflammation. The inflammasome becomes activated and initiates conversion of pro–IL-18 and pro–IL1-β to their mature forms to be released from the cell. NF-κB translocates to the nucleus, which also initiates the production and release of other cytokines. When cells are treated with rhPRG4, these inflammatory cascades are halted. rhPRG4 strongly binds to both TLR2 and TLR4 as an antagonist and competitor with other ligands. rhRPG4 also becomes internalized into the cell via CD44, allowing rhRPG4 to both prevent activation of the inflammasome and translocation of NF-κB, thereby preventing the formation of cytokines.

that sepsis is challenging to treat is the delay between the time the patient presents with symptoms to the time that white blood cell, blood cultures, and serum lactate test results are received, resulting in a delay of diagnosis.[67] Currently, results can take up to 72 hours and the tests are unreliable for sepsis diagnostics.[67,68] Currently, broad-spectrum antibiotics, vasopressors, and drugs to treat hypotension are administered to patients with suspected sepsis. Patients treated more quickly are likely to have a more positive outcome.[65,69] Even with current sepsis treatments, there is still a 30% death rate of patients with sepsis, indicating the need for more effective treatments.[70]

Therefore, new biomarkers and detection techniques for earlier identification of sepsis are needed.[71–74] A new report details an antibody based small microelectrode biosensor to test levels of the cytokine IL-6 within as little as 2.5 minutes, a significant improvement in treatment time for septic patients.[70] The biosensor can also be engineered to test multiple biomarkers at the same time, which would significantly improve patient wait times and treatment paradigms.[72] Other types of biosensors have also been explored, including electrochemical, optical, and microfluidic-based sensors.[75] The issues with biosensors, however, include high cost, low sensitivity, and short shelf-life all, of which create a hindrance for use in the clinic.[75] Once the logistical issues are removed, however, biosensors will become a critical piece of sepsis diagnosis in the future.

Cytokine Role in Sepsis: Role of interleukin-6 in sepsis

The glycoprotein IL-6 is a cytokine that is released during the body's inflammatory response resulting from pathogen invasion or tissue damage.[76,77] IL-6 is secreted from many different cell types, including leukocytes, vascular endothelial cells, mesenchymal cells, fibroblasts, osteoblasts and tumor cells.[78] IL-6 is produced and released via stimulation by other cytokines, such as IL-1β and TNF-α, via the host cell's initial recognition of pathogen-associated molecular patterns through pathogen-recognition receptors, or from damage-associated molecular pattern and acts as a warning signal to other cells.[76,79] IL-6 is typically thought of as a proinflammatory cytokine but does function in the anti-inflammatory pathway as well.[77] When IL-6 expression and secretion becomes dysregulated, severe immune-related disorders develop, one of them being sepsis.[79] Therefore, drugs, biologics and therapeutics that are able to block secretion and/or binding of IL-6 to its receptors have become a major research focus.[79]

Sepsis has 2 phases: the hyperinflammatory phase and the immunosuppressive phase, both of which contain different cytokine spikes.[80] There are several cytokines that can be tested as biomarkers of the severity of a sepsis infection, although IL-6 is considered one of the best early biomarkers for prognosis of both adult and neonate patients with a severe sepsis infection and/or septic shock.[74,81–85]

Therefore, based on the aforementioned information, IL-6 stood out as an important marker for early cellular inflammatory responses to which lubricin could make a potential therapeutic impact if it were able to reduce IL-6 protein and gene expression.

RESULTS FROM THE AUTHORS' LABORATORY

Due to lubricin's role in the inflammatory pathways involving CD44, TLR4, and NLRP3, as discussed previously, the authors' laboratory has identified lubricin as a possible therapeutic for patients with sepsis due to its ability to lower both protein levels and gene expression of IL-6 in human umbilical vascular endothelial cells (HUVECs) and in human lung microvascular endothelial cells (HLMVECs).[86] HUVECs and HLMVECs were treated with LPS to induce a high inflammatory state, resulting in significantly increased IL-6 protein levels and gene expression, both of which were reversed to control levels with 50 μg/ mL, 100 μg/mL, and 150 μg/mL rhPRG4 treatment.[86] Moreover, HLMVECs were treated with plasma from septic patients to induce an inflammatory response and rhPRG4 significantly lowered IL-6 protein levels in approximately 75% of the patients.[86]

Because lubricin biosynthesis is down-regulated by various cytokines, including IL-1β and TNF-α, it is possible lubricin could serve not only as a therapeutic but also as a biomarker of inflammation and infections, including sepsis.[62]

SUMMARY

Lubricin's original role in the reduction of joint friction has evolved to a multitude of reports on the nontribologic functions of lubricin, notably within inflammatory pathways. Lubricin is an antagonist of TLR2 and TLR4, which is one mechanism of its role in reducing inflammation. Moreover, lubricin also interacts with CD44 in order to block NF-κB translocation into the nucleus and formation of the NLRP3 inflammasome. Therefore, these results led to further research into lubricin as an anti-inflammatory and possible biomarker of sepsis. Lubricin effectively decreased protein levels and gene expression of IL-6, a prominent sepsis biomarker. The authors conclude that lubricin has the potential to be an effective therapeutic for many diseases with underlying inflammation, including but not limited to sepsis.

REFERENCES

1. Swann DA, Slayter HS, Silver FH. The molecular structure of lubricating glycoprotein-I, the boundary lubricant for articular cartilage. J Biol Chem 1981; 256(11):5921–5.
2. Swann DA, Sotman S, Dixon M, et al. The isolation and partial characterization of the major glycoprotein (LGP-I) from the articular lubricating fraction from bovine synovial fluid. Biochem J 1977;161(3):473–85.
3. Swann DA, Hendren RB, Radin EL, et al. The lubricating activity of synovial fluid glycoproteins. Arthritis Rheum 1981;24(1):22–30.
4. Swann DA, Silver FH, Slayter HS, et al. The molecular structure and lubricating activity of lubricin isolated from bovine and human synovial fluids. Biochem J 1985;225(1):195–201.
5. Jay GD, Britt DE, Cha CJ. Lubricin is a product of megakaryocyte stimulating factor gene expression by human synovial fibroblasts. J Rheumatol 2000;27(3): 594–600.
6. Ikegawa S, Sano M, Koshizuka Y, et al. Isolation, characterization and mapping of the mouse and human PRG4 (proteoglycan 4) genes. Cytogenet Cell Genet 2000;90(3–4):291–7.
7. Jay GD, Tantravahi U, Britt DE, et al. Homology of lubricin and superficial zone protein (SZP): products of megakaryocyte stimulating factor (MSF) gene expression by human synovial fibroblasts and articular chondrocytes localized to chromosome 1q25. J Orthop Res 2001;19(4):677–87.
8. Lord MS, Estrella RP, Chuang CY, et al. Not all lubricin isoforms are substituted with a glycosaminoglycan chain. Connect Tissue Res 2012;53(2):132–41.
9. Rhee DK, Marcelino J, Baker M, et al. The secreted glycoprotein lubricin protects cartilage surfaces and inhibits synovial cell overgrowth. J Clin Invest 2005;115(3): 622–31.
10. Marcelino J, Carpten JD, Suwairi WM, et al. CACP, encoding a secreted proteoglycan, is mutated in camptodactyly-arthropathy-coxa vara-pericarditis syndrome. Nat Genet 1999;23(3):319–22.
11. Bao JP, Chen WP, Wu LD. Lubricin: a novel potential biotherapeutic approaches for the treatment of osteoarthritis. Mol Biol Rep 2011;38(5):2879–85.
12. Bahabri SA, Suwairi WM, Laxer RM, et al. The camptodactyly-arthropathy-coxa vara-pericarditis syndrome: clinical features and genetic mapping to human chromosome 1. Arthritis Rheum 1998;41(4):730–5.
13. Hill A, Waller KA, Cui Y, et al. Lubricin restoration in a mouse model of congenital deficiency. Arthritis Rheumatol 2015;67(11):3070–81.
14. Waller KA, Zhang LX, Jay GD. Friction-induced mitochondrial dysregulation contributes to joint deterioration in Prg4 knockout mice. Int J Mol Sci 2017;18(6) [pii: E1252].
15. Waller KA, Zhang LX, Elsaid KA, et al. Role of lubricin and boundary lubrication in the prevention of chondrocyte apoptosis. Proc Natl Acad Sci U S A 2013;110(15): 5852–7.
16. Elsaid KA, Zhang L, Waller K, et al. The impact of forced joint exercise on lubricin biosynthesis from articular cartilage following ACL transection and intra-articular lubricin's effect in exercised joints following ACL transection. Osteoarthritis Cartilage 2012;20(8):940–8.
17. Mobasheri A, Batt M. An update on the pathophysiology of osteoarthritis. Ann Phys Rehabil Med 2016;59(5–6):333–9.

18. Flannery CR, Zollner R, Corcoran C, et al. Prevention of cartilage degeneration in a rat model of osteoarthritis by intraarticular treatment with recombinant lubricin. Arthritis Rheum 2009;60(3):840–7.

19. Young AA, McLennan S, Smith MM, et al. Proteoglycan 4 downregulation in a sheep meniscectomy model of early osteoarthritis. Arthritis Res Ther 2006; 8(2):R41.

20. Neu CP, Reddi AH, Komvopoulos K, et al. Increased friction coefficient and superficial zone protein expression in patients with advanced osteoarthritis. Arthritis Rheum 2010;62(9):2680–7.

21. Ruan MZ, Erez A, Guse K, et al. Proteoglycan 4 expression protects against the development of osteoarthritis. Sci Transl Med 2013;5(176):176ra34.

22. Ruan MZ, Cerullo V, Cela R, et al. Treatment of osteoarthritis using a helper-dependent adenoviral vector retargeted to chondrocytes. Mol Ther Methods Clin Dev 2016;3:16008.

23. Smolen JS, Aletaha D, McInnes IB. Rheumatoid arthritis. Lancet 2016; 388(10055):2023–38.

24. Scott DL, Wolfe F, Huizinga TW. Rheumatoid arthritis. Lancet 2010;376(9746): 1094–108.

25. Kosinska MK, Ludwig TE, Liebisch G, et al. Articular joint lubricants during osteoarthritis and rheumatoid arthritis display altered levels and molecular species. PLoS One 2015;10(5):e0125192.

26. Elsaid KA, Jay GD, Warman ML, et al. Association of articular cartilage degradation and loss of boundary-lubricating ability of synovial fluid following injury and inflammatory arthritis. Arthritis Rheum 2005;52(6):1746–55.

27. Lord MS, Farrugia BL, Rnjak-Kovacina J, et al. Current serological possibilities for the diagnosis of arthritis with special focus on proteins and proteoglycans from the extracellular matrix. Expert Rev Mol Diagn 2015;15(1):77–95.

28. Schmidt TA, Sullivan DA, Knop E, et al. Transcription, translation, and function of lubricin, a boundary lubricant, at the ocular surface. JAMA Ophthalmol 2013; 131(6):766–76.

29. Greenwood-Van Meerveld B, Mohammadi E, Latorre R, et al. Preclinical animal studies of intravesical recombinant human proteoglycan 4 as a novel potential therapy for diseases resulting from increased bladder permeability. Urology 2018;116:230.e1–7.

30. Holtmann GJ, Ford AC, Talley NJ. Pathophysiology of irritable bowel syndrome. Lancet Gastroenterol Hepatol 2016;1(2):133–46.

31. Ogawa T, Ishizuka O, Ueda T, et al. Current and emerging drugs for interstitial cystitis/bladder pain syndrome (IC/BPS). Expert Opin Emerg Drugs 2015;20(4): 555–70.

32. Greenwood-Van Meerveld B, Mohammadi E, Tyler K, et al. Mechanisms of visceral organ crosstalk: importance of alterations in permeability in rodent models. J Urol 2015;194(3):804–11.

33. Menzies D, Ellis H. Intestinal obstruction from adhesions–how big is the problem? Ann R Coll Surg Engl 1990;72(1):60–3.

34. Gutt CN, Oniu T, Schemmer P, et al. Fewer adhesions induced by laparoscopic surgery? Surg Endosc 2004;18(6):898–906.

35. Oh J, Kuan KG, Tiong LU, et al. Recombinant human lubricin for prevention of postoperative intra-abdominal adhesions in a rat model. J Surg Res 2017; 208:20–5.

36. Messmer EM. The pathophysiology, diagnosis, and treatment of dry eye disease. Dtsch Arztebl Int 2015;112(5):71–81 [quiz 2].

37. Mayo clinic. Dry eyes. 2019. Available at: https://www.mayoclinic.org/diseases-conditions/dry-eyes/symptoms-causes/syc-20371863. Accessed February 12, 2019.
38. Millsop JW, Wang EA, Fazel N. Etiology, evaluation, and management of xerostomia. Clin Dermatol 2017;35(5):468–76.
39. Maslinska M, Przygodzka M, Kwiatkowska B, et al. Sjogren's syndrome: still not fully understood disease. Rheumatol Int 2015;35(2):233–41.
40. Lambiase A, Sullivan BD, Schmidt TA, et al. A two-week, randomized, double-masked study to evaluate safety and efficacy of lubricin (150 mug/mL) eye drops versus Sodium Hyaluronate (HA) 0.18% eye drops (Vismed(R)) in patients with moderate dry eye disease. Ocul Surf 2017;15(1):77–87.
41. Hamm-Alvarez SF, Janga SR, Edman MC, et al. Tear cathepsin S as a candidate biomarker for Sjogren's syndrome. Arthritis Rheumatol 2014;66(7):1872–81.
42. Regmi SC, Samsom ML, Heynen ML, et al. Degradation of proteoglycan 4/lubricin by cathepsin S: potential mechanism for diminished ocular surface lubrication in Sjogren's syndrome. Exp Eye Res 2017;161:1–9.
43. Alquraini A, Garguilo S, D'Souza G, et al. The interaction of lubricin/proteoglycan 4 (PRG4) with toll-like receptors 2 and 4: an anti-inflammatory role of PRG4 in synovial fluid. Arthritis Res Ther 2015;17:353.
44. Al-Sharif A, Jamal M, Zhang LX, et al. Lubricin/proteoglycan 4 binding to CD44 receptor: a mechanism of the suppression of proinflammatory cytokine-induced synoviocyte proliferation by lubricin. Arthritis Rheumatol 2015;67(6):1503–13.
45. Culty M, Nguyen HA, Underhill CB. The hyaluronan receptor (CD44) participates in the uptake and degradation of hyaluronan. J Cell Biol 1992;116(4):1055–62.
46. Hua Q, Knudson CB, Knudson W. Internalization of hyaluronan by chondrocytes occurs via receptor-mediated endocytosis. J Cell Sci 1993;106(Pt 1):365–75.
47. Underhill CB, Thurn AL, Lacy BE. Characterization and identification of the hyaluronate binding site from membranes of SV-3T3 cells. J Biol Chem 1985;260(13): 8128–33.
48. Johnson P, Ruffell B. CD44 and its role in inflammation and inflammatory diseases. Inflamm Allergy Drug Targets 2009;8(3):208–20.
49. Rampanelli E, Dessing MC, Claessen N, et al. CD44-deficiency attenuates the immunologic responses to LPS and delays the onset of endotoxic shock-induced renal inflammation and dysfunction. PLoS One 2013;8(12):e84479.
50. Wang Q, Teder P, Judd NP, et al. CD44 deficiency leads to enhanced neutrophil migration and lung injury in Escherichia coli pneumonia in mice. Am J Pathol 2002;161(6):2219–28.
51. van der Windt GJ, van 't Veer C, Florquin S, et al. CD44 deficiency is associated with enhanced Escherichia coli-induced proinflammatory cytokine and chemokine release by peritoneal macrophages. Infect Immun 2010;78(1):115–24.
52. Sarkar A, Chanda A, Regmi SC, et al. Recombinant human PRG4 (rhPRG4) suppresses breast cancer cell invasion by inhibiting TGFβ Hyaluronan-CD44 signalling pathway. PLoS One 2019;14(7):1–29.
53. Chen K, Huang J, Gong W, et al. Toll-like receptors in inflammation, infection and cancer. Int Immunopharmacol 2007;7(10):1271–85.
54. Takeda K, Akira S. Toll-like receptors in innate immunity. Int Immunol 2005; 17(1):1–14.
55. Patra MC, Choi S. Recent progress in the development of Toll-like receptor (TLR) antagonists. Expert Opin Ther Pat 2016;26(6):719–30.

56. Gao W, Xiong Y, Li Q, et al. Inhibition of toll-like receptor signaling as a promising therapy for inflammatory diseases: a journey from molecular to nano therapeutics. Front Physiol 2017;8:508.
57. Lawrence T. The nuclear factor NF-kappaB pathway in inflammation. Cold Spring Harb Perspect Biol 2009;1(6):a001651.
58. Li Q, Verma IM. NF-kappaB regulation in the immune system. Nat Rev Immunol 2002;2(10):725–34.
59. Qadri M, Jay GD, Zhang LX, et al. Recombinant human proteoglycan-4 reduces phagocytosis of urate crystals and downstream nuclear factor kappa B and inflammasome activation and production of cytokines and chemokines in human and murine macrophages. Arthritis Res Ther 2018;20(1):192.
60. Afonina IS, Zhong Z, Karin M, et al. Limiting inflammation-the negative regulation of NF-kappaB and the NLRP3 inflammasome. Nat Immunol 2017;18(8):861–9.
61. He Y, Hara H, Nunez G. Mechanism and regulation of NLRP3 inflammasome activation. Trends Biochem Sci 2016;41(12):1012–21.
62. Jones AR, Flannery CR. Bioregulation of lubricin expression by growth factors and cytokines. Eur Cell Mater 2007;13:40–5 [discussion: 5].
63. Flannery CR, Hughes CE, Schumacher BL, et al. Articular cartilage superficial zone protein (SZP) is homologous to megakaryocyte stimulating factor precursor and is a multifunctional proteoglycan with potential growth-promoting, cytoprotective, and lubricating properties in cartilage metabolism. Biochem Biophys Res Commun 1999;254(3):535–41.
64. Singer M, Deutschman CS, Seymour CW, et al. The third international consensus definitions for sepsis and septic shock (Sepsis-3). Jama 2016;315(8):801–10.
65. Toledo AG, Golden G, Campos AR, et al. Proteomic atlas of organ vasculopathies triggered by Staphylococcus aureus sepsis. Nature Comm, in press.
66. Gotts JE, Matthay MA. Sepsis: pathophysiology and clinical management. BMJ 2016;353:i1585.
67. Calandra T, Cohen J. The international sepsis forum consensus conference on definitions of infection in the intensive care unit. Crit Care Med 2005;33(7):1538–48.
68. Rhee C, Murphy MV, Li L, et al. Lactate testing in suspected sepsis: trends and predictors of failure to measure levels. Crit Care Med 2015;43(8):1669–76.
69. Dellinger RP, Levy MM, Rhodes A, et al. Surviving sepsis campaign: international guidelines for management of severe sepsis and septic shock, 2012. Intensive Care Med 2013;39(2):165–228.
70. CDC. Sepsis. 2017. Available at: https://www.cdc.gov/sepsis/datareports/index.html. Accessed February 15, 2019.
71. Bloos F, Reinhart K. Rapid diagnosis of sepsis. Virulence 2014;5(1):154–60.
72. Russell C, Ward AC, Vezza V, et al. Development of a needle shaped microelectrode for electrochemical detection of the sepsis biomarker interleukin-6 (IL-6) in real time. Biosens Bioelectron 2019;126:806–14.
73. Ricarte-Bratti JP, Brizuela NY, Jaime-Albarran N, et al. IL-6, MMP 3 and prognosis in previously healthy sepsis patients. Rev Fac Cien Med Univ Nac Cordoba 2017;74(2):99–106.
74. Biron BM, Ayala A, Lomas-Neira JL. Biomarkers for sepsis: what is and what might be? Biomark Insights 2015;10s4:BMI.S29519.
75. Kumar S, Tripathy S, Jyoti A, et al. Recent advances in biosensors for diagnosis and detection of sepsis: a comprehensive review. Biosens Bioelectron 2019;124-125:205–15.

76. Tanaka T, Narazaki M, Kishimoto T. IL-6 in inflammation, immunity, and disease. Cold Spring Harb Perspect Biol 2014;6(10):a016295.
77. Scheller J, Chalaris A, Schmidt-Arras D, et al. The pro- and anti-inflammatory properties of the cytokine interleukin-6. Biochim Biophys Acta 2011;1813(5):878–88.
78. Kobeissi Z, Zanotti-Cavazzoni S. Biomarkers of sepsis Marshall JC, for the international sepsis forum (Li Ka Shing Knowledge Inst, Toronto, Ontario, Canada, St. Michael's Hosp, Toronto, Ontario, Canada, Univ of Toronto, Toronto, Ontario, Canada; Friedrich-Schiller Univ, Jena, Germany) Crit Care Med 37: 2290-2298, 2009. Year Book. Crit Care Med 2010;2010:227–8.
79. Tanaka T, Narazaki M, Kishimoto T. Immunotherapeutic implications of IL-6 blockade for cytokine storm. Immunotherapy 2016;8(8):959–70.
80. Tamayo E, Fernandez A, Almansa R, et al. Pro- and anti-inflammatory responses are regulated simultaneously from the first moments of septic shock. Eur Cytokine Netw 2011;22(2):82–7.
81. Rios-Toro JJ, Marquez-Coello M, Garcia-Alvarez JM, et al. Soluble membrane receptors, interleukin 6, procalcitonin and C reactive protein as prognostic markers in patients with severe sepsis and septic shock. PLoS One 2017;12(4):e0175254.
82. Andaluz-Ojeda D, Bobillo F, Iglesias V, et al. A combined score of pro- and anti-inflammatory interleukins improves mortality prediction in severe sepsis. Cytokine 2012;57(3):332–6.
83. Gogos CA, Drosou E, Bassaris HP, et al. Pro- versus anti-inflammatory cytokine profile in patients with severe sepsis: a marker for prognosis and future therapeutic options. J Infect Dis 2000;181(1):176–80.
84. Franco DM, Arevalo-Rodriguez I, i Figuls MR, et al. Interleukin-6 for diagnosis of sepsis in critically ill adult patients. Cochrane Database Syst Rev 2015;(7):CD011811.
85. Sun B, Liang LF, Li J, et al. A meta-analysis of interleukin-6 as a valid and accurate index in diagnosing early neonatal sepsis. Int Wound J 2019;16(2):527–33.
86. Richendrfer H, Schmidt TM, Levy MM, et al. Recombinant human proteoglycan-4 (rhPRG4) decreases IL-6 in human endothelial cells with a sepsis phenotype. Las Vegas (NV): Society of Academic Emergency Medicine; 2019.

Check Point Inhibitors and Their Role in Immunosuppression in Sepsis

Michelle E. Wakeley, MD[a], Chyna C. Gray, BA[b],
Sean F. Monaghan, MD[c,d], Daithi S. Heffernan, MD, AFRCSI[e,f],
Alfred Ayala, PhD[g],*

KEYWORDS

- Checkpoint regulators • Immunosuppression • Sepsis • PD-1 • CTLA-4 • VISTA
- HVEM

KEY POINTS

- Checkpoint regulators are a diverse group of membrane bound proteins, with varied expression and notable redundancy, which dictate immune cell response to antigen presentation.
- Septic immunosuppression predisposing patients to secondary infection after a primary infectious insult is mediated, at least in part, by checkpoint regulators.
- Checkpoint regulators have been manipulated in animal models improving outcomes after septic insult but have not been successfully harnessed as therapeutic targets in humans.

Disclosure Statement: The authors report no proprietary or commercial interest in any product mentioned or concept discussed in this article.

Funding Sources: This work was supported by the National Institutes of Health (grant numbers R35 GM118097 [A. Ayala], R25 GM083270 [C.C. Gray], P20GM103652 [S.F. Monaghan], and K08-GM110495 [D.S. Heffernan]) as well as a Post-doctoral fellowship award from the National Institutes of Health (MEW) [grant number T32 GM065085].

[a] Division of Surgical Research, Department of Surgery, Brown University, Rhode Island Hospital, Room 242 Aldrich Building, 593 Eddy Street, Providence, RI 02903, USA; [b] Molecular Biology, Cell Biology and Biochemistry Department, Brown University, Rhode Island Hospital, Room 244 Aldrich Building, 593 Eddy Street, Providence, RI 02903, USA; [c] Division of Surgical Research, Department of Surgery, Brown University, Rhode Island Hospital, Room 211 Middle House, 593 Eddy Street, Providence, RI 02903, USA; [d] Division of Trauma and Surgical Critical Care, Department of Surgery, Brown University, Rhode Island Hospital, Room 211 Middle House, 593 Eddy Street, Providence, RI 02903, USA; [e] Division of Surgical Research, Department of Surgery, Brown University, Rhode Island Hospital, Room 205 Middle House, 593 Eddy Street, Providence, RI 02903, USA; [f] Division of Trauma and Surgical Critical Care, Department of Surgery, Brown University, Rhode Island Hospital, Room 205 Middle House, 593 Eddy Street, Providence, RI 02903, USA; [g] Division of Surgical Research, Department of Surgery, Brown University, Rhode Island Hospital, Room 227 Aldrich Building, 593 Eddy Street, Providence, RI 02903, USA

* Corresponding author.

E-mail address: aayala@lifespan.org

INTRODUCTION

Sepsis is a life-threatening organ dysfunction, which results from a dysregulated host response to infection, and it remains a common, deadly, and expensive problem.[1] Treatment advances ranging from measured resuscitation strategies to broad-spectrum antibiotics have improved the morbidity and mortality associated with sepsis. Despite these advances, approximately 50,000 cases occur annually in the United States, and sepsis remains the leading cause of death in the noncoronary intensive care units, costing more than $24 billion as of 2014.[2,3] In response to septic insults, a profound immune activation occurs as the body attempts to corral the infectious source. The result of such extreme immune activation is a multifactorial disharmony of immune cells. This disruption of immune homeostasis results in circulating immune cell influx into distal organs, leading to multiorgan failure.[4] This necessary balance between activation and suppression is mediated by immune checkpoint regulators. These regulators are implicated in multiple instances of immune imbalance, including in sepsis.

The immune system utilizes checkpoint regulators to balance immune activity throughout the body. Checkpoint regulators are membrane-bound proteins that serve as a second signal to direct the immune response to a particular antigen (**Fig. 1**).[5] An antigen bound by major histocompatibility complex (MHC) class I or II receptors on an antigen-presenting cell (APC) is presented to a T-cell receptor (TCR), acting as the first signal. The second signal, from a checkpoint regulator, is necessary to instruct the T cell on how to respond to this antigen. Without such signals, the immune response is attenuated or absent. These proteins further allow for modification of the immune response over time, enabling different immune cells to respond to various environmental cues in unique ways.[6,7] Stimulatory signals from regulators can lead to activation and subsequent cell and humoral–mediated immunity, whereas inhibitory signals can lead to anergic T cells unable to respond to further signals.[8]

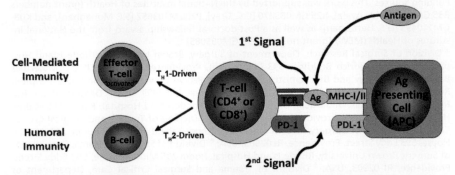

Fig. 1. Checkpoint regulators serve as a necessary second signal for immune responses: Checkpoint regulators are membrane bound proteins, which serve as a second signal to direct the immune response to a particular antigen. When an antigen is present it is bound by MHC class I or II receptors on an APC and presented to a TCR. After this, a second signal, from a checkpoint regulator, is necessary to instruct the T cell on how to respond to this antigen, shown here as the Programmed Cell Death 1 (PD-1)/Programmed Cell Death Ligand 1 (PDL-1) interaction. Stimulatory signals from regulators can lead to activation, and subsequent cell and humorally mediated immunity, whereas inhibitory signals can lead to anergic T cells unable to respond to further signals.

In the setting of overwhelming infection, checkpoint regulators serve as key mediators of the immune dysfunction that portends a risk of secondary infection. These regulators promote tolerance and can inhibit further immune reactivity to an infectious stimulus, traits that can be detrimental in the setting of overly profound infection.[7] It has been demonstrated that alteration in signaling through a variety of such regulators can alter outcomes after sepsis in animal models, and this has introduced new therapeutic targets that are beginning to be tested in clinical settings.[9] These regulatory systems are made up of a variety of proteins with nonredundant spatial and temporal functions, yet their ultimate signaling outcomes demonstrate substantial redundancy. The purpose of such repetition is incompletely understood. With a more complete understanding of these immune policing proteins, it is thought that their power might be harnessed to better treat patients enduring septic insults.[10] This article elaborates on the roles of diverse checkpoint regulators, such as programmed cell death-1 (PD-1), V-domain immunoglobulin (Ig) suppressor of T-cell activation (VISTA), cytotoxic T-lymphocyte–associated protein 4 (CTLA-4), and herpes virus entry mediator (HVEM), in immune regulation after sepsis and their contribution to postseptic immunosuppression.

PROGRAMMED CELL DEATH-1 (*PDCD1*)

PD-1 is an immune checkpoint protein first identified as a classical programmed cell death–induced gene, *Pdcd1*. PD-1 bears a variable Ig (IgV) domain and belongs to the B7-CD28 superfamily of checkpoint proteins. Both PD-1 and its ligands are expressed on a variety of immune cell types, and the PD-1 signaling pathway uniquely allows for maintenance of both central and peripheral tolerance by limiting the activation of T cells.[11]

PROGRAMMED CELL DEATH-1 AND ITS LIGANDS
Nonredundant Signaling Pathway

PD-1 signals as a receptor tyrosine kinase. Its cytoplasmic domain contains an immunoreceptor tyrosine-based switch motif (ITSM) domain and an immunoreceptor tyrosine-based inhibitory motif (ITIM) domain.[12] After ligation to the PD-1 ligands, the ITSM and ITIM domains are phosphorylated and Src homology region 2 domain-containing phosphatases (SHPs) 1 and 2 dock at the ITSM domain. On activation by PD-1, SHP-2 dephosphorylates kinases, phosphoinositide 3-kinase (PI3K) and zeta-chain-associated protein kinase 70 (ZAP70) to inhibit the Protein Kinase B (Akt) and extracellular signal-regulated kinase/mitogen-activated protein kinase (ERK/MAPK) pathways, as shown in **Fig. 2**.[13–15] Both TCR antigen stimulation and PD-1 ligation are requisite for PD-1–mediated suppression.[16]

Broad Expression Patterns Promote Tolerance

PD-1 is expressed on conventional T (Tconv) cells, regulatory T cells (Tregs), natural killer (NK) T cells, B cells, dendritic cells (DCs), and macrophages.[17,18] Transcription factors, such as NFAT2, STATs, Notch, and FoxO1, bind the *Pdcd1* promoter to transiently up-regulate PD-1 expression after TCR-antigen stimulation.[19–21] The expression of PD-1 during antigen stimulation sets a threshold for reactivation of lymphocytes.[14] As lymphocyte stimulation subsides, PD-1 expression is down-regulated by Blimp-1 and T-bet transcription factors to prevent overt T-cell exhaustion.[22,23]

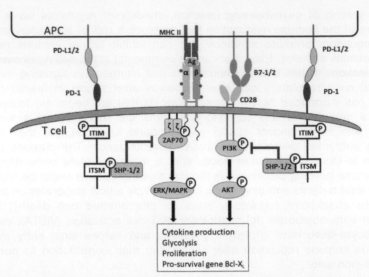

Fig. 2. PD-1 exerts intrinsic suppression of T-cell activity proximal to the TCR: ligation of PD-1 with its ligands results in recruitment of SHPs to the phosphorylated ITSM domain where they become functionally active. ZAP70 associates with the CD3-zeta chain and PI3K associates with the CD28 cytoplasmic tail on TCR stimulation and CD28 ligation. ZAP70 is an AP that recruits and stabilizes a kinase complex to initiate the ERK/MAPK pathway. PI3K serves as the initial kinase in the Akt pathway. Active SHP-1/2 dephosphorylate ZAP70 and PI3K; thus, inhibiting these kinase pathways and preventing T-cell activity, proper metabolic activity, T-cell survival via expression of b-cell lymphoma-extra large (Bcl-XL), and proliferation.

PD-L1 (B7-H1) and PD-L2 (B7-DC) are type 1 transmembrane proteins and CD28-B7 family members containing an extracellular region with IgV-like and constant Ig (IgC)-like domains. PD-L1 and PD-L2 compete for PD-1 binding with different affinities, and both bind additional ligand-specific partners B7-1 and repulsive guidance molecule b, respectively.[24,25] The differential cell-specific and tissue-specific expression patterns and competing molecular mechanisms of PD-L1 and PD-L2 promotes dynamic activity of PD-1 based on spatial and temporal context.[26]

PD-L1 is broadly expressed on both lymphoid and nonlymphoid cells in peripheral tissues, mediating PD-1 activation at sites of infection. PD-L1 is constitutively expressed at high levels by naïve CD4+ T cells, CD8+ T cells, B cells, DCs, and macrophages. On activation of lymphoid cells, PD-L1 surface expression is up-regulated and induced on monocytes.[27] Nonlymphoid cells, including cardiac endothelium, lung, placenta, kidney, salivary gland, glial cells, muscle cells, epithelial cells, and liver nonparenchymal cells, express PD-L1 constitutively as well.[28] These expression patterns ensure that activated T cells are systemically regulated to maintain peripheral tolerance.[26] PD-L2 is more tightly regulated with weaker expression on a smaller subset of cells and high binding specificity to PD-1. PD-L2 expression is induced specifically on activated bone marrow–derived DCs and macrophages found in the liver, lung, and spleen. Despite the differences between these ligands, they share some expression characteristics. Both PD-Ls are expressed on tumor cells, although PD-L1 expression extends to hematopoietic and nonhematopoietic tumors, and PD-L2 is largely restricted to leukemias. In addition, PD-L1/2 expression on splenic DCs is up-regulated by interferon-gamma (IFN-γ), granulocyte-macrophage colony-stimulating factor, and interleukin (IL)-4.[27] PD-1 and its ligands mediate interactions between both immune and nonimmune cell types to prevent autoreactivity in the periphery. The expansive influence of the PD-1 pathway has been exploited, however, to curtail immune surveillance in cancer and chronic viral infections. This pathway also has demonstrated detrimental activity in other diseases, such as sepsis and acute lung injury (ALI).

THE ROLE OF PROGRAMMED CELL DEATH-1 IN IMMUNOPATHOLOGY
Sepsis

As discussed previously, sepsis is characterized by systemic immune dysfunction. As with other immune-related diseases, such as cancer and chronic viral infection, T-cell anergy is implicated in sepsis development. The large impact that lymphocyte regulation and activity have in immune dysfunction prompted Huang and colleagues[29] to investigate the role of PD-1 in sepsis progression. This group found that adult *PD-1$^{-/-}$* mice have a survival advantage after intra-abdominal septic insult via the cecal ligation and puncture (CLP) procedure. The PD-1–deficient mice maintained macrophage function, demonstrating improved bacterial clearance and reduced inflammatory cytokine production. The survival results were recapitulated in a neonatal murine sepsis model using the neonatal cecal slurry technique. PD-1 deficiency promoted neonatal survival compared with wild-type (WT) controls but did not alter bactericidal efficacy.[30]

Monaghan and colleagues[31] expanded on the adult murine findings by analyzing the PD-1 expression patterns and cytokine profile of patients with septic shock. In septic patients, PD-1 was significantly up-regulated on circulating monocytes, granulocytes, and lymphocytes compared with healthy controls. This up-regulation positively correlated to IFN-γ, IL-4, and IL-2 levels, which are associated with the T helper cell 1/2 response and cytokine storm. The up-regulation of PD-1 surface expression and cytokine production also correlated with the severity of illness as determined by the Acute Physiology And Chronic Health Evaluation (APACHE) II score.[32] Thus, the increase in disease severity (APACHE II >20) associated with PD-1 overexpression demonstrates the potential of PD-1 blockade as a therapeutic intervention for sepsis.[31]

Acute Lung Injury and Respiratory Distress Syndrome

ALI can develop after an infectious insult ranging from sepsis, trauma, shock, or pneumonia and can progress into the more severe acute respiratory distress syndrome (ARDS). ALI/ARDS development is largely induced by neutrophils, lung epithelial, and lung endothelial cells. Because PD-1 and its ligands exert suppressive function in the periphery, it was postulated that this pathway may play a role in ALI/ARDS.[33] In a murine model of indirect ALI (iALI), PD-1 was up-regulated on several immune populations, such as T cells (CD4$^+$), tissue-resident DCs (CD11c$^+$), and Gr1$^+$ cells in the lung. This result was also mirrored in ARDS patients with a significant increase in PD-1 expressing CD3$^+$ T cells in the blood compared with healthy controls. In ARDS patients, the level of tumor necrosis factor (TNF)-α found in the bronchoalveolar lavage fluid and immune cell apoptosis was significantly higher. The loss of lung barrier function due to apoptosis of epithelial and endothelial cells is another phenotype of ALI/ARDS patients, implicating TNF-α further in the development of this disease. In *PD-1−/−* mice, pathologic indices of ARDS, such as TNF-α levels, tissue congestion, neutrophil influx in the lungs, and immune cell apoptosis were significantly lower than WT mice. PD-1–deficient mice also demonstrated a survival advantage compared with WT mice (70% vs 31.25%). These murine and human results further support a role for PD-1 in the development of ALI/ARDS.[33]

Viral Control

Evading immune surveillance is a phenomenon that is typically associated with cancer. Antitumoral immunity can be dampened by exploiting negative checkpoint pathways, allowing tumors to expand and thrive in the host. The PD-1/PD-L1 pathway has been targeted pharmacologically as an anticancer treatment with great efficacy, resulting in the development of multiple Food and Drug Administration approved PD-1 inhibitors.[34] This method of immune evasion is not limited to cancer. Human rhinovirus is among the most common infections and has evolved a mechanism to escape the immune response through the PD-1/PD-L1 pathway. Kirchberger and colleagues[35] demonstrated that human rhinovirus induces PD-L1 expression on DCs, blunting the ability to stimulate T cells and promoting T-cell tolerance. In line with the known PD-1/PD-L1 function, T cells were also reduced to a hypoproliferative state. These results support a clear role for the PD-1/PD-L1 pathway in sepsis, ARDS, and chronic infections.

V-DOMAIN IMMUNOGLOBULIN SUPPRESSOR OF T-CELL ACTIVATION (*VSIR*)

VISTA, also commonly referred to as Programmed cell death-1 homolog (PD-1H), is a negative checkpoint regulator that is encoded by the *vsir* gene, belongs to the B7-CD28 family. It contains an IgV domain, a transmembrane domain, a cytoplasmic tail, and an extracellular domain homologous to PD-L1. Despite belonging to the B7-CD28 family, VISTA has several unique characteristics that are not shared with other family members.[36] For instance, the cytoplasmic tail lacks both an ITIM and ITSM domain but contains proline residues, additional cysteines, and potential protein kinase C binding sites. It is theorized, based on these characteristics, that VISTA signals through a nonredundant pathway that remains undefined.[37] Another unique characteristic of VISTA is its receptor and ligand-like structure, expression, and function.[38] Acting as a receptor and ligand, VISTA inhibits T-cell proliferation, production of cytokines, such as IL-2, and IFN-γ, and chemokine production after TCR activation.[39] Through this inhibition, VISTA promotes peripheral tolerance.[36]

V-DOMAIN IMMUNOGLOBULIN SUPPRESSOR OF T-CELL ACTIVATION AS A RECEPTOR AND A LIGAND
V-domain Immunoglobulin Suppressor of T-cell Activation–V-domain Immunoglobulin Suppressor of T-cell Activation Interaction Promotes Context Dependent Regulation

VISTA is almost exclusively expressed on hematopoietic lineages, such as neutrophils, monocytes, DCs, and macrophages at high levels. VISTA is also constitutively expressed at lower levels on naïve CD4$^+$ T cells, CD8$^+$ T cells, Tregs, and tumor-infiltrating lymphocytes.[40] When expressed on Tconv cells, such as CD4$^+$ T cells, VISTA functions as a receptor and inhibits antigen-specific proliferation, cytokine, and chemokine production through cell intrinsic regulation.[38] VISTA can also act as a ligand when expressed on APCs and Tregs. The VISTA ligand exerts cell extrinsic regulation of Tconv cells by interacting with the uncharacterized VISTA receptor on T cells to suppress activation.[41]

The proposed VISTA-VISTA interaction between Tconv cells and Tregs also could promote the differentiation and suppressive function of Tregs.[39] VISTA also seems to have a stimulatory role when expressed as a receptor on myeloid cells by enhancing inflammatory cytokine production and antigen presentation.[37] Thus, the VISTA receptor inhibits Tconv cells whereas the VISTA ligand stimulates APC and Treg function. The ability to function as a ligand and a receptor depending on cellular context demonstrates the multifaceted, dynamic regulatory role of VISTA.

V-domain Immunoglobulin Suppressor of T-cell Activation–V-set and Immunoglobulin Domain Containing 3 Interaction Represents a Novel Checkpoint Pathway

In addition to VISTA-VISTA interactions, a new VISTA ligand has been identified. V-set and Ig domain containing 3 (VSIG-3) is a ligand in the Ig family and functionally interacts with VISTA expressed on T cells.[36] VSIG-3 is expressed in the brain, kidney, skeletal muscles, and germinal centers. It is also overexpressed in hepatic, colorectal, and gastric cancers.[42] VSIG-3 is a homophilic adhesion molecule and shares structural homology with B7 family members. Association between the VSIG-3 and VISTA ectodomains suppresses the T-cell response and cytokine and chemokine production.[36] In parallel with other checkpoint proteins discussed thus far, VISTA activity also can exacerbate immune-related pathologies.

THE ROLE OF V-DOMAIN IMMUNOGLOBULIN SUPPRESSOR OF T-CELL ACTIVATION IN IMMUNOPATHOLOGY
Sepsis

Although VISTA has mostly been discussed in the context of cancer and autoimmune disease, some recent work by Bharaj and colleagues[43] demonstrated that monocytes up-regulate VISTA after CLP in humanized bone marrow, liver, thymus (BLT) mice. BLT mice have severe immunodeficient nonobese diabetic phenotypes and produce inflammatory monocytes. After CLP in BLT mice, VISTA expression was significantly up-regulated on monocytes. These results support a role for VISTA in activating monocytes and contributing to the inflammatory response during sepsis progression.

Chronic Viral Infection (Human Immunodeficiency Virus)

As discussed previously, PD-1 plays an important role in chronic viral and bacterial infections. VISTA is no exception. In vitro treatment with Toll-like receptor (TLR) 3 and TLR5 correlated with significant VISTA up-regulation in circulating CD14+ monocytes and macrophages. TLR3 and TLR5 are virus-associated and bacteria-associated agonists, respectively. Based on these preliminary data, Bharaj and colleagues[37] also investigated VISTA in the context of human immunodeficiency virus (HIV)-infected patients. This research group found significant up-regulation of VISTA on monocytes associated with enhanced cytokine secretion in these individuals. It seems that the VISTA ligand plays a stimulatory role when expressed on monocytes during chronic viral infection. The differential role of VISTA as a ligand and receptor based on cell-type and disease context, further highlight the complex regulatory function of this checkpoint protein.

CYTOTOXIC T-LYMPHOCYTE–ASSOCIATED PROTEIN 4

CTLA-4 is a negative checkpoint regulator that was first identified as a homolog to costimulatory protein CD28 and belongs to the Ig superfamily.[44] CD28 and CTLA-4 are founding members of the CD28-B7 family and serve as the paradigm for immune checkpoint pathways. Both regulators bind B-cell activation antigens (B7-1/CD80 and B7-2/CD86) and are expressed on the surface of T cells. B7-1 and B7-2 expression is restricted to lymphoid tissues. B7-1 expression is induced in T cells, B cells, monocytes, and DCs. B7-2 is constitutively expressed on B cells, DCs, and monocytes. After activation, B7-2 is also up-regulated on B cells, DCs, and monocytes and induced on T cells.[45] Despite structural similarity and shared ligands, CTLA-4 is a coinhibitory protein whereas CD28 is costimulatory. CTLA-4 has higher affinity and avidity to B7s so it competes against CD28 to suppress activated T cells.[46]

COMPLEX MOLECULAR MECHANISMS OF CYTOTOXIC T–ASSOCIATED PROTEIN 4–MEDIATED SUPPRESSION

Cytotoxic T-lymphocyte–Associated Protein 4 and CD28 Target the Same Signaling Pathway

Both CTLA-4 and CD28 associate with serine/threonine Protein Phosphatase 2A (PP2A) to regulate T-cell activation. CTLA-4, however, is able to regulate T cells through cell intrinsic and extrinsic inhibition, as seen in **Figs. 3**A and B. When the TCR is stimulated, CTLA-4 recruits PP2A,[47] inhibiting the Akt tyrosine kinase cascade responsible for potentiating T-cell activation.[47,48] This T-cell intrinsic mechanism targets Akt pathway kinases that are distal to the membrane whereas PD-1 targets this pathway proximal to the TCR (see **Figs. 2** and **3**A). In addition to Akt pathway inhibition, CTLA-4 competes for B7 binding to inhibit CD28 stimulatory activity and further suppress T-cell activation.[46]

CTLA-4 also suppresses CD4$^+$ and CD8$^+$ T-cell activity through cell extrinsic mechanisms. Interaction of CTLA-4 with B7-1/B7-2 promotes trans-endocytosis to sequester these ligands from APCs, preventing CD28 binding, thereby inhibiting T-cell activation. Constitutively expressed CTLA-4 also enhances the suppressive function of Tregs to further inhibit Tconv activation.[49] Phosphorylated CTLA-4 also enhances the production of signaling molecules by T cells. This down-regulates B7 expression in the APC and reduces the ability of APCs to stimulate T cells (see **Fig 3**B).[50] The multiple molecular mechanisms by which CTLA-4 suppresses effector T cells demonstrates the importance of this regulatory pathway in maintaining immune tolerance.

Cytotoxic T-lymphocyte–Associated Protein 4 Expression Is Not Restricted to Lymphoid Cells

Unlike CD28, which is constitutively expressed on T cells, CTLA-4 expression is induced in naïve T cells on TCR stimulation and constitutively expressed on Tregs. CTLA-4 is also expressed on B cells, NK cells, NK T cells, and DCs.[51,52] This restricted expression can be attributed to strict regulation through multiple mechanisms, including transcriptional control, post-transcriptional modifications, and intracellular trafficking of CTLA-4. NFAT and Foxp3 are transcription factors that induce CTLA-4 transcription in Tconv cells and Tregs, respectively.[53,54] MicroRNA activity and the post-transcriptional modifications of the CTLA-4 3' UTR regulate CTLA-4 mRNA stability. These transcriptional and post-transcriptional mechanisms provide temporal control of CTLA-4 surface expression.[55,56]

Intracellular trafficking regulates CTLA-4 surface expression via endocytic and secretory pathways, polarizing CTLA-4 surface expression to the immune synapse and maintaining spatial control of CTLA-4 activity.[57,58] In CD4$^+$ T cells, CTLA-4 is localized within secretory lysosomes. Within these lysosomes, CTLA-4 is rapidly degraded when it is not being actively transcribed. When the TCR is stimulated, CTLA-4 gene expression is induced, intracellular CTLA-4 accumulates, and lysosomes secrete CTLA-4 to the cell surface.[57] In CD8$^+$ T cells, intracellular trafficking of CTLA-4 is mediated through endocytic pathways.[58] In activated T cells, the

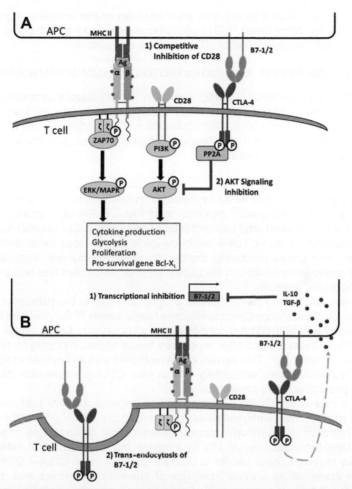

Fig. 3. CTLA-4 suppresses T cells through both T-cell intrinsic and extrinsic mechanisms: (A). On TCR activation, CTLA-4 is expressed on the T cell surface and exerts cell intrinsic inhibition. CTLA-4 outcompetes CD28 for the B7-1/2 ligands, resulting in reduced CD28 stimulatory activity. CTLA-4 also recruits the phosphatase PP2A to its phosphorylated cytoplasmic tail. Active PP2A dephosphorylates Akt, preventing downstream signaling, thus inhibiting T-cell activity, proliferation, and survival. (B) After CTLA-4 phosphorylation and ligation, a signal cascade is initiated by which IL-10, TGF-β, and soluble CTLA-4 (not shown) are up-regulated. These signaling molecules are endocytosed by the APC and inhibit the transcription of B7-1 and B7-2, reducing the amount of B7-1/2 surface expression by APCs and preventing CD28 stimulation. When CTLA-4 binds to B7-1/2, it can also trigger trans-endocytosis of these ligands. This reduces the surface expression of B7-1/2 on the APC and further hinders the ability of CD28 to be stimulatory.

LRBA protein promotes migration of CTLA-4 containing endosomes to the plasma membrane.[59] Once expressed proximal to the TCR, CTLA-4 effectively suppresses T-cell function.[47] To limit its activity and overall abundance in the absence of TCR stimulation, CTLA-4 is negatively regulated by clathrin-associated adaptor proteins AP-1 and AP-2. In resting T cells, AP-1 and AP-2 interact with the unphosphorylated cytoplasmic tail of CTLA-4 to promote internalization of this receptor into the lysosomal network for degradation.[59] This phosphorylation-dependent trafficking allows for rapid and dynamic regulation of CTLA-4 at the cell surface.

CYTOTOXIC T-LYMPHOCYTE–ASSOCIATED PROTEIN 4 IN IMMUNOPATHOLOGY

CTLA-4 has been implicated in multiple roles in human disease processes varying from autoimmune phenomena to oncologic pathogenesis to infectious immunosuppression. Similarly to other checkpoint regulators, it often mediates overly robust tolerance of abnormal signals in the setting of profound disease, preventing necessary immune responsiveness to threat.

Sepsis

CTLA-4 has been implicated as a key mediator in septic immunosuppression. Early work by Inoue and colleagues[60] demonstrated that CTLA-4 up-regulation on CD4, CD8, and Tregs increased after experimental sepsis using a CLP model. Administration of intraperitoneal anti–CTLA-4 antibody generated a dose-dependent survival benefit, with low doses producing profoundly improved survival associated with decreased septic-induced splenic apoptosis. High-dose CTLA-4 was less protective, inducing increased mortality.[60]

CTLA-4 has additionally demonstrated a significant role in the pathophysiology of both primary and secondary *Candida albicans* fungal sepsis.[61] Survival was improved in mice treated with anti–CTLA-4 antibody both after primary fungal sepsis, induced through tail vein injection, and after secondary fungal sepsis, modeled by tail vein injection 72 hours after CLP. This benefit was associated with an increase in splenocyte derived IFN-γ production, suggesting that in vivo CTLA-4 expression inhibits this necessary protective IFN-γ phenotype.

CTLA-4's role in septic immunosuppression extends to viral pathogens, with significant roles in the pathogenesis of 2 contemporary and highly morbid viruses, HIV and hepatitis C. Although current antiretroviral therapy has dramatically improved long-term outcomes in HIV by suppressing viral replication, latent stores of HIV have proved a major barrier to ultimate disease cure. CTLA-4 CD4$^+$ T cells have been identified as a major reservoir of latent viral particles and, therefore, a target for future therapeutics.[62] Furthermore, specific genetic variants of CTLA-4 have been associated with chronic hepatitis C infection, suggesting that some variants may predispose individuals to risk of chronic conversion on viral exposure.[63]

Cytotoxic T-lymphocyte–Associated Protein 4 in Critical Illness

Patients who are critically ill from nonseptic sources are known to be similarly at risk of secondary infections. For example, patients with acute liver failure frequently overexpress CTLA-4 on circulating T cells compared with healthy controls.[64] Furthermore, T cells isolated from patients with acute liver failure were hypo proliferative when challenged with CD3 or antigen stimulation. Serum from these patients possessed increased amounts of soluble B7, which was shown to induce CTLA-4 up-regulation in healthy control T cells.[64] This implicates CTLA-4 as a prime mediator of decreased innate immune responses to infectious challenges in critical illness.

HERPES VIRUS ENTRY MEDIATOR

HVEM is a type I transmembrane receptor member of the tumor necrosis factor receptor superfamily (TNFRSF), first discovered by Montgomery and colleagues[65] as the necessary cell surface receptor for herpes simplex virus (HSV)-1 entry.[66] It was separately identified in an expressed sequence tag survey seeking additional members of the TNFRSF.[67] The TNFRSF consists of 10 cell-surface proteins that regulate immune development and homeostasis. HVEM contains 4 cysteine-rich domains (CRDs) in its extracellular region, as depicted in **Fig. 4**A, a characteristic feature of TNFRSF utilized for ligand engagement. The cytoplasmic region of HVEM associates with tumor necrosis factor receptor-associated factor (TRAF) 1, TRAF2, TRAF3, TRAF5, and Stat3, and, when transfected, cells demonstrate significant activation of nuclear factor (NF)-κB, Jun N-terminal kinase, and AP-1.[67,68]

Unlike many other checkpoint regulators whose expression is confined to immune cells, HVEM is expressed diffusely on multiple tissue types as well as many immune cell subsets. Northern blot survey of human tissue types demonstrated HVEM expression in most tissues, with the highest levels in adult spleen, peripheral blood leukocytes, fetal lung, and kidney.[67] Immune cell characterization demonstrated

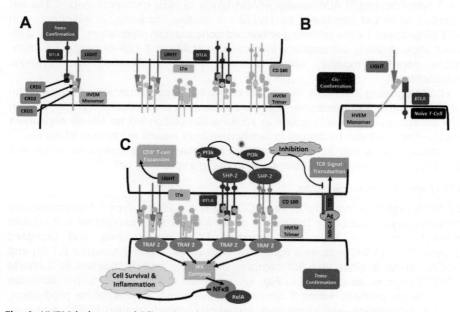

Fig. 4. HVEM behaves as bidirectional switch based on environmental signals. (*A*) HVEM associates with LIGHT, LTα, BTLA, and CD160 in trimeric confirmations when expressed in *trans* confirmation. LIGHT and LTα associate with CRD2/3 binding domains, whereas BTLA and CD160 associate with CRD1. All ligands associate with HVEM in a trimeric confirmation, generating a 3:3:3 complex of 3 HVEM molecules with 3 BTLA or CD160 molecules and 3 LIGHT or LTα molecules. (*B*) HVEM interacts with coexpressed BTLA to from an inert complex when both are expressed in their *cis*-confirmation, most commonly on naïve T cells. In this formation HVEM can still associate with soluble LIGHT or LTα at its exposed CRD1 binding domain, yet no downstream signal is generated from the interaction. (*C*) When HVEM is expressed in the *trans* confirmation on the membrane, ligation of LIGHT, LTα, BTLA, or CD160 results in TRAF2 recruitment within the HVEM-expressing cell. TRAF2 activates an IκB kinase complex, which, in turn, activates the RelA form of NF-κB to promote cell survival. Within BTLA and CD160–expressing cells, ligation of HVEM results in ITIM phosphorylation, recruiting SHP1 and SHP2, ultimately resulting in inhibitory signaling interrupting TCR signal transduction via dephosphorylation of PI3k-PKB pathway. Despite apparent absence of intracellular signaling motifs, LIGHT ligation of HVEM stimulates CD8+ T-cell expansion.

monomeric HVEM expression on T cells, B cells, NK cells, DCs, and myeloid cells.[7] Specifically, human naïve and memory B cells express high levels of HVEM whereas germinal center B cells lack HVEM expression, and T cells constitutively express HVEM, unique from other TNFRs.[7]

HERPES VIRUS ENTRY MEDIATOR AND ITS LIGANDS
Herpes Virus Entry Mediator Behaves as Both a Receptor and a Ligand, with Variable Downstream Effects

HVEM has a total of 5 described ligands, including members both within and outside of the TNFSF, a unique trait not possessed by other TNFRSF members.[7] Ig family ligands include B-lymphocyte and T-lymphocyte attenuator (BTLA) and CD160, whereas TNFSF ligands include lymphotoxin alpha (LTα) and LIGHT (homologous to lymphotoxin, exhibits inducible expression, and competes with HSV glycoprotein D for binding to herpesvirus entry mediator, a receptor expressed on T lymphocytes).[69] Additionally, HVEM binds to HSV glycoprotein-D.[65] The net function of HVEM, illustrated by HVEM $^{-/-}$ murine modeling, is inhibitory, with HVEM-deficient T cells exhibiting enhanced concanavalin stimulation.[70] HVEM deficient mice similarly demonstrate increased mortality in T-cell–dependent autoimmune hepatitis models, with increased T-cell proliferation and cytokine production.[70]

HVEM signaling is variable, dependent on the ligand interacted with, the orientation of HVEM within the membrane, and the surrounding environment.[69] HVEM-binding TNFSF members generally results in immune stimulation via an NF-κB dependent mechanism, whereas binding of Ig family members results in immune inhibition.[7,71] In addition to its role as a receptor, HVEM behaves as a ligand for BTLA and CD160, inducing inhibitory signaling within the Ig-expressing cells.[72]

LIGHT and Lymphotoxin Alpha

LIGHT is also known as TNFSF14 or CD258. It is a 29-kD, type II transmembrane protein and member of the TNF family, which formulates a homotrimer and exhibits highest expression in spleen, immature DCs, granulocytes, and activated T cells.[7,66,73] LIGHT acts as a ligand for both lymphotoxin-β receptor (LTβR) and HVEM, which it binds in a 3:3 complex of trimeric LIGHT attached to 3 HVEM CRD2/3 regions, as depicted in **Fig. 4**A.[7,73] When binding LTβR, LIGHT activates a cell death pathway within T lymphocytes, resulting in chemokine production, TRAF2 degradation, and caspase-8 activation.[71] When binding HVEM, however, LIGHT stimulates a robust stimulatory signal, which, after TRAF2 recruitment, results in NF-κB activation, and promoting cell survival, depicted in **Fig. 4**C.[71]

LTα is a compact trimer that is assembled from subunits expressed by B cells, T cells, and NK cells.[7,66] Lacking a transmembrane domain, LTα is secreted in its homotrimeric form and binds to HVEM in a stimulatory manner similar to LIGHT, resulting in NF-κB recruitment and cell survival, depicted in **Fig. 4**C.[66] Like LIGHT, LTα binds to the CRD2/3 of the inner surface of HVEM forming a 3:3 complex on the membrane, as depicted in **Fig. 4**A.[7]

B-lymphocyte and T-lymphocyte Attenuator and CD160

A member of the Ig superfamily, BTLA possesses an intermediate-type Ig fold in its ectodomain and 2 cytosolic ITIM inhibitory signaling domains.[72,74] BTLA expression is highest in spleen, lymph nodes, activated T cells, and resting B-cells.[7] BTLA engagement by HVEM results ITIM activation, inducing SHP-1/2 phosphatase recruitment, and subsequent attenuation of IL-2 within the BTLA-expressing cell.[72,74] Within the HVEM-expressing cell, BTLA engagement mirrors the stimulatory LIGHT and LTα pathway, resulting in NF-κB activation, depicted in **Fig. 4C**.[69] This is supported by evidence that BTLA binding to HVEM promotes survival and memory generation in CD8[+] T cells.[72] Given that the net function of HVEM signaling is inhibitory, the ultimate signal generated from BTLA and CD160 ligation remains unclear. Evidence points to inhibition, yet no mechanism connecting the known stimulatory activation of NF-κB to an inhibitory end result has been discovered.[7] It is this behavior, with inhibition when acting as a ligand, but stimulation while acting as receptor, that leads to the description of HVEM as a bidirectional switch.

CD160 was the last of HVEM's ligands to be discovered, identified through an attempt to isolate NK cell–specific receptors.[7] It is a member of the Ig superfamily of receptors and contains a glycosylphosphatidylinositol anchor and single IgV-like domain.[75] It is expressed highly in spleen, small intestine, and peripheral blood leukocytes, NK cells, and γδT cells.[7] BTLA and CD160 both associate with the CRD1 domain of HVEM, as depicted in **Fig. 4A**, demonstrating competitive binding. Mutagenesis studies have demonstrated, however, that the 2 possess overlapping but not identical binding domains within this CRD1 region.[76]

Ligand Binding Can Occur Simultaneously

HVEM's binding complexity is increased by the discovery that its orientation within the membrane alters its binding site availability, affecting the manner in which it interacts with available ligands.[77] Like other members of the TNF family, HVEM orients into a trimer within the membrane meaning it forms 3:3 complexes with many of its ligands.[7] With its multiple CRDs located on alternate faces of the trimer complex, this allows HVEM to bind both at its CRD1 and CRD2/3 regions simultaneously, forming complexes with 3 LIGHT or LTα molecules bound to one face and 3 BTLA or CD160 to the other when HVEM is expressed in its *trans* confirmation.[7] In addition to these complexes, HVEM and BTLA can be coexpressed on single cells, forming a stable complex, with both proteins expressed in the *cis*-confirmation on the membrane, shown in **Fig. 4B**.[77] This is seen almost exclusively in naïve T cells, where HVEM seems to associate with LIGHT, but no down-stream signaling, either stimulatory nor inhibitory, is noted within the cells.[77] It is thought that this *cis*-complex competitively inhibits HVEM activation with the surrounding environmental ligands, maintaining T-cell naïveté.

HERPES VIRUS ENTRY MEDIATOR S ROLE IN SEPTIC IMMUNOSUPPRESSION

HVEM's role in septic immunosuppression is best characterized by its behavior at mucosal barriers, but it has also been implicated in more systemic roles in iALI, viral illness, and nonseptic systemic critical illnesses, such as liver failure.[78–80] Unlike other checkpoint regulators, HVEM has been implicated both in septic immunosuppressive roles, mediating inappropriate levels of tolerance, and as a mechanism of excessive immune activation, responsible for tissue injury. This represents a physical manifestation of its unique bidirectional behavior, making it an interesting therapeutic target allowing more context specificity.

Herpes Virus Entry Mediator is Essential to Mucosal Immunity

The mucosal surfaces serve as a primary entry site for many infectious threats, and the immune presence within these tissues is extensive. An investigation of innate lymphoid cell (ILC) checkpoint regulation demonstrated that HVEM signaling within the ILC3 subset was both necessary and sufficient to generate an appropriate

IFN-γ response to protect against *Yersinia enterocolitica* infection.[81] Improved survival, via IFN-γ production, was mediated through the HVEM-LIGHT axis, with no affect from BTLA or CD160.

Shui and colleagues[68] echoed HVEM's invaluable role in mucosal barrier signaling utilizing intestinal *Citrobacter rodentium* and *Streptococcus pneumoniae* pulmonary infection models. HVEM stimulation, by either BTLA or CD160, in colonic epithelial cells induced STAT3 phosphorylation and innate inflammatory responses, such as IL-6, CXCL1, and CCL20 production. *HVEM* $^{-/-}$ mice survived significantly worse than WT when subjected to *C rodentium* infection, a surrogate for enteropathogenic *Escherichia coli* infection. These mice also had higher bacterial burden and lower STAT3 activation. They established this effect was mediated exclusively through CD160 interaction using *BTLA* $^{-/-}$, *LIGHT* $^{-/-}$, and CD160 antibody administration.[68] Their results were confirmed in mice subjected to a *S pneumoniae* pulmonary infection model where again the HVEM-CD160 axis was essential to survival and bacterial clearance. In both examples, the HVEM axis defends mucosal barriers against infection, with blockade of deletion resulting in decreased mucosal barrier defense, as is common after sepsis.

Herpes Virus Entry Mediator in Respiratory Immunity

The role of HVEM in immune dysfunction in respiratory tissues has been similarly well established. In a murine model of *Chlamydia psittaci* respiratory infection *LIGHT* $^{-/-}$ mice demonstrated a profound survival deficit with increased weight loss, higher bacterial burden, and heightened severity of lung tissue injury.[82] Lung tissue from these mice demonstrated decreased IFN-γ, TNF-α, and IL-12 mRNA levels, with elevated Treg abundance. Mice subjected to iALI using a double hit model of hemorrhage followed by CLP up-regulate HVEM expression in lung tissue.[78] Administration of intra-tracheal HVEM siRNA attenuated this increased HVEM expression and conveyed a transient early survival benefit.[78] Similar to *LIGHT* $^{-/-}$ mice, HVEM siRNA–treated mice had reduced cytokine and chemokine levels in respiratory mucosa, suggesting that HVEM signaling was necessary for this local inflammatory response, an example of inappropriate immune activation after sepsis. Together, these examples demonstrate that the HVEM pathway, although necessary for response to respiratory infectious threats, can be inappropriately activated by distant infectious challenges, resulting in inappropriate tissue injury.

Herpes Virus Entry Mediator and Herpes Simplex Virus-1

In addition to allowing cell entry for HSV-1, HVEM mediates HSV-1's ability to chronically infect individuals by influencing the Treg population.[80] After HSV infection, there is marked expansion of Treg populations and HVEM is up-regulated on CD4$^+$FoxP3$^+$ Tregs after HSV infection. *HVEM* $^{-/-}$ are more susceptible to HSV ocular disease and these mice had reduced T-cell expansion compared with WT mice.[80] This suggests that HVEM regulation of Treg expansion initially aids in control of the infection and direct tissue injury but may ultimately enable a definitive reservoir for chronic HSV infection.

Herpes Virus Entry Mediator Expression in Critically Ill Patients

Expression of HVEM and its major ligand BTLA was explored in critically ill surgical patients by Shubin and colleagues[83,84] demonstrating BTLA up-regulation on CD4$^+$ T cells, monocytes, and granulocytes and similar HVEM up-regulation on granulocytes and monocytes in septic patients. Nonseptic critically ill patients with greater than 80% BTLA expression on CD4$^+$ T cells were at increased risk of developing secondary infection.[84] Also, *BTLA* $^{-/-}$ mice demonstrate a survival benefit over WT controls with improved bacterial clearance after CLP.[83] Finally, critically ill patients with Hepatitis B-induced acute on chronic liver failure were shown to coexpress HVEM, BTLA, and fibrinogen-like protein (a virus induced molecule) on liver macrophages, implying absence of HVEM signaling by HVEM-BTLA complexing may play a role in Hepatitis pathogenesis and acute reactivation.[79]

SUMMARY

Checkpoint regulators are crucial in producing an appropriate and controlled immune response to insults. Their expansive roles in immune modulation, described previously, highlights their essential function. Their powerful role is often mistakenly used, however, to reduce immune reactions when true nonself threats exist or to activate immune responses in the absence of infectious pathogens, resulting in tissue injury. The immense role of checkpoint regulators in immune dysfunction, especially during sepsis progression, makes them an attractive target for therapeutic interventions.

Multiple clinical trials have been undertaken to investigate blockade of various checkpoint regulators during sepsis. Unfortunately, all reported clinical trials have demonstrated lackluster results thus far. The most recent trial of immunotherapy in sepsis, utilizing an anti–PD-L1 antibody in septic patients, demonstrated no change in mortality or cytokine levels. A modest increase in monocyte human leukocyte antigen-DR expression was obtained with anti–PD-L1 but only at higher doses.[85] Earlier immunotherapy trials demonstrated similarly disappointing results, as treatment with), granulocyte-macrophage colony-stimulating factor provided no survival benefit and only a modest reduction in ventilatory days.[86] Treatment with IFN-γ correlates with decreased TNF-α response to lipopolysaccharide stimulation and is Food and Drug Administration approved for treatment of fungal sepsis in patients with chronic granulomatous disease. Despite this small success, no broadly applicable immunomodulatory agent is approved for use in sepsis treatment at this time.[10]

These underwhelming results may be due in part to the reliance on animal modeling to study these complex molecular mechanisms with limited confirmation from human sampling. Furthermore, the lack of specific septic patient criteria makes it difficult to select ideal patient cohorts for treatment as has successfully been done in cancer clinical trials. Finally, failures in sepsis clinical trials may stem from targeting single regulators in isolation, ignoring how molecules endogenously act in concert. The family of checkpoint regulators is extensive, diverse, and important. Many of these regulators, however, have overlapping roles without an obvious indication for such redundancy. Thus, a more thorough understanding of the behavior and hierarchy of checkpoint regulators in sepsis may afford a more effective combinatorial therapeutic approach.

REFERENCES

1. Singer M, Deutschman CS, Seymour CW, et al. The Third International Consensus Definitions for sepsis and septic shock (Sepsis-3). JAMA 2016;315(8):801–10.
2. Murphy SL, Xu J, Kochanek KD. Deaths: preliminary data for 2010. Natl Vital Stat Rep 2012;60:1–52.
3. Rhee C, Murphy MV, Li LL, et al. Comparison of Trends in sepsis incidence and coding using administrative claims versus objective clinical data. Clin Infect Dis 2015;60(1):88–95.
4. Boomer JS, To K, Chang KC, et al. Immunosuppression in patients who die of sepsis and multiple organ failure. JAMA 2011;306(23):2594–605.

5. Bretscher P, Cohn M. A theory of self-nonself discrimination. Science 1970; 169(3950):1042–9.

6. Lafferty KJ, Cunningham AJ. A new analysis of allogeneic interactions. Aust J Exp Biol Med Sci 1975;53(1):27–42.

7. Cai G, Freeman GJ. The CD160, BTLA, LIGHT/HVEM pathway: a bidirectional switch regulating T-cell activation. Immunol Rev 2009;229(1):244–58.

8. Wherry EJ, Blattman JN, Murali-Krishna K, et al. Viral persistence alters CD8 T-cell immunodominance and tissue distribution and results in distinct stages of functional impairment. J Virol 2003;77(8):4911–27.

9. Biron BM, Ayala A, Lomas-Neira JL. Biomarkers for sepsis: what is and what might be? Biomark Insights 2015;10:7–17.

10. Hotchkiss RS, Monneret G, Payen D. Immunosuppression in sepsis: a novel understanding of the disorder and a new therapeutic approach. Lancet Infect Dis 2013;13(3):260–8.

11. Okazaki T, Honjo T. The PD-1-PD-L pathway in immunological tolerance. Trends Immunol 2006;27(4):195–201.

12. Ishida Y, Agata Y, Shibahara K, et al. Induced expression of PD-1, a novel member of the immunoglobulin gene superfamily, upon programmed cell death. EMBO J 1992;11(11):3887–95.

13. So L, Fruman DA. PI3K signalling in B- and T-lymphocytes: new developments and therapeutic advances. Biochem J 2012;442(3):465–81.

14. Freeman GJ, Long AJ, Iwai Y, et al. Engagement of the PD-1 immunoinhibitory receptor by a novel B7 family member leads to negative regulation of lymphocyte activation. J Exp Med 2000;192(7):1027–34.

15. Parry RV, Chemnitz JM, Frauwirth KA, et al. CTLA-4 and PD-1 receptors inhibit T-cell activation by distinct mechanisms. Mol Cell Biol 2005;25(21):9543–53.

16. Chemnitz JM, Parry RV, Nichols KE, et al. SHP-1 and SHP-2 associate with immunoreceptor tyrosine-based switch motif of programmed death 1 upon primary human T cell stimulation, but only receptor ligation prevents T cell activation. J Immunol 2004;173(2):945–54.

17. Chang WS, Kim JY, Kim YJ, et al. Cutting edge: programmed death-1/ programmed death ligand 1 interaction regulates the induction and maintenance of invariant NKT cell anergy. J Immunol 2008;181(10):6707–10.

18. Liu Y, Yu Y, Yang S, et al. Regulation of arginase I activity and expression by both PD-1 and CTLA-4 on the myeloid-derived suppressor cells. Cancer Immunol Immunother 2009;58(5):687–97.

19. Austin JW, Lu P, Majumder P, et al. STAT3, STAT4, NFATc1, and CTCF regulate PD-1 through multiple novel regulatory regions in murine T cells. J Immunol 2014;192(10):4876–86.

20. Cho HY, Lee SW, Seo SK, et al. Interferon-sensitive response element (ISRE) is mainly responsible for IFN-alpha-induced upregulation of programmed death-1 (PD-1) in macrophages. Biochim Biophys Acta 2008;1779(12):811–9.

21. Mathieu M, Cotta-Grand N, Daudelin JF, et al. Notch signaling regulates PD-1 expression during CD8(+) T-cell activation. Immunol Cell Biol 2013;91(1):82–8.

22. Lu P, Youngblood BA, Austin JW, et al. Blimp-1 represses CD8 T cell expression of PD-1 using a feed-forward transcriptional circuit during acute viral infection. J Exp Med 2014;211(3):515–27.

23. Kao C, Oestreich KJ, Paley MA, et al. Transcription factor T-bet represses expression of the inhibitory receptor PD-1 and sustains virus-specific CD8+ T cell responses during chronic infection. Nat Immunol 2011;12(7):663–71.

24. Butte MJ, Keir ME, Phamduy TB, et al. Programmed death-1 ligand 1 interacts specifically with the B7-1 costimulatory molecule to inhibit T cell responses. Immunity 2007;27(1):111–22.
25. Xiao Y, Yu S, Zhu B, et al. RGMb is a novel binding partner for PD-L2 and its engagement with PD-L2 promotes respiratory tolerance. J Exp Med 2014; 211(5):943–59.
26. Ghiotto M, Gauthier L, Serriari N, et al. PD-L1 and PD-L2 differ in their molecular mechanisms of interaction with PD-1. Int Immunol 2010;22(8):651–60.
27. Yamazaki T, Akiba H, Iwai H, et al. Expression of programmed death 1 ligands by murine T cells and APC. J Immunol 2002;169(10):5538–45.
28. Iwai Y, Terawaki S, Ikegawa M, et al. PD-1 inhibits antiviral immunity at the effector phase in the liver. J Exp Med 2003;198(1):39–50.
29. Huang X, Venet F, Wang YL, et al. PD-1 expression by macrophages plays a pathologic role in altering microbial clearance and the innate inflammatory response to sepsis. Proc Natl Acad Sci U S A 2009;106(15):6303–8.
30. Young WA, Fallon EA, Heffernan DS, et al. Improved survival after induction of sepsis by cecal slurry in PD-1 knockout murine neonates. Surgery 2017;161(5): 1387–93.
31. Monaghan SF, Thakkar RK, Tran ML, et al. Programmed death 1 expression as a marker for immune and physiological dysfunction in the critically ill surgical patient. Shock 2012;38(2):117–22.
32. Knaus WA, Draper EA, Wagner DP, et al. APACHE II: a severity of disease classification system. Crit Care Med 1985;13(10):818–29.
33. Monaghan SF, Thakkar RK, Heffernan DS, et al. Mechanisms of indirect acute lung injury: a novel role for the coinhibitory receptor, programmed death-1. Ann Surg 2012;255(1):158–64.
34. Gong J, Chehrazi-Raffle A, Reddi S, et al. Development of PD-1 and PD-L1 inhibitors as a form of cancer immunotherapy: a comprehensive review of registration trials and future considerations. J Immunother Cancer 2018;6(1):8.
35. Kirchberger S, Majdic O, Steinberger P, et al. Human rhinoviruses inhibit the accessory function of dendritic cells by inducing sialoadhesin and B7-H1 expression. J Immunol 2005;175(2):1145–52.
36. Wang J, Wu G, Manick B, et al. VSIG-3 as a ligand of VISTA inhibits human T-cell function. Immunology 2019;156(1):74–85.
37. Bharaj P, Chahar HS, Alozie OK, et al. Characterization of programmed death-1 homologue-1 (PD-1H) expression and function in normal and HIV infected individuals. PLoS One 2014;9(10):e109103.
38. Wang L, Rubinstein R, Lines JL, et al. VISTA, a novel mouse Ig superfamily ligand that negatively regulates T cell responses. J Exp Med 2011;208(3):577–92.
39. Le Mercier I, Chen W, Lines JL, et al. VISTA regulates the development of protective antitumor immunity. Cancer Res 2014;74(7):1933–44.
40. Lines JL, Pantazi E, Mak J, et al. VISTA is an immune checkpoint molecule for human T cells. Cancer Res 2014;74(7):1924–32.
41. Flies DB, Han X, Higuchi T, et al. Coinhibitory receptor PD-1H preferentially suppresses CD4(+) T cell-mediated immunity. J Clin Invest 2014;124(5):1966–75.
42. Watanabe T, Suda T, Tsunoda T, et al. Identification of immunoglobulin superfamily 11 (IGSF11) as a novel target for cancer immunotherapy of gastrointestinal and hepatocellular carcinomas. Cancer Sci 2005;96(8):498–506.
43. Bharaj P, Ye C, Petersen S, et al. Gene array analysis of PD-1H overexpressing monocytes reveals a pro-inflammatory profile. Heliyon 2018;4(2):e00545.

44. Williams AF, Barclay AN. The immunoglobulin superfamily—domains for cell surface recognition. Annu Rev Immunol 1988;6:381–405.

45. Collins M, Ling V, Carreno BM. The B7 family of immune-regulatory ligands. Genome Biol 2005;6(6):223.

46. Linsley PS, Brady W, Urnes M, et al. CTLA-4 is a second receptor for the B cell activation antigen B7. J Exp Med 1991;174(3):561–9.

47. Chuang E, Fisher TS, Morgan RW, et al. The CD28 and CTLA-4 receptors associate with the serine/threonine phosphatase PP2A. Immunity 2000;13(3):313–22.

48. Kane LP, Weiss A. The PI-3 kinase/Akt pathway and T cell activation: pleiotropic pathways downstream of PIP3. Immunol Rev 2003;192:7–20.

49. Wang XB, Kakoulidou M, Giscombe R, et al. Abnormal expression of CTLA-4 by T cells from patients with myasthenia gravis: effect of an AT-rich gene sequence. J Neuroimmunol 2002;130(1–2):224–32.

50. Qureshi OS, Zheng Y, Nakamura K, et al. Trans-endocytosis of CD80 and CD86: a molecular basis for the cell-extrinsic function of CTLA-4. Science 2011; 332(6029):600–3.

51. Kaufman KA, Bowen JA, Tsai AF, et al. The CTLA-4 gene is expressed in placental fibroblasts. Mol Hum Reprod 1999;5(1):84–7.

52. Wang XB, Giscombe R, Yan Z, et al. Expression of CTLA-4 by human monocytes. Scand J Immunol 2002;55(1):53–60.

53. Gibson HM, Hedgcock CJ, Aufiero BM, et al. Induction of the CTLA-4 gene in human lymphocytes is dependent on NFAT binding the proximal promoter. J Immunol 2007;179(6):3831–40.

54. Zheng Y, Josefowicz SZ, Kas A, et al. Genome-wide analysis of Foxp3 target genes in developing and mature regulatory T cells. Nature 2007;445(7130): 936–40.

55. de Jong VM, Zaldumbide A, van der Slik AR, et al. Post-transcriptional control of candidate risk genes for type 1 diabetes by rare genetic variants. Genes Immun 2013;14(1):58–61.

56. Sonkoly E, Janson P, Majuri ML, et al. MiR-155 is overexpressed in patients with atopic dermatitis and modulates T-cell proliferative responses by targeting cytotoxic T lymphocyte-associated antigen 4. J Allergy Clin Immunol 2010;126(3): 581–9.e1-20.

57. Iida T, Ohno H, Nakaseko C, et al. Regulation of cell surface expression of CTLA-4 by secretion of CTLA-4-containing lysosomes upon activation of CD4+ T cells. J Immunol 2000;165(9):5062–8.

58. Linsley PS, Bradshaw J, Greene J, et al. Intracellular trafficking of CTLA-4 and focal localization towards sites of TCR engagement. Immunity 1996;4(6):535–43.

59. Lo B, Zhang K, Lu W, et al. AUTOIMMUNE DISEASE. Patients with LRBA deficiency show CTLA4 loss and immune dysregulation responsive to abatacept therapy. Science 2015;349(6246):436–40.

60. Inoue S, Bo L, Bian J, et al. Dose-dependent effect of anti-CTLA-4 on survival in sepsis. Shock 2011;36(1):38–44.

61. Chang KC, Burnham CA, Compton SM, et al. Blockade of the negative co-stimulatory molecules PD-1 and CTLA-4 improves survival in primary and secondary fungal sepsis. Crit Care 2013;17(3):R85.

62. McGary CS, Deleage C, Harper J, et al. CTLA-4(+)PD-1(-) memory CD4(+) T cells critically contribute to viral persistence in antiretroviral therapy-suppressed, SIV-infected rhesus macaques. Immunity 2017;47(4):776–88.e5.

63. Sepahi S, Pasdar A, Gerayli S, et al. CTLA-4 gene haplotypes and the risk of chronic hepatitis C infection; a case control study. Rep Biochem Mol Biol 2017; 6(1):51–8.
64. Khamri W, Abeles RD, Hou TZ, et al. Increased expression of cytotoxic T-lymphocyte-associated protein 4 by T cells, induced by B7 in sera, reduces adaptive immunity in patients with acute liver failure. Gastroenterology 2017; 153(1):263–76.e8.
65. Montgomery RI, Warner MS, Lum BJ, et al. Herpes simplex virus-1 entry into cells mediated by a novel member of the TNF/NGF receptor family. Cell 1996;87(3): 427–36.
66. Mauri DN, Ebner R, Montgomery RI, et al. LIGHT, a new member of the TNF superfamily, and lymphotoxin alpha are ligands for herpesvirus entry mediator. Immunity 1998;8(1):21–30.
67. Marsters SA, Ayres TM, Skubatch M, et al. Herpesvirus entry mediator, a member of the tumor necrosis factor receptor (TNFR) family, interacts with members of the TNFR-associated factor family and activates the transcription factors NF-kappaB and AP-1. J Biol Chem 1997;272(22):14029–32.
68. Shui JW, Larange A, Kim G, et al. HVEM signalling at mucosal barriers provides host defence against pathogenic bacteria. Nature 2012;488(7410):222–5.
69. Cheung TC, Steinberg MW, Oborne LM, et al. Unconventional ligand activation of herpesvirus entry mediator signals cell survival. Proc Natl Acad Sci U S A 2009; 106(15):6244–9.
70. Wang Y, Subudhi SK, Anders RA, et al. The role of herpesvirus entry mediator as a negative regulator of T cell-mediated responses. J Clin Invest 2005;115(3): 711–7.
71. Bechill J, Muller WJ. Herpesvirus entry mediator (HVEM) attenuates signals mediated by the lymphotoxin beta receptor (LTbetaR) in human cells stimulated by the shared ligand LIGHT. Mol Immunol 2014;62(1):96–103.
72. Steinberg MW, Huang Y, Wang-Zhu Y, et al. BTLA interaction with HVEM expressed on CD8(+) T cells promotes survival and memory generation in response to a bacterial infection. PLoS One 2013;8(10):e77992.
73. Rooney IA, Butrovich KD, Glass AA, et al. The lymphotoxin-beta receptor is necessary and sufficient for LIGHT-mediated apoptosis of tumor cells. J Biol Chem 2000;275(19):14307–15.
74. Watanabe N, Gavrieli M, Sedy JR, et al. BTLA is a lymphocyte inhibitory receptor with similarities to CTLA-4 and PD-1. Nat Immunol 2003;4(7):670–9.
75. Giustiniani J, Bensussan A, Marie-Cardine A. Identification and characterization of a transmembrane isoform of CD160 (CD160-TM), a unique activating receptor selectively expressed upon human NK cell activation. J Immunol 2009;182(1): 63–71.
76. Kojima R, Kajikawa M, Shiroishi M, et al. Molecular basis for herpesvirus entry mediator recognition by the human immune inhibitory receptor CD160 and its relationship to the cosignaling molecules BTLA and LIGHT. J Mol Biol 2011; 413(4):762–72.
77. Cheung TC, Oborne LM, Steinberg MW, et al. T cell intrinsic heterodimeric complexes between HVEM and BTLA determine receptivity to the surrounding microenvironment. J Immunol 2009;183(11):7286–96.
78. Cheng T, Bai J, Chung CS, et al. Herpes virus entry mediator (HVEM) expression promotes inflammation/organ injury in response to experimental indirect-acute lung injury. Shock 2019;51(4):487–94.

79. Xu H, Cao D, Guo G, et al. The intrahepatic expression and distribution of BTLA and its ligand HVEM in patients with HBV-related acute-on-chronic liver failure. Diagn Pathol 2012;7:142.
80. Sharma S, Rajasagi NK, Veiga-Parga T, et al. Herpes virus entry mediator (HVEM) modulates proliferation and activation of regulatory T cells following HSV-1 infection. Microbes Infect 2014;16(8):648–60.
81. Seo GY, Shui JW, Takahashi D, et al. LIGHT-HVEM signaling in innate lymphoid cell subsets protects against enteric bacterial infection. Cell Host Microbe 2018;24(2):249–60.e4.
82. Cai H, Chen S, Xu S, et al. Deficiency of LIGHT signaling pathway exacerbates Chlamydia psittaci respiratory tract infection in mice. Microb Pathog 2016;100:250–6.
83. Shubin NJ, Chung CS, Heffernan DS, et al. BTLA expression contributes to septic morbidity and mortality by inducing innate inflammatory cell dysfunction. J Leukoc Biol 2012;92(3):593–603.
84. Shubin NJ, Monaghan SF, Heffernan DS, et al. B and T lymphocyte attenuator expression on CD4+ T-cells associates with sepsis and subsequent infections in ICU patients. Crit Care 2013;17(6):R276.
85. Hotchkiss RS, Colston E, Yende S, et al. Immune checkpoint inhibition in sepsis: a phase 1b randomized, placebo-controlled, single ascending dose study of anti-programmed cell death-ligand 1 (BMS-936559). Crit Care Med 2019;47(5):632–42.
86. Meisel C, Schefold JC, Pschowski R, et al. Granulocyte-macrophage colony-stimulating factor to reverse sepsis-associated immunosuppression: a double-blind, randomized, placebo-controlled multicenter trial. Am J Respir Crit Care Med 2009;180(7):640–8.

Biomarker Panels in Critical Care

Susan R. Conway, MD[a,b,*], Hector R. Wong, MD[c,d]

KEYWORDS

- Biomarker panels • Critical care • Sepsis

KEY POINTS

- In critical care, clinicians often are presented with patients at the extremes of disease, who may not neatly fit one clinical diagnosis.
- The spectrum of critical illness includes heterogeneous syndromes, defined clinically, and encompassing a range of underlying molecular mechanisms.
- Given rapid advances in the technologies available for biomarker discovery and validation, biomarkers, specifically biomarker panels, show great promise for helping us diagnose and treat heterogeneous syndromes.

INTRODUCTION

In medicine, clinical and radiographic features often are relied upon to direct diagnosis and treatment. Ideally, clinical assessment is combined with molecular, biochemical, and/or microbiological data to make diagnoses precise and to target treatments to patients. In critical care, patients often present at the extremes of disease and may not neatly fit one clinical diagnosis. Moreover, the spectrum of critical illness includes heterogeneous syndromes, defined clinically, and likely encompassing a range of underlying molecular mechanisms. As such, despite sound preclinical investigation and hypothesis-driven approaches based on the best current understanding of the field, it has been difficult to identify a gold standard for the diagnosis of these conditions and to develop effective treatments for them. In order to more effectively care for patients with critical illness, it will be important to better delineate the boundaries between critical disease processes based on underlying mechanisms of disease. This

[a] Division of Critical Care Medicine, Children's National Medical Center, 111 Michigan Avenue Northwest, Washington, DC 20010, USA; [b] Department of Pediatrics, George Washington University School of Medicine, Washington, DC, USA; [c] Division of Critical Care Medicine, Cincinnati Children's Hospital Medical Center, Cincinnati Children's Research Foundation, 3333 Burnet Avenue, Cincinnati, OH 45229, USA; [d] Department of Pediatrics, University of Cincinnati College of Medicine, Cincinnati, OH, USA
* Corresponding author. Division of Critical Care Medicine, Children's National Medical Center, 111 Michigan Avenue Northwest, Washington, DC 20010.
E-mail address: sconway@childrensnational.org

Crit Care Clin 36 (2020) 89–104
https://doi.org/10.1016/j.ccc.2019.08.007
0749-0704/20/© 2019 Elsevier Inc. All rights reserved.
criticalcare.theclinics.com

will allow more precise targeting of treatments and should also advance understanding of the relevant disease processes. Given rapid advances in the technologies available for biomarker discovery and validation, biomarkers, specifically biomarker panels, show great promise for helping us accomplish this task.

BIOMARKER DEFINITION AND CHARACTERISTICS

A 2001 consensus definition states that a biomarker is "a characteristic that is objectively measured and evaluated as an indicator of normal biological processes, pathogenic processes, or pharmacologic responses to a therapeutic intervention."[1] Accordingly, although biomarkers are commonly conceptualized as laboratory values that correlate with a particular disease state, they may be understood not only as laboratory values but also as clinical measurements. Biomarkers can be subdivided into 4 broad classes depending on their use: diagnostic, monitoring, surrogate, and stratification.[2,3] Diagnostic biomarkers are intended to aid in diagnosis of disease. Monitoring biomarkers are used to track response to therapeutic intervention. Surrogate biomarkers can serve as proxy outcome endpoints in clinical trials, theoretically reducing the number of patients needed to identify significant responses to interventions under investigation. Lastly, stratification biomarkers are used to subdivide groups of patients with a particular diagnosis based on prognosis or mortality risk. Stratification biomarkers may also classify patients based on underlying biological commonalities.

Within this framework, one can identify important characteristics of a biomarker with clinical utility. First, biomarkers must have clinically useful test characteristics. Ideally the area under the receiver operating characteristic curve (AUROC) should approach 1 and must be greater than 0.5 for any biomarker used to distinguish between disease states. Cutoff points may be chosen to maximize sensitivity or specificity, depending on the intended use of the biomarker. Biomarkers that display useful test characteristics must also be relatively easy to obtain, rapidly measureable, and generalizable. In general, ability to measure and interpret a biomarker early in the progression of disease is useful, so that it can be used to direct treatment and potentially alter the course of disease.[4,5] As developments in genomics, proteomics, and metabolomics have enhanced discovery of new biomarkers, the issues of rapid measurability and feasibility for clinical use have become increasingly relevant. In particular, as biomarker panels are developed to augment useful test characteristics in the setting of heterogeneous critical illnesses, it becomes necessary to develop platforms that make these panels available in real-time in the clinical setting.[6,7]

BIOMARKER PANELS

Although individual biomarkers remain integral to the practice of critical care, single measurements are unlikely to fully capture the biological complexity of critical illness to an extent that decreases their clinical utility. Procalcitonin (PCT), for example, has shown clinical utility in guiding antibiotic usage in the setting of lower respiratory tract infections,[8,9] but its predictive and prognostic capacity in sepsis is controversial.[10–13] Among other factors, interpretation of PCT is complicated by confounders affecting its concentration other than presence of infection. Additionally, assessment of its diagnostic capacity has been limited by the lack of a robust confirmatory test for infection in the setting of suspected sepsis. These issues are common in the setting of heterogeneous critical illnesses and lend themselves to the use of biomarker panels rather than individual biomarkers. Kofoed and colleagues,[14] for example, constructed a biomarker panel to diagnose bacterial infection in sepsis comprising 6 biomarkers, including PCT, and found that the 6-marker panel had a significantly higher AUROC than any of its individual components.

There are 2 general approaches to biomarker discovery: hypothesis-based and unbiased. In the hypothesis-based approach, candidate biomarkers are identified based on knowledge of a disease process and then their test characteristics determined. Although this approach is less likely to yield false-positive results, given that it is rooted in a biologically plausible hypothesis, it is also limited by current understanding of the field. The unbiased, or data-driven, approach to discovery is rooted in the ability to generate large amounts of transcriptomic, proteomic, or metabolomic data. These data can be used to identify thousands of genes, proteins, or metabolites that are differentially expressed among patients.[15,16] This allows for rapid discovery of a large number of candidate biomarkers not limited by current understanding of the field. Data-driven approaches can also aid in hypothesis generation, identifying previously unconsidered genes, proteins, and pathways of interest for basic science and translational research.[17] Because biomarker discovery rooted in omics generates a large amount of data, it is more likely to yield false-positive results. In addition, analytical and dimensionality reduction techniques become important when faced with a large data set.

Biomarker panels may combine known biomarkers using a hypothesis-driven approach or they may be generated using data-driven techniques. Data-driven approaches generally begin with a training or discovery cohort that is used to generate a large data set of candidate biomarkers. Bioinformatic techniques, including clustering and iterative regression, are then used to organize these data and yield groups of patients with similarities in candidate biomarker values. Subsequent correlation with clinical parameters in the training cohort can determine whether the derived subgroups are clinically relevant. When biomarker panels are derived using this approach, both generalizability and reproducibility must be considered carefully. This is due to the risk of false positives with an unbiased approach and the risk of propagating imprecision throughout all of biomarker discovery if there are flaws in initial generation of the training data set. Perhaps most importantly, the techniques used to derive biomarker panels risk over-fitting the training cohort, decreasing generalizability. For this reason, ideal studies reporting biomarker panels must not only involve discovery of candidate biomarkers but also validation in an independent patient cohort.[18]

DIAGNOSTIC BIOMARKER PANELS FOR SEPSIS

Sepsis remains a leading cause of morbidity and mortality among critically ill patients.[19–21] Hundreds of clinical trials based on sound preclinical research have failed to show clear benefit of treatments targeting sepsis pathophysiology,[22,23] such that the mainstays of treatment remain early recognition and resuscitation, antibiotics, and supportive care.[24,25] The reasons for these failures are undoubtedly complex but certainly involve the now well-recognized heterogeneity among septic patients.[26] Such heterogeneity is likely caused by baseline genetic variation affecting the host response to infection,[27,28] along with differences in host response related to age,[29] comorbidity, and potentially the infecting pathogen. Given this, biomarker research in sepsis has focused, in part, on more effectively stratifying patients based on prognosis and sepsis subtype. These markers could be used not only to inform treatment decisions but also to enrich clinical trials based on prognosis and underlying molecular mechanism of disease. In addition, biomarker development has aimed at more effectively diagnosing sepsis among patients with signs of systemic inflammation. Such markers could decrease unnecessary exposure to antibiotics and allow more effective targeting of antibiotics at the infecting pathogen. They also could decrease confounders in clinical trials by limiting enrollment of patients with noninfectious systemic inflammation. Importantly, advances in polymerase chain reaction (PCR)-based, mass spectrometry–based, and next-generation sequencing–based techniques may accomplish some of these goals by more rapidly and sensitively identifying microbial pathogens.[28,30]

A large proportion—47% in a recent study of 7 million patients in the United States from 2001 to 2010—of sepsis cases admitted to the ICU remain culture negative.[31] Moreover, the ability to identify which of these patients are infected based on clinical features is poor.[32] Clearly, improved diagnostics are needed to distinguish between sterile inflammation, viral infection, and bacterial infection in patients with suspected sepsis. Several groups have used high-throughput transcriptomic techniques to identify molecular signatures specific to the host response to infection. McHugh and colleagues[33] used microarrays on whole blood-derived RNA from 74 septic cases and 31 postsurgical controls to derive SeptiCyte LAB (Immunexpress, Inc, Seattle, WA), a 4-gene classifier composed of RNA biomarkers for distinguishing infectious from noninfectious etiologies of systemic inflammation. They used this panel to derive a quantitative score, the SeptiScore, which distinguished infectious from noninfectious inflammation with an AUROC of 0.89 (95% CI, 0.85–0.93) in the more heterogeneous of their 2 validation cohorts. They further validated the Septi-Score in a prospective observational trial, where it yielded an AUROC of 0.82 to 0.89 for diagnosing infectious inflammation compared with retrospective physician diagnosis by 3 experts.[34] Sweeney and colleagues[35] also used genome-wide expression analysis to identify an 11-gene panel, which they converted to an infection z score, for distinguishing sterile from infectious inflammation. They used publicly available gene expression data in a multicohort approach to improve the generalizability of their findings, and time-matched trauma/systemic inflammatory reponse syndrome controls during discovery to limit confounders introduced by temporal changes in gene expression after injury. In a separate study also based in multicohort genome-wide expression analysis, the same group identified a 7-gene panel to discriminate between viral and bacterial infections. They then combined their 11-gene and 7-gene panels to derive an antibiotics decision model that identified bacterial infection, with sensitivity and specificity of 94% and 59.8%, respectively.[36] This antibiotics decision model is currently being evaluated (Timothy E. Sweeney, MD, PhD, personal communication, 2019). A 2-biomarker panel—the FAIM3:PLAC8 ratio—initially derived by Scicluna and colleagues[37] to identify adult patients with community-acquired pneumonia (CAP) on intensive care init (ICU) admission, has also shown diagnostic utility in discriminating between patients with sepsis and sterile inflammation.[38] To benchmark current diagnostic tools in sepsis, Sweeney and colleagues[38] used publicly available gene expression data to evaluate the performance of their 11-gene panel, which they termed the Sepsis MetaScore, SeptiCyte LAB, and the FAIM3:PLAC8 ratio. They found that although the 3 panels showed similar diagnostic performance overall, there were cohort-specific decreases in AUROC suggesting the need for further prospective testing to clarify the strengths and weaknesses of all 3 panels. In addition to identifying the presence of infection, some studies have focused on classifying infecting pathogens based on host responses. These studies have generally used relatively small cohorts and results have been mixed.[39] Larger studies may identify panels that distinguish between gram-negative and gram-positive infections or provide even more specific pathogen identification based on a characteristic host response.[40,41]

PROGNOSTIC BIOMARKER PANELS FOR SEPSIS

Among patients diagnosed with sepsis, stratification according to prognosis has become an important clinical and research goal, for the reasons discussed previously. Prognostic biomarkers currently in clinical use include serum lactate and procalcitonin.[13,42,43] No biomarker panels currently are used in the clinical setting for patient stratification, but prognostic panels have shown promise in the research setting. Several trials have identified biomarker panels for use in the emergency department to identify septic patients at increased risk for mortality or complicated course.[44–46] This early risk stratification might allow for more rapid intervention and triage to the appropriate level of care. Panels drawn early in ICU admission could be used in a similar way. Langley and colleagues[47] used mass spectrometry to semiquantitatively evaluate the metabolome of septic patients and found significant differences in greater than 100 metabolites between survivors and nonsurvivors on arrival to the emergency department and at 24 hours postadmission. The group then selected 4 clinical parameters and 12 metabolites as candidate prognostic biomarkers. Clinical parameters were chosen based on prior clinical analyses, and metabolites were chosen based on both the magnitude of difference between survivors and nonsurvivors and existence of a plausible biological link to outcome in sepsis. They used penalized predictor reduction to derive a 7-marker panel, including 5 metabolites and 2 clinical parameters. This clinicometabolomic panel displayed strong prognostic discrimination between survivors and nonsurvivors in the discovery cohort and in independent validation cohorts. Wong and colleagues[15] also derived an early risk stratification tool termed, the Pediatric Sepsis Biomarker Risk Panel (PERSEVERE), for pediatric patients admitted to the ICU with septic shock. The group used genome-wide expression profiling to identify gene probes with outcome predictive strength in pediatric septic shock.[2,48] They then applied the criteria that candidate probes translate to readily measured serum proteins with a biologically plausible link to sepsis pathology to identify 12 candidate protein biomarkers. Using classification and regression tree (CART) analysis, they narrowed these 12 candidate biomarkers to the 5-protein decision tree, PERSEVERE, that identified patients at risk of death with sensitivity and specificity of 89% and 64%, respectively, in their test cohort.[15] The group has subsequently improved on the initial model by adding and pruning nodes with subsequent validation cohorts, resulting in the most recent model, PERSEVERE-XP, which yielded an AUROC of 0.96 (95% CI, 0.91–1.0) for differentiating between survivors and nonsurvivors in a test cohort.[17,49] Although PERSEVERE can function as a dichotomous test for survival versus nonsurvival among pediatric septic shock patients, it also can be viewed as a mortality risk continuum. Those patients classified by PERSEVERE as moderate risk or high risk who survive demonstrate increased rates of complicated course and longer ICU stays than low-risk patients, indicating that they are likely a sicker group of patients. This risk continuum could be used for prognostic enrichment of clinical trials as well as for benchmarking clinical performance in treating septic shock patients.[50,51]

Sweeney and colleagues[52] have sought to improve generalizability of biomarker panels by using broad arrays of public and privately held gene expression data, and by inviting multiple scientific groups to participate in model building. When they used this approach to identify biomarker panels for 30-day mortality prediction in sepsis, 3 invited groups developed 4 models using different methods. These were tested in independent validation cohorts and showed generally preserved prognostic power with summary AUROCs ranging from 0.75 to 0.87. Although each panel comprised unique genes, the combination of all 4 models into an ensemble model failed to improve prognostic performance, suggesting that each might represent a ceiling to prognostic accuracy inherent in the data used. This approach illustrates the importance of collaboration in model development and public availability of gene expression data so that reliability of biomarker panels can be established.[53]

BIOMARKER PANELS FOR IDENTIFYING SEPSIS SUBTYPES

Apart from stratification based on prognosis, there is also great interest in stratifying sepsis based on biological commonalities. Sepsis subtypes can be identified based on clinical characteristics or on molecular signatures, which may relate to underlying mechanisms of disease.[54,55] The general idea here is to generate more homogenous subgroups of patients with sepsis, who share underlying biological mechanisms that could potentially be targeted in a more specific manner. Most recent research into identifying subtypes of sepsis has focused on transcriptomic identification of subtypes, followed by analysis to determine whether these molecular subtypes carry a clinically relevant phenotype. Using transcriptomic analysis of peripheral blood leukocytes from patients enrolled in the UK Genomic Advances in Sepsis (UK GAinS) study, Davenport and colleagues[56] identified 2 clinically relevant subtypes of adult patients with sepsis due to CAP, termed, sepsis response signature 1 (SRS1) and SRS2. They found that SRS1 patients displayed immunosuppressed features including endotoxin tolerance, T-cell exhaustion and HLA class II downregulation, along with higher 14-day mortality (hazard ratio [HR] 2.8; 95% CI, 1.5–5.1) compared with SRS2 patients. When they applied a sparse response model to the greater than 3000 genes differentially expressed between SRS groups, they identified a 7-gene panel that reliably predicted SRS assignment. In a subsequent study, the group found that the same SRS groups could be identified in patients with sepsis due to fecal peritonitis and that variation among patients with CAP and fecal peritonitis depended more on SRS group membership than on source of infection.[57] Scicluna and colleagues[58] applied similar transcriptomic analysis in a discovery and 2 validation cohorts, including a cohort from the UK GAinS study. They identified 4 rather than 2 endotypes, termed Mars1 through Mars4, but identified patterns similar to those found by Davenport and colleagues.

Mars1, not unlike SRS1, was consistently associated with the highest 28-day mortality (HR 1.86–2.02 across the discovery and validation cohorts compared with Mars2-4 combined) and decreased expression of genes involved in innate and adaptive immune functions. Mars3 assignment was associated with low risk of mortality and increased expression of genes involved in adaptive immune function. When analyzed in the UK GAinS cohort, Mars3 and SRS2 membership showed significant overlap. Among pediatric septic shock patients, Wong and colleagues[59] derived 2 sepsis subclasses, termed endotype A and endotype B, that differed both in transcriptomic signature and in clinical phenotype. Endotype A patients displayed decreased expression of genes involved in adaptive immunity and response to corticosteroids compared with endotype B. They also showed higher illness severity, higher rates of organ dysfunction, and higher mortality than endotype B patients. To simplify patient stratification by endotype, they used CART methodology to narrow their original 100 endotype-defining genes to a 4-gene decision tree that reliably identified endotype A patients in a test cohort.[60]

Given the seeming overlap in underlying pathology and clinical phenotype between SRS1 and endotype A, Burnham and colleagues[57] investigated their similarity using comparative differential gene expression analysis. They found that the genes defining SRS assignment did not overlap with pediatric endotype-defining genes, although they did find some overlap in pathway enrichment between the 2 groups. Wong and colleagues[61] performed retrospective analysis of publicly available transcriptomic data from septic adults and found only a weak positive relationship between endotype assignment and SRS membership. When they performed multivariable logistic regression, however, they found that interactions between endotype A membership, SRS1 membership, and age were associated with mortality, and that patients classified as both SRS1 and endotype A had the highest mortality. Scicluna and colleagues[58] identified Mars1, Mars2, and Mars4 transcriptomic signatures in a pediatric septic shock cohort but were unable to reliably identify Mars3. They found no association between Mars subtype and mortality in this pediatric cohort. These analyses suggest that although there is likely some clinically relevant overlap, there also are marked differences in the septic transcriptomic response between adults and children. These differences may lead to important new discoveries related to the effects of development and aging on sepsis pathology.

BIOMARKER PANELS FOR ACUTE RESPIRATORY DISTRESS SYNDROME

Acute respiratory distress syndrome (ARDS), like sepsis, is defined clinically and represents a syndrome with heterogeneous pathophysiology, mortality risk and response to treatment modalities.[62] Direct versus indirect causes of lung injury, degree of systemic inflammation, and extent of fibroproliferation are all known to differ among patients meeting clinical criteria for ARDS and may alter prognosis and response to therapeutics.[63-65] As such, it is desirable to identify markers that subdivide patients with ARDS along biologically and clinically relevant lines.[62,66,67] Although transcriptomic approaches have not yet been employed in this context, data from large clinical trials, including ARMA and ALVEOLI, have been mined retrospectively to identify subphenotypes of ARDS with specific biomarker signatures.[65,68] Using latent class analysis (LCA) based on presenting clinical data and measured biomarkers, Calfee and colleagues[65] identified 2 distinct subphenotypes that differed in degree of systemic inflammation and response to ventilator strategy, independent of ARDS severity. These subphenotypes could be reliably distinguished using a 3-biomarker panel— interleukin (IL)-6, tumor necrosis factor receptor-1, and vasopressor use—and have since been reproduced in follow-up studies.[63,64] In a separate retrospective study, when patients were subdivided according to mechanism of lung injury, those with direct lung injury had significantly higher levels of surfactant protein D (a marker of epithelial injury) and lower angiopoietin-2, von Willebrand factor, IL-6, and IL-8 (markers of systemic inflammation and endothelial injury) than patients with indirect lung injury.[68] This suggests that patients with direct versus indirect lung injury might respond differently to therapeutics targeting the epithelium versus the endothelium and that these factors should be considered when designing clinical trials.[68] Several other individual biomarkers have been shown to have prognostic or predictive value in ARDS. Soluble receptor for glycation end-products, angiopoietin-2, soluble intercellular adhesion molecule-1, surfactant proteins A and D, type III procollagen, Clara cell protein 16, IL-6, and IL-8 have all been associated with either underlying pathophysiology or risk of mortality or multiorgan dysfunction.[65,69-77] Although these markers may identify important differences in underlying pathophysiology among ARDS patients, they have not undergone rigorous testing in a way that would confirm their accuracy, precision, and generalizability for clinical use. Moreover, given the complexity of ARDS, it seems likely that biomarkers panels, rather than single biomarkers, will maximize utility in guiding ARDS treatment and clinical trial enrollment.

Two recent studies highlight the importance of establishing biomarker panels to subdivide ARDS patients.[63,64] Both also serve as verification of the subphenotypes initially derived by Calfee and colleagues[65] using the ARMA and ALVEOLI cohorts. In a secondary analysis of the HARP-2 trial—a multicenter randomized controlled trial of simvastatin versus placebo for early-onset ARDS treatment—Calfee and colleagues[63,65] again identified 2 subphenotypes differing in their degree of systemic inflammation. Although the HARP-2 trial failed to show benefit with simvastatin treatment of the entire cohort, secondary analysis showed that patients within the hyperinflammatory subphenotype had significantly improved survival with simvastatin treatment compared with those given placebo ($P = .008$).[63] In another secondary analysis of the Fuids and Catheters Treatment Trial (FACTT), the same group performed LCA and again identified a hyperinflammatory and a hypoinflammatory subphenotype. Response to fluid management strategy was significantly different between subphenotypes. Mortality decreased with a fluid-conservative management strategy in the hypoinflammatory group but increased with the same strategy in the hyperinflammatory group. A biomarker panel consisting of IL-8, bicarbonate level and tumor necrosis factor receptor-1 distinguished the subphenotypes with an area under the curve of 0.95, and was verified in 2 previously used cohorts from the ARMA and ALVEOLI trials.[64] Importantly, the FACTT trial found no difference in mortality based on fluid management strategy, but it did find an overall decrease in ventilator-free days using a fluid conservative strategy. Because of this, the current recommendation is to manage ARDS patients not in shock with a fluid conservative strategy. It is possible that these recommendations should be tailored more specifically based on ARDS subtype. Given these findings on secondary analysis of clinical trials, it is apparent that subphenotype should be considered in the design of new clinical trials in ARDS. In order to accomplish this, robust biomarker panels to rapidly and reliably subclassify ARDS patients must be developed and prospectively validated.[78]

BIOMARKER PANELS FOR ACUTE KIDNEY INJURY

AKI is a common problem among critically ill patients and is associated with increased risk of mortality, along with short-term and long-term morbidity.[79–83] Given the potential for early intervention—with limitation of nephrotoxins, conservative fluid management strategies, and possibly early initiation of renal replacement therapy[84–88]—efforts at improving outcomes in AKI have focused in part on early identification of at-risk patients, along with timely diagnosis of those who have already developed kidney injury.[89] These efforts have historically been hampered by the lack of a consensus definition for AKI, although the adoption of Kidney Disease Improving Global Outcomes (KDIGO) guidelines has improved diagnostic consistency and, therefore, reproducibility of clinical research in the field.[90] The KDIGO definition, along with other commonly accepted diagnostic criteria, depends on a combination of urine output and serum creatinine measurements for diagnosis. Although these clearly have predictive and prognostic value in the setting of AKI, they are also relatively late markers of kidney injury[91] and can be confounded by baseline creatinine value, patient fluid and nutritional status, and co-occurring critical illness.[80,92–94] In addition, serum creatinine is a marker of kidney function—a surrogate measure of glomerular filtration rate—and does not correlate with kidney injury per se. New biomarker strategies have aimed at identifying earlier markers that are more directly linked to tubular injury, along with subdividing AKI patients according to the etiology of their injury.[95,96]

Among the early biomarkers of kidney injury specifically linked to tubular damage are the urinary biomarkers neutrophil gelatinase–associated lipocalin (NGAL), liver fatty acid binding protein, IL-18, and kidney injury molecule-1.[97–100] Additionally, urinary tissue inhibitor of metalloproteinase-2 and insulinlike growth factor-binding protein 7 sensitively detect early acute tubular injury[101] and are now Food and Drug Administration–approved as NephroCheck (Biomerieux, Marcy-l'Etoile, France), a biomarker panel for early detection of AKI. Because of their mechanistic link to kidney injury, these biomarkers show promise in discriminating between intrinsic kidney injury and prerenal azotemia.[95,102] They also have both predictive and prognostic value. Early identification of kidney injury without change in creatinine has led to the description of a new subset of patients with subclinical AKI. Subclinical AKI has been associated with development of traditionally defined AKI, prolonged duration and severity of AKI, and increased risk of mortality.[103,104] Using hypothesis-driven approaches to biomarker panel development, several groups have shown improved diagnostic and prognostic performance when individual biomarkers of kidney injury are combined with each other or with clinical risk scores.[100,101,105–108] Basu and colleagues[105] developed a clinical risk score, the renal angina index (RAI), to determine which patients are at increased risk of AKI on admission to the ICU. In their analysis of 242 patients admitted to the PICU with sepsis, this score performed better than any single biomarker in predicting severe AKI. Inclusion of NGAL, matrix metalloproteinase-8 (MMP-8), or elastase-2 (Ela-2) measurements with the RAI improved its classification with net reclassification indices (NRIs) of 0.512, 0.428, and 0.545, respectively. The inclusion of both Ela-2 and NGAL improved diagnostic accuracy with an NRI of 0.871. This suggests that a combination of clinical and biochemical biomarkers may be useful in identifying patients at the highest risk for severe renal injury in the ICU.

Data-driven approaches to biomarker discovery may allow for subdivision of patients with AKI to better target management strategies according to the cause of their injury.[109–113] Transcriptomic analysis of pediatric septic shock patients identified 21 unique gene probes linked to septic shock–associated AKI (SSAKI). Two of these probes—MMP-8 and Ela-2—showed high sensitivity for diagnosing SSAKI.[111] Similar identification of context-specific markers may be useful for improving diagnostic precision of AKI in critically ill patients. The discovery of such biomarkers may also point to differences in underlying mechanisms of AKI depending on the clinical context. In an effort to subdivide patients with AKI, Bhatraju and colleagues[114] used LCA of AKI cohorts to identify 2 distinct subphenotypes that differ in mortality risk, endothelial dysfunction and inflammation. When they applied these subphenotypes to the Vasopressin in Septic Shock Trial, they found that vasopressin compared with norepinephrine was associated with decreased mortality in subphenotype 1 but not in subphenotype 2.[115] This suggests that accurate subclassification of patients with AKI may have profound implications for therapeutic decision-making and enrollment in clinical trials.

TRANSLATIONAL CONSIDERATIONS

Although biomarker panels could be used to guide treatment decisions and enrollment in clinical trials, they have yet to be widely applied in the clinical setting. Barriers to clinical application include questions regarding the generalizability of derived panels and the lack of clinically feasible platforms to provide the rapid results needed in the critical care setting.[116] Among the common approaches to improving generalizability are the use of broadly inclusive discovery cohorts and independent validation cohorts. Publicly available gene expression data allow for multicohort analyses that should improve the robustness of biomarker panels, although the use of these data requires careful attention to normalization techniques.[18,53] Public databases often also lack details on potentially confounding clinical factors. Prospective testing and regular benchmarking of currently available models, with revisions according to the results, should strengthen the performance of biomarker panels. In addition, rather than focusing exclusively on generalizability, development of context-specific biomarkers may be necessary under some circumstances.[50,117]

In order to make biomarker panels clinically useful, point-of-care platforms that provide interpretable results in a clinically relevant timeframe must be developed. Although system-wide approaches, such as microarrays, have been integral to the development of biomarker panels, they currently are too slow for use at the bedside. To overcome this problem, many groups have used variable reduction to derive representative groups of biomarkers that predict system-wide results.[33,34,47,57,58,60] Point-of-care tests, such as reverse transcriptase–PCR, using predispensed reagents and user-friendly interfaces, can then be employed to generate more rapid results.[33] Aside from their 4-gene decision tree, Wong and colleagues[6,7,60,118] developed 2 platforms with which to translate pediatric endotype assignment to the clinical setting. These include (1) provider-based interpretation of computer-generated gene expression mosaics that visually display the 100-gene endotype signatures in recognizable color-coded maps and (2) a gene expression score that distinguishes between endotypes based on decreased variability in gene expression among endotype A patients. If transcriptomic data become available in a clinically useful timeframe, such platforms will be necessary to make the results interpretable by the clinicians who use them.

SUMMARY

In order to improve outcomes among critically ill patients, efforts to protocolize care must be balanced with a need to target pathology-specific interventions at the patients who will benefit from them.[119] Given the heterogeneity that complicates therapeutic interventions in the critically ill, patient stratification according to prognosis and pathology has become a priority.[25,78] Such stratification should allow design of more informative clinical trials, along with guiding interventions toward those who are expected to benefit from them most. In the future, biomarker panels and the platforms that support them may allow for characterization and monitoring of each individual patient response, such that treatment can be guided by their specific pathophysiology, an approach termed, theranostics. For now, the goal should be 2-fold: (1) to direct research into the molecular mechanisms underlying critical illness using the wealth of information obtained from omic approaches to biomarker discovery and (2) to prospectively test biomarker panels and the platforms that support them in the clinical setting, thus moving closer to a precision medicine approach to the practice of critical care.

REFERENCES

1. Biomarkers Definitions Working Group.. Biomarkers and surrogate endpoints: preferred definitions and conceptual framework. Clin Pharmacol Ther 2001; 69(3):89–95.
2. Kaplan JM, Wong HR. Biomarker discovery and development in pediatric critical care medicine. Pediatr Crit Care Med 2011;12(2):165–73.
3. Marshall JC, Reinhart K, International Sepsis Forum. Biomarkers of sepsis. Crit Care Med 2009;37(7):2290–8.
4. van Engelen TSR, Wiersinga WJ, Scicluna BP, et al. Biomarkers in sepsis. Crit Care Clin 2018;34(1):139–52.
5. Casserly B, Read R, Levy MM. Multimarker panels in sepsis. Crit Care Clin 2011; 27(2):391–405.

6. Wong HR, Cvijanovich NZ, Anas N, et al. Developing a clinically feasible personalized medicine approach to pediatric septic shock. Am J Respir Crit Care Med 2015;191(3):309–15.

7. Wong HR, Wheeler D, Tegtmeyer K, et al. Toward a clinically feasible gene expression-based subclassification strategy for septic shock: proof of concept. Crit Care Med 2010;38(10):1955–61.

8. Huang DT, Yealy DM, Filbin MR, et al. Procalcitonin-guided use of antibiotics for lower respiratory tract infection. N Engl J Med 2018;379(3):236–49.

9. Schuetz P, Muller B, Christ-Crain M, et al. Procalcitonin to initiate or discontinue antibiotics in acute respiratory tract infections. Evid Based Child Health 2013; 8(4):1297–371.

10. Wacker C, Prkno A, Brunkhorst FM, et al. Procalcitonin as a diagnostic marker for sepsis: a systematic review and meta-analysis. Lancet Infect Dis 2013; 13(5):426–35.

11. Reinhart K, Meisner M. Biomarkers in the critically ill patient: procalcitonin. Crit Care Clin 2011;27(2):253–63.

12. Lautz AJ, Dziorny AC, Denson AR, et al. Value of procalcitonin measurement for early evidence of severe bacterial infections in the pediatric intensive care unit. J Pediatr 2016;179:74–81.e2.

13. Schuetz P, Birkhahn R, Sherwin R, et al. Serial procalcitonin predicts mortality in severe sepsis patients: results from the multicenter procalcitonin MOnitoring SEpsis (MOSES) study. Crit Care Med 2017;45(5):781–9.

14. Kofoed K, Andersen O, Kronborg G, et al. Use of plasma C-reactive protein, procalcitonin, neutrophils, macrophage migration inhibitory factor, soluble urokinase-type plasminogen activator receptor, and soluble triggering receptor expressed on myeloid cells-1 in combination to diagnose infections: a prospective study. Crit Care 2007;11(2):R38.

15. Wong HR, Salisbury S, Xiao Q, et al. The pediatric sepsis biomarker risk model. Crit Care 2012;16(5):R174.

16. Skibsted S, Shapiro NI. Transcriptomics may pave the biomarker road in sepsis*. Crit Care Med 2014;42(4):974–5.

17. Wong HR, Cvijanovich NZ, Anas N, et al. Improved risk stratification in pediatric septic shock using both protein and mRNA biomarkers. PERSEVERE-XP. Am J Respir Crit Care Med 2017;196(4):494–501.

18. Sweeney TE, Khatri P. Generalizable biomarkers in critical care: toward precision medicine. Crit Care Med 2017;45(6):934–9.

19. Martin GS, Mannino DM, Eaton S, et al. The epidemiology of sepsis in the United States from 1979 through 2000. N Engl J Med 2003;348(16):1546–54.

20. Paoli CJ, Reynolds MA, Sinha M, et al. Epidemiology and costs of sepsis in the United States-an analysis based on timing of diagnosis and severity level. Crit Care Med 2018;46(12):1889–97.

21. Singer M, Deutschman CS, Seymour CW, et al. The third international consensus definitions for sepsis and septic shock (Sepsis-3). JAMA 2016;315(8):801–10.

22. Marshall JC. Why have clinical trials in sepsis failed? Trends Mol Med 2014; 20(4):195–203.

23. Opal SM, Dellinger RP, Vincent JL, et al. The next generation of sepsis clinical trial designs: what is next after the demise of recombinant human activated protein C?*. Crit Care Med 2014;42(7):1714–21.

24. Rhodes A, Evans LE, Alhazzani W, et al. Surviving sepsis campaign: international guidelines for management of sepsis and septic shock: 2016. Intensive Care Med 2017;43(3):304–77.

25. Cohen J, Vincent JL, Adhikari NK, et al. Sepsis: a roadmap for future research. Lancet Infect Dis 2015;15(5):581–614.
26. Iskander KN, Osuchowski MF, Stearns-Kurosawa DJ, et al. Sepsis: multiple abnormalities, heterogeneous responses, and evolving understanding. Physiol Rev 2013;93(3):1247–88.
27. Sorensen TI, Nielsen GG, Andersen PK, et al. Genetic and environmental influences on premature death in adult adoptees. N Engl J Med 1988;318(12): 727–32.
28. Goh C, Knight JC. Enhanced understanding of the host-pathogen interaction in sepsis: new opportunities for omic approaches. Lancet Respir Med 2017;5(3): 212–23.
29. Wynn JL, Cvijanovich NZ, Allen GL, et al. The influence of developmental age on the early transcriptomic response of children with septic shock. Mol Med 2011; 17(11–12):1146–56.
30. Holcomb ZE, Tsalik EL, Woods CW, et al. Host-based peripheral blood gene expression analysis for diagnosis of infectious diseases. J Clin Microbiol 2017;55(2):360–8.
31. Gupta S, Sakhuja A, Kumar G, et al. Culture-negative severe sepsis: nationwide trends and outcomes. Chest 2016;150(6):1251–9.
32. Klein Klouwenberg PM, Cremer OL, van Vught LA, et al. Likelihood of infection in patients with presumed sepsis at the time of intensive care unit admission: a cohort study. Crit Care 2015;19:319.
33. McHugh L, Seldon TA, Brandon RA, et al. A molecular host response assay to discriminate between sepsis and infection-negative systemic inflammation in critically ill patients: discovery and validation in independent cohorts. PLoS Med 2015;12(12):e1001916.
34. Miller RR 3rd, Lopansri BK, Burke JP, et al. Validation of a host response assay, SeptiCyte LAB, for discriminating sepsis from systemic inflammatory response syndrome in the ICU. Am J Respir Crit Care Med 2018;198(7):903–13.
35. Sweeney TE, Shidham A, Wong HR, et al. A comprehensive time-course-based multicohort analysis of sepsis and sterile inflammation reveals a robust diagnostic gene set. Sci Transl Med 2015;7(287):287ra71.
36. Sweeney TE, Wong HR, Khatri P. Robust classification of bacterial and viral infections via integrated host gene expression diagnostics. Sci Transl Med 2016; 8(346):346ra91.
37. Scicluna BP, Klein Klouwenberg PM, van Vught LA, et al. A molecular biomarker to diagnose community-acquired pneumonia on intensive care unit admission. Am J Respir Crit Care Med 2015;192(7):826–35.
38. Sweeney TE, Khatri P. Benchmarking sepsis gene expression diagnostics using public data. Crit Care Med 2017;45(1):1–10.
39. Tang BM, McLean AS, Dawes IW, et al. Gene-expression profiling of gram-positive and gram-negative sepsis in critically ill patients. Crit Care Med 2008; 36(4):1125–8.
40. Ramilo O, Allman W, Chung W, et al. Gene expression patterns in blood leukocytes discriminate patients with acute infections. Blood 2007;109(5):2066–77.
41. Feezor RJ, Oberholzer C, Baker HV, et al. Molecular characterization of the acute inflammatory response to infections with gram-negative versus gram-positive bacteria. Infect Immun 2003;71(10):5803–13.
42. Nichol AD, Egi M, Pettila V, et al. Relative hyperlactatemia and hospital mortality in critically ill patients: a retrospective multi-centre study. Crit Care 2010; 14(1):R25.

43. Wacharasint P, Nakada T, Boyd JH, et al. Normal-range blood lactate concentration in septic shock is prognostic and predictive. Shock 2012;38(1):4–10.
44. Shapiro NI, Trzeciak S, Hollander JE, et al. A prospective, multicenter derivation of a biomarker panel to assess risk of organ dysfunction, shock, and death in emergency department patients with suspected sepsis. Crit Care Med 2009;37(1):96–104.
45. Schuetz P, Hausfater P, Amin D, et al. Biomarkers from distinct biological pathways improve early risk stratification in medical emergency patients: the multinational, prospective, observational TRIAGE study. Crit Care 2015;19:377.
46. Kutz A, Hausfater P, Amin D, et al. The TRIAGE-ProADM score for an early risk stratification of medical patients in the emergency department - development based on a multi-national, prospective, observational study. PLoS One 2016; 11(12):e0168076.
47. Langley RJ, Tsalik EL, van Velkinburgh JC, et al. An integrated clinico-metabolomic model improves prediction of death in sepsis. Sci Transl Med 2013;5(195):195ra95.
48. Standage SW, Wong HR. Biomarkers for pediatric sepsis and septic shock. Expert Rev Anti Infect Ther 2011;9(1):71–9.
49. Wong HR, Weiss SL, Giuliano JS, et al. Testing the prognostic accuracy of the updated pediatric sepsis biomarker risk model. PLoS One 2014;9(1):e86242.
50. Wong HR, Cvijanovich NZ, Anas N, et al. Pediatric sepsis biomarker risk model-II: redefining the pediatric sepsis biomarker risk model with septic shock phenotype. Crit Care Med 2016;44(11):2010–7.
51. Wong HR, Atkinson SJ, Cvijanovich NZ, et al. Combining prognostic and predictive enrichment strategies to identify children with septic shock responsive to corticosteroids. Crit Care Med 2016;44(10):e1000–3.
52. Sweeney TE, Perumal TM, Henao R, et al. A community approach to mortality prediction in sepsis via gene expression analysis. Nat Commun 2018;9(1):694.
53. Sweeney TE, Azad TD, Donato M, et al. Unsupervised analysis of transcriptomics in bacterial sepsis across multiple datasets reveals three robust clusters. Crit Care Med 2018;46(6):915–25.
54. Alder MN, Lindsell CJ, Wong HR. The pediatric sepsis biomarker risk model: potential implications for sepsis therapy and biology. Expert Rev Anti Infect Ther 2014;12(7):809–16.
55. Knox DB, Lanspa MJ, Kuttler KG, et al. Phenotypic clusters within sepsis-associated multiple organ dysfunction syndrome. Intensive Care Med 2015; 41(5):814–22.
56. Davenport EE, Burnham KL, Radhakrishnan J, et al. Genomic landscape of the individual host response and outcomes in sepsis: a prospective cohort study. Lancet Respir Med 2016;4(4):259–71.
57. Burnham KL, Davenport EE, Radhakrishnan J, et al. Shared and distinct aspects of the sepsis transcriptomic response to fecal peritonitis and pneumonia. Am J Respir Crit Care Med 2017;196(3):328–39.
58. Scicluna BP, van Vught LA, Zwinderman AH, et al. Classification of patients with sepsis according to blood genomic endotype: a prospective cohort study. Lancet Respir Med 2017;5(10):816–26.
59. Wong HR, Cvijanovich NZ, Lin R, et al. Identification of pediatric septic shock subclasses based on genome-wide expression profiling. BMC Med 2009;7:34.
60. Wong HR, Sweeney TE, Lindsell CJ. Simplification of a septic shock endotyping strategy for clinical application. Am J Respir Crit Care Med 2017;195(2):263–5.
61. Wong HR, Sweeney TE, Hart KW, et al. Pediatric sepsis endotypes among adults with sepsis. Crit Care Med 2017;45(12):e1289–91.

62. Coiffard B, Papazian L. Time to evaluate biomarkers for use in directing treatment strategies in ARDS patients. Intensive Care Med 2018;44(9):1553–5.
63. Calfee CS, Delucchi KL, Sinha P, et al. Acute respiratory distress syndrome subphenotypes and differential response to simvastatin: secondary analysis of a randomised controlled trial. Lancet Respir Med 2018;6(9):691–8.
64. Famous KR, Delucchi K, Ware LB, et al. Acute respiratory distress syndrome subphenotypes respond differently to randomized fluid management strategy. Am J Respir Crit Care Med 2017;195(3):331–8.
65. Calfee CS, Delucchi K, Parsons PE, et al. Subphenotypes in acute respiratory distress syndrome: latent class analysis of data from two randomised controlled trials. Lancet Respir Med 2014;2(8):611–20.
66. Shankar-Hari M, McAuley DF. Divide and conquer: identifying acute respiratory distress syndrome subphenotypes. Thorax 2017;72(10):867–9.
67. Ware LB, Koyama T, Billheimer DD, et al. Prognostic and pathogenetic value of combining clinical and biochemical indices in patients with acute lung injury. Chest 2010;137(2):288–96.
68. Calfee CS, Janz DR, Bernard GR, et al. Distinct molecular phenotypes of direct vs indirect ARDS in single-center and multicenter studies. Chest 2015;147(6):1539–48.
69. Jabaudon M, Blondonnet R, Roszyk L, et al. Soluble receptor for advanced glycation end-products predicts impaired alveolar fluid clearance in acute respiratory distress syndrome. Am J Respir Crit Care Med 2015;192(2):191–9.
70. Mrozek S, Jabaudon M, Jaber S, et al. Elevated plasma levels of sRAGE are associated with nonfocal CT-based lung imaging in patients with ARDS: a prospective multicenter study. Chest 2016;150(5):998–1007.
71. Yehya N, Thomas NJ, Meyer NJ, et al. Circulating markers of endothelial and alveolar epithelial dysfunction are associated with mortality in pediatric acute respiratory distress syndrome. Intensive Care Med 2016;42(7):1137–45.
72. Agrawal A, Matthay MA, Kangelaris KN, et al. Plasma angiopoietin-2 predicts the onset of acute lung injury in critically ill patients. Am J Respir Crit Care Med 2013;187(7):736–42.
73. Cheng IW, Ware LB, Greene KE, et al. Prognostic value of surfactant proteins A and D in patients with acute lung injury. Crit Care Med 2003;31(1):20–7.
74. Eisner MD, Parsons P, Matthay MA, et al. Plasma surfactant protein levels and clinical outcomes in patients with acute lung injury. Thorax 2003;58(11):983–8.
75. Forel JM, Guervilly C, Hraiech S, et al. Type III procollagen is a reliable marker of ARDS-associated lung fibroproliferation. Intensive Care Med 2015;41(1):1–11.
76. Kropski JA, Fremont RD, Calfee CS, et al. Clara cell protein (CC16), a marker of lung epithelial injury, is decreased in plasma and pulmonary edema fluid from patients with acute lung injury. Chest 2009;135(6):1440–7.
77. Calfee CS, Eisner MD, Parsons PE, et al. Soluble intercellular adhesion molecule-1 and clinical outcomes in patients with acute lung injury. Intensive Care Med 2009;35(2):248–57.
78. Prescott HC, Calfee CS, Thompson BT, et al. Toward smarter lumping and smarter splitting: rethinking strategies for sepsis and acute respiratory distress syndrome clinical trial design. Am J Respir Crit Care Med 2016;194(2):147–55.
79. Kaddourah A, Basu RK, Bagshaw SM, et al. Epidemiology of acute kidney injury in critically ill children and young adults. N Engl J Med 2017;376(1):11–20.
80. Rewa O, Bagshaw SM. Acute kidney injury-epidemiology, outcomes and economics. Nat Rev Nephrol 2014;10(4):193–207.

81. Uber AM, Sutherland SM. Acute kidney injury in hospitalized children: consequences and outcomes. Pediatr Nephrol 2018. [Epub ahead of print].
82. Sovik S, Isachsen MS, Nordhuus KM, et al. Acute kidney injury in trauma patients admitted to the ICU: a systematic review and meta-analysis. Intensive Care Med 2019;45(4):407–19.
83. Kaddourah A, Basu RK, Goldstein SL, et al. Oliguria and acute kidney injury in critically ill children: implications for diagnosis and outcomes. Pediatr Crit Care Med 2019;20(4):332–9.
84. Alobaidi R, Morgan C, Basu RK, et al. Association between fluid balance and outcomes in critically ill children: a systematic review and meta-analysis. JAMA Pediatr 2018;172(3):257–68.
85. Wang N, Jiang L, Zhu B, et al. Fluid balance and mortality in critically ill patients with acute kidney injury: a multicenter prospective epidemiological study. Crit Care 2015;19:371.
86. Selewski DT, Askenazi DJ, Bridges BC, et al. The impact of fluid overload on outcomes in children treated with extracorporeal membrane oxygenation: a multicenter retrospective cohort study. Pediatr Crit Care Med 2017;18(12):1126–35.
87. Shiao CC, Huang TM, Spapen HD, et al. Optimal timing of renal replacement therapy initiation in acute kidney injury: the elephant felt by the blindmen? Crit Care 2017;21(1):146.
88. Barbar SD, Clere-Jehl R, Bourredjem A, et al. Timing of renal-replacement therapy in patients with acute kidney injury and sepsis. N Engl J Med 2018; 379(15):1431–42.
89. Mekontso Dessap A, Ware LB, Bagshaw SM. How could biomarkers of ARDS and AKI drive clinical strategies? Intensive Care Med 2016;42(5):800–2.
90. Sutherland SM, Byrnes JJ, Kothari M, et al. AKI in hospitalized children: comparing the pRIFLE, AKIN, and KDIGO definitions. Clin J Am Soc Nephrol 2015;10(4):554–61.
91. Pickering JW, Endre ZH. GFR shot by RIFLE: errors in staging acute kidney injury. Lancet 2009;373(9672):1318–9.
92. Doi K, Yuen PS, Eisner C, et al. Reduced production of creatinine limits its use as marker of kidney injury in sepsis. J Am Soc Nephrol 2009;20(6):1217–21.
93. Macedo E, Bouchard J, Soroko SH, et al. Fluid accumulation, recognition and staging of acute kidney injury in critically-ill patients. Crit Care 2010;14(3):R82.
94. Xu X, Nie S, Zhang A, et al. A new criterion for pediatric AKI based on the reference change value of serum creatinine. J Am Soc Nephrol 2018;29(9):2432–42.
95. Parikh CR, Mansour SG. Perspective on clinical application of biomarkers in AKI. J Am Soc Nephrol 2017;28(6):1677–85.
96. Kashani K, Cheungpasitporn W, Ronco C. Biomarkers of acute kidney injury: the pathway from discovery to clinical adoption. Clin Chem Lab Med 2017;55(8): 1074–89.
97. Zappitelli M, Washburn KK, Arikan AA, et al. Urine neutrophil gelatinase-associated lipocalin is an early marker of acute kidney injury in critically ill children: a prospective cohort study. Crit Care 2007;11(4):R84.
98. Parikh CR, Jani A, Melnikov VY, et al. Urinary interleukin-18 is a marker of human acute tubular necrosis. Am J Kidney Dis 2004;43(3):405–14.
99. Han WK, Bailly V, Abichandani R, et al. Kidney Injury Molecule-1 (KIM-1): a novel biomarker for human renal proximal tubule injury. Kidney Int 2002;62(1):237–44.
100. Deng Y, Chi R, Chen S, et al. Evaluation of clinically available renal biomarkers in critically ill adults: a prospective multicenter observational study. Crit Care 2017;21(1):46.

101. Kashani K, Al-Khafaji A, Ardiles T, et al. Discovery and validation of cell cycle arrest biomarkers in human acute kidney injury. Crit Care 2013;17(1):R25.
102. Singer E, Elger A, Elitok S, et al. Urinary neutrophil gelatinase-associated lipocalin distinguishes pre-renal from intrinsic renal failure and predicts outcomes. Kidney Int 2011;80(4):405–14.
103. Hall IE, Coca SG, Perazella MA, et al. Risk of poor outcomes with novel and traditional biomarkers at clinical AKI diagnosis. Clin J Am Soc Nephrol 2011; 6(12):2740–9.
104. Coca SG, Nadkarni GN, Garg AX, et al. First post-operative urinary kidney injury biomarkers and association with the duration of AKI in the TRIBE-AKI cohort. PLoS One 2016;11(8):e0161098.
105. Basu RK, Wang Y, Wong HR, et al. Incorporation of biomarkers with the renal angina index for prediction of severe AKI in critically ill children. Clin J Am Soc Nephrol 2014;9(4):654–62.
106. Gunnerson KJ, Shaw AD, Chawla LS, et al. TIMP2*IGFBP7 biomarker panel accurately predicts acute kidney injury in high-risk surgical patients. J Trauma Acute Care Surg 2016;80(2):243–9.
107. Pipili C, Ioannidou S, Tripodaki ES, et al. Prediction of the renal replacement therapy requirement in mechanically ventilated critically ill patients by combining biomarkers for glomerular filtration and tubular damage. J Crit Care 2014;29(4):692.e7-13.
108. Wang JJ, Chi NH, Huang TM, et al. Urinary biomarkers predict advanced acute kidney injury after cardiovascular surgery. Crit Care 2018;22(1):108.
109. Marx D, Metzger J, Pejchinovski M, et al. Proteomics and metabolomics for AKI diagnosis. Semin Nephrol 2018;38(1):63–87.
110. Kellum JA, Prowle JR. Paradigms of acute kidney injury in the intensive care setting. Nat Rev Nephrol 2018;14(4):217–30.
111. Basu RK, Standage SW, Cvijanovich NZ, et al. Identification of candidate serum biomarkers for severe septic shock-associated kidney injury via microarray. Crit Care 2011;15(6):R273.
112. Jones TF, Bekele S, O'Dwyer MJ, et al. MicroRNAs in acute kidney injury. Nephron 2018;140(2):124–8.
113. Ge QM, Huang CM, Zhu XY, et al. Differentially expressed miRNAs in sepsis-induced acute kidney injury target oxidative stress and mitochondrial dysfunction pathways. PLoS One 2017;12(3):e0173292.
114. Bhatraju PK, Mukherjee P, Robinson-Cohen, et al. Acute kidney injury subphenotypes based on creatinine trajectory identifies patients at increased risk of death. Crit Care 2016;20(1):372.
115. Bhatraju PK, Zelnick LR, Herting J, et al. Identification of acute kidney injury subphenotypes with differing molecular signatures and response to vasopressin therapy. Am J Respir Crit Care Med 2019;199(7):863–72.
116. Maslove DM, Wong HR. Gene expression profiling in sepsis: timing, tissue, and translational considerations. Trends Mol Med 2014;20(4):204–13.
117. Wong HR, Lindsell CJ, Pettila V, et al. A multibiomarker-based outcome risk stratification model for adult septic shock*. Crit Care Med 2014;42(4):781–9.
118. Wong HR, Cvijanovich NZ, Allen GL, et al. Validation of a gene expression-based subclassification strategy for pediatric septic shock. Crit Care Med 2011;39(11):2511–7.
119. Ahasic AM, Christiani DC. Personalized critical care medicine: how far away are we? Semin Respir Crit Care Med 2015;36(6):809–22.

Metabolomics and the Microbiome as Biomarkers in Sepsis

Jisoo Lee, MD[a,b,*], Debasree Banerjee, MD, MS[a,b]

KEYWORDS

- Metabolomics • Pharmaco-metabonomics • Microbiome • Gut microbiota
- Dysbiosis • Personalized medicine

KEY POINTS

- Technologic advancements in mass spectrometry offer opportunities to study metabolite profiles using targeted and untargeted approaches.
- Metabolomics provides new ways of exploring the diagnosis, mechanism, and prognosis of sepsis via novel biomarkers.
- The use of pharmaco-metabonomics in predicting drug response may enable patient stratification and precision medicine.
- Microbiome composition changes dramatically in sepsis, as the diversity of microbiota decreases, and potential pathogens become dominant.
- Understanding the complex interactions of the host's metabolomics and microbiome can provide novel preventive and therapeutic strategies against sepsis.

INTRODUCTION

Sepsis remains a clinical challenge to physicians and researchers alike, given its heterogeneity in presentation, from diagnosis, pharmacologic and nonpharmacological interventions, and prognostication. Sepsis is defined as a "life-threatening organ dysfunction due to a dysregulated host response to infection."[1] Decades of research in sepsis has revealed that the pathways and outcomes of sepsis is largely affected by the interactions of 2 factors: the host genetics and environmental factors. Advances in technology have allowed us to delve further into the cellular and subcellular pathologic changes that occur in a septic host. The study of "Omics" comprises genomics,

Disclosure Statement: None.
[a] Division of Pulmonary, Critical Care and Sleep Medicine, The Warren Alpert School of Medicine at Brown University, Providence, RI, USA; [b] Division of Pulmonary, Critical Care & Sleep Medicine, Rhode Island Hospital, POB Suite 224, 595 Eddy Street, Providence, RI 02903, USA
* Corresponding author. Division of Pulmonary, Critical Care, & Sleep Medicine, Rhode Island Hospital, POB Suite 224, 595 Eddy Street, Providence, RI 02903.
E-mail address: jisoo_lee@brown.edu

Crit Care Clin 36 (2020) 105–113
https://doi.org/10.1016/j.ccc.2019.08.008
0749-0704/20/© 2019 Elsevier Inc. All rights reserved.

transcriptomics, proteomics, and metabolomics, and refers to the systemic measurement of an entire class of biochemical species at the DNA, RNA, protein, and metabolite levels.[2] The host's genome, transcriptome, and proteome are all reflected in the metabolome, a snapshot of the metabolites in the host at any specific time point during the disease process.[3] Similarly, emerging technologies have allowed more in-depth understanding of environmental factors that influence sepsis outcome, particularly the microbiome and its role in nosocomial and opportunistic infection, a well-described sequelae of sepsis. Metabolomics and the study of the microbiome together provide new possibilities in the quest for personalized medicine in sepsis through the integration of host and environmental factors.

THE DEFINITION OF METABOLOMICS

Metabolomics is the study of the metabolome, which is a collection of small molecules produced by cells that are responsible for metabolic processes in organisms.[4] Metabolomics is a relatively new concept that has appeared in the past decade. Metabolomics, unlike genomics, transcriptomics, and proteomics, serve as direct biomarkers of biochemical activity, and are thus easier to directly correlate with phenotypes.[5]

There are targeted and untargeted approaches to studying the metabolome. The targeted metabolomics studies focus on measuring a specified number of metabolites in the pathway of interest.[5] This approach allows researchers to ask a specific biochemical question based on a hypothesis. Although it is an effective way to obtain deeper insights of a specific hypothesis, the success of the study depends on the strength of preexisting data and knowledge.[6] The untargeted metabolomics, or "global metabolomics," on the other hand, uses an unbiased screening method to identify thousands of metabolites in a single experiment, and thus enables exploratory studies of unknown metabolites.[7] The metabolic profile is then compared in 2 conditions or across a population in order to discover a novel metabolite.[6] The untargeted approach allows a broad and comprehensive inspection into the metabolome. **Fig. 1** describes the workflow of targeted and untargeted approaches of liquid chromatography–mass spectrometry (LC-MS), one of the tools used to identify metabolites from specimens.[5]

Metabolomics is increasingly used in a wide variety of research, such as to identify biomarkers, identify drug activities, or drug-induced toxicity and metabolism.[8] The application of metabolomics in various scientific fields is depicted in **Fig. 2**.[6]

THE PLATFORMS OF METABOLOMICS

There are several platforms that enable metabolomics experiments. In targeted metabolomics, triple quadrupole mass spectrometry is used to target a list of metabolites to be screened for a disease or biochemical pathway.[5] This is a highly sensitive method that enables absolute quantification of low-concentration metabolites.[5] In untargeted metabolomics, platforms such as nuclear magnetic resonance (NMR), gas chromatography-mass spectrometry (GC-MS), and LC-MS are used. Each of these platforms have strengths and weaknesses, as shown in **Table 1**. These platforms are often used in various combinations in experiments.

NMR spectroscopy measures the signals from the nuclei of isotopes of certain atoms, such as hydrogen-1 (^1H), and it can elucidate more detailed molecular structures of compounds in the solution state compared with mass spectrometry.[4,7] NMR enables real-time reaction monitoring at controlled temperatures[6]; however, it has lower sensitivity compared with mass spectrometry. Mass spectrometry measures the mass-to-charge ratio of charged molecules or molecular fragments, and

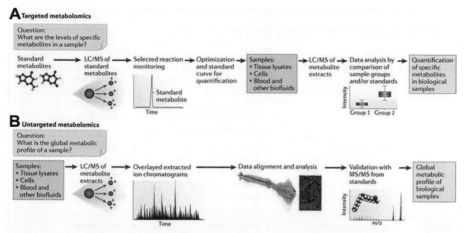

Fig. 1. The targeted and untargeted workflow for LC-MS–based metabolomics. (*A*) Targeted methods are established based on standard metabolites. The metabolites are then extracted from samples such as tissue lysates, cells, or blood and other biofluids. The metabolites are analyzed, and the data output provides quantification of these metabolites by comparing to the previously built standard methods. (*B*) Untargeted method takes the biologic samples, such as tissue lysates, cells, or blood and other biofluids, which are separated using liquid chromatography. These samples are subsequently analyzed by mass spectrometry for data acquisition. The results are processed by bioinformatic software to generate global metabolic profile of biological samples. (*From* Patti GJ, Yanes O, Siuzdak G. Innovation: Metabolomics: the apogee of the omics trilogy. Nat Rev Mol Cell Biol. 2012 Mar 22;13(4):263-9. https://doi.org/10.1038/nrm3314; with permission.)

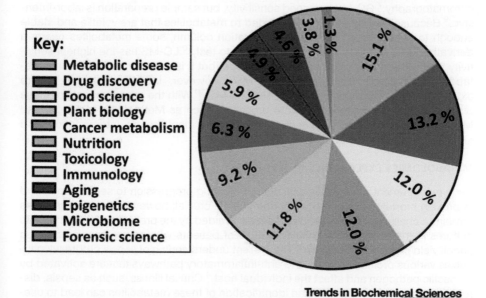

Fig. 2. The distribution of recent publications on applications of metabolomics by scientific field. (*From* Liu X, Locasale JW. Metabolomics: A Primer. Trends Biochem Sci. 2017 Apr;42(4):274-284. https://doi.org/10.1016/j.tibs.2017.01.004. Epub 2017 Feb 11; with permission.)

Table 1
Platforms of metabolomics: the mechanism, pros, and cons

	NMR	GC-MS	LC-MS
Mechanism	Measures the signals from the nuclei of isotopes of atoms	Measures the mass-to-charge ratio of charged metabolites; metabolites are separated by gas chromatography	Measures the mass-to-charge ratio of charged molecules; metabolites are separated by liquid chromatography
Pros	• Real-time measurements • Nondestructive • More detailed molecular structures • Quantitative	• Good sensitivity • Broad metabolite detection coverage • Good for analysis of gases or volatile metabolites	• Highest sensitivity • Broad metabolite detection coverage • Easy sample preparation
Cons	• Low sensitivity	• Destructive • Labor-intensive sample preparation • Limited to volatile metabolites • Potential noise from derivatization • Nonquantitative	• Destructive • Limited to organic compounds that form molecular ions • Nonquantitative

Abbreviations: GC-MS, gas chromatography–mass spectrometry; LC-MS, liquid chromatography–mass spectrometry; NMR, nuclear magnetic resonance.

identifies the ionized metabolites by separating technology involving gas or liquid chromatography.[7] GC-MS has good sensitivity, but sample preparation is labor-intensive.[9] Because the use of GC-MS is limited to metabolites that are volatile and stable enough to pass through the heated separation column, some metabolites needs a derivatization process to make them suitable to test.[10] LC-MS has the highest sensitivity with wider metabolite detection coverage, but it is more difficult to identify metabolites compared with NMR or GC-MS[9]; however, LC-MS does not require extraction or derivatization processes like GC-MS.[10] With the advancements of these platforms and metabolomic software programs such as MathDAMP, MetAlign, and MzMine, there has been significant progress in the identification, interpretation, and analysis of massive metabolomic profiles.[5]

METABOLOMICS EXPERIMENTS IN SEPSIS

Early management of sepsis is critical in preventing progression to septic shock and improving mortality. Therefore, early detection is crucial; however, diagnosing sepsis remains a challenge. The diagnosis of sepsis is aided by the presence of microbiologic cultures in the body, but only 30% to 40% of patients with severe sepsis or septic shock yield positive test results.[11] The current understanding of sepsis progression involves various proinflammatory and anti-inflammatory pathways that are activated by a specific pathogen and affect the individual host.[4] Critical illness, such as sepsis, disrupts the metabolomic profile, and identification of these metabolites can lead to useful innovations to detect and treat sepsis.[3]

In humans, serum, plasma and urine samples can be used to study the metabolome. In the article by Su and colleagues,[12] a total of 65 patients (35 patients with sepsis, 15 patients with systemic inflammatory response syndrome [SIRS], and 15 healthy subjects) were studied to identify and differentiate metabolic biomarkers involved in the different stages of sepsis. Patients' serum samples from venipuncture were used to measure metabolites by LC-MS technique. The investigators found that the metabolic profiling of the healthy controls, patients with SIRS, and patients with sepsis were markedly different. Patients with sepsis had significantly lower levels of lactitol dehydrate and S-phenyl-D-cysteine and higher levels of S-(3-methylbutanoyl)-dihydrolipoamide-E and N-nonanoyl glycine, when compared with patients with SIRS. Although further studies are required for validation, the identification of these metabolites can provide the basis for future study in distinguishing sterile from infected inflammatory responses in patients. This study also showed that 2-phenylacetamide, dimethylysine, glyceryl-phosphoryl-ethanolamine, and D-cysteine were related to the severity of sepsis. Furthermore, 4 metabolites, S-(3-methylbutanoyl)-dihydrolipoamide-E, PG (22:2(13Z,16Z)0:0), glycerophosphocholine, and S-succinyl-glutathione, were elevated within the 48 hours before death, indicating their possible use in predicting mortality.

Another study by Stringer and colleagues[13] used NMR spectroscopy to study the metabolome of patients with sepsis-induced acute lung injury. This study looked at 6 healthy controls and 13 patients with sepsis-induced acute lung injury (ALI), and identified 4 metabolites that were significantly different. Total glutathione associated with oxidant stress, adenosine associated with the loss of ATP homeostasis, phosphatidylserine associated with apoptosis, were all significantly elevated in the sepsis-induced ALI group compared with the healthy control group. On the other hand, sphingomyelin, which is associated with disruption of endothelial barrier function, was significantly decreased in the sepsis-induced ALI group compared with the healthy control group.

Schmerler and colleagues[14] used targeted metabolomics to identify lipids that could differentiate sepsis from SIRS. The LC-MS platform was used to study a total of 186 metabolites from 6 analyte classes (acylcarnitines, amino acids, biogenic amines, glycerophospholipids, sphingolipids, and carbohydrates) were determined in 74 patients with SIRS and 69 patients with sepsis. This study determined that the activities of acylcarnitine C10:1 and glycerophospholipid PCaaC32:0 were significantly different in patients with sepsis compared with patients with SIRS. Using the 2 markers, C10:1 and PCaaC32:0, the investigators were able to correctly classify SIRS and sepsis in 80% of patients in the training set and 70% of patients in the test set for validation.

METABOLOMICS IN THERAPEUTIC OUTCOMES OF SEPSIS

Metabolomics has been widely explored in evaluating therapeutic outcomes. Drug effects are widely varied in individuals, which is determined not only by the genetic variation but also by environmental influences such as nutritional status, gut microbiota, age, illness, and drug-drug interactions.[10] Although pharmacogenomics has led to significant improvements in correlating drugs responses with host genetic polymorphisms,[15] pharmacogonomics does not take environmental factors into account. The "pharmaco-metabonomic" approach is defined as "the prediction of the outcome of a drug or xenobiotic intervention in an individual based on a mathematical model of pre-intervention metabolite signatures."[10] The pharmaco-metabonomics has the potential to identify metabolites that could predict responses of clinical drugs based on the individual's baseline metabolic profile. Furthermore, comparing the metabolic profiles of an individual's pretreatment and posttreatment can reveal novel drug mechanisms and their metabolic pathways.[8] The advancements in the metabolomics and pharmaco-metabonomics may lead to tailored therapy, enabling optimization of therapeutic outcome.[7]

The clinical application of pharmaco-metabonomics is exemplified by a study by Clayton and colleagues.[16] In this study, ^{1}H NMR spectroscopy was used to compare the urinary metabolite profiles in 99 healthy male volunteers before and after a standard dose of acetaminophen. The investigators found that elevated levels of predose *para*-cresol sulfate was associated with decreased postdose ratios of acetaminophen sulfate to acetaminophen glucuronide. *Para*-cresol is thought to originate from bacteria in the gut microbiome, and thus the investigators conclude that individual's gut microbiome with different levels of *para*-cresol leads to different systemic effect of acetaminophen. This illustrates how pharmaco-metabonomics enables deeper insight into the interplay of metabolomics and microbiome in the efficacy of drug treatment.

Despite recent advancements of technologies enabling rapid and efficient profiling of the metabolome, there are many limitations of metabolomics at this time, which include lack of validation, limited clinical experience and research data, and dearth of standardized technologies and software used as a gold standard for the study of the metabolome.

MICROBIOME IN SEPSIS

Although metabolomics increases the depth of understanding of the host's response to disease, understanding its relationship with environmental factors (ie, microbiome) is equally crucial in developing targeted therapies. The microbiome of an individual changes according to the severity of the illness.[17] It has been shown that when the diverse and balanced gut microbiota is disturbed, it leads to altered host immunity to pathogens, causing increased susceptibility of sepsis.[18] This is described as "dysbiosis," which is a state that the composition and diversity of microbiome is distorted.[19]

Dysbiosis of the gut microbiome affects sepsis outcomes. The upper gastrointestinal (GI) tract becomes a reservoir of pathogens, such as *Escherichia coli*, *Pseudomonas aeruginosa*, *Enterococcus*, as it loses acidity for protective microbiomes.[17] In the lower GI tract, the diversity of the microbiome decreases, and the intestinal mucus layer is thinned and disrupted and allows for pathogens to grow in abundance.[17] The bacterial content of the gut determines the severity of systemic injury in sepsis. The inflammation and injury sustained by organs is lessened when the bacterial burden is lowered. Lowering bacterial burden is done primarily by defecation, however this process is slowed in critical illness due to disturbances of glucose and electrolyte levels, endogenous opioid production, as well as by therapeutic interventions such as sedatives, opioids, and catecholamines.[17]

The respiratory microbiome is also severely altered in patients with sepsis. The oropharyngeal microbes migrate to the lungs in critical illness, and the pathogenic bacteria of the oropharynx such as *Klebsiella pneumoniae*, *Pseudomonas aeruginosa* and Proteobacteria increase the risk of infection in the lungs.[17,20] Normal lungs are usually not a favorable place for microbes given the lack of nutrition and presence of a lipid-rich surfactant.[17] As the alveoli become filled with oropharyngeal microbes, the lungs become a reservoir and source of nutrition for the pathogens to disrupt the systemic immunity. Furthermore, during lung injury from critical illness such as sepsis or acute respiratory distress syndrome, the surfactant becomes inactivated, mucociliary clearance is impaired, and the influx of edema creates steep oxygen gradients, which all help facilitate bacterial growth.[17,21–23] Thus, in the lungs in critical illness, there is increased migration of microbiota from the gut to the lungs, decreased elimination, and increased growth of potential pathogens. Molecular stress signals from catecholamines and inflammatory cytokines also increase the likelihood of the growth of pathogens. Increased alveolar catecholamine concentrations were shown to correlate with the disruption of microbiome in human bronchoalveolar lavage samples, thus creating dominant species, such as *Pseudomonas aeruginosa, Streptococcus pneumoniae, Staphylococcus aureus*, and *Klebsiella pneumoniae*.[17]

Microbiota of patients alter significantly with disease severity and pharmacologic and nonpharmacological interventions and procedures done to the patient. Understanding the relationships of microbiota and host resistance can lead to significant innovations to preventive and therapeutic strategies against sepsis.

MICROBIOME MODULATION IN SEPSIS MANAGEMENT

There are attempts to use microbiome modulation for sepsis management in several stages; prevention, treatment, and recovery.[18] In a systemic review and meta-analysis of 30 trials of 2972 patients,[24] it showed that probiotics were associated with reduced infection. The study also noted a reduction in the incidence of ventilator-associated pneumonia, but did not see any effect on mortality, length of stay, or diarrhea.

Synbiotics, which is "a combination of probiotics and prebiotics: dietary components that enhance the growth of these species," is a promising therapy to restore dysbiosis.[19] A randomized, double-blinded placebo-controlled trial in rural India looked at more than 4500 infants at least 35 weeks of gestation without signs of sepsis or other morbidity and administered oral symbiotic preparation of *Lactobacillus plantarum* and a fructooligosaccharide versus placebo.[25] Administration of the symbiotic preparation resulted in a significant reduction in the primary outcome (the combination of sepsis and death). This study also showed that the treatment group had significantly reduced incidence of lower respiratory tract infections, as well as culture-positive and culture-negative sepsis.

Decolonization strategies, such as selective decolonization of the digestive tract (SDD), selective oropharyngeal decontamination (SOD), and topical oropharyngeal chlorhexidine were studied to determine its effect on mortality.[26] SDD uses nonabsorbable antibiotics, such as polymyxin, tobramycin, and amphotericin, that are applied as a paste during routine mouth care, in combination with a short course of intravenous antibiotics.[26] SOD applies the antibiotic paste to the oropharynx only without empirical intravenous antibiotics. The systemic review and meta-analysis of Price and colleagues[26] revealed that SDD and SOD had favorable effects on mortality in adults patients in the intensive care units, however chlorhexidine was associated with increased mortality.

Fecal microbiota transplantation (FMT) is another means of trying to regain homeostasis of the microbiome and is commonly used in recurrent *Clostridium difficile* infection. Its use has been expanded and explored in the treatment of diarrhea and sepsis as well. A case report from China showed that FMT was successful in treating septic shock and diarrhea in a 44-year-old woman who presented with polymicrobial septic shock in the setting of severe watery diarrhea.[27] The analysis of patient's fecal microbiota before FMT showed significant intestinal microbiota dysbiosis with dominant pathogenic Proteobacteria. After the FMT, there was a significant modification in the patient's microbiota, with enrichment of commensal Firmicutes and depletion of opportunistic Proteobacteria and thus restoring the disrupted microbiota. Another ongoing study is aiming to find the efficacy of auto-FMT for prevention of infection in a cohort of patients receiving allo-hematopoietic cell transplantation (clinicaltrials.-gov: NCT02269150).

SUMMARY

Although there have been significant improvements in sepsis management and out-comes, understanding the pathophysiology and mechanism of sepsis progression as well as attempts to personalize sepsis treatment remain a big challenge. Metabolomics provides a unique approach to study the impact of sepsis on the host's metabolite profiles at specific time points during illness. Furthermore, the dysbiosis caused in the host's microbiome severely affects the host's vulnerability to pathogens and thus the severity of sepsis. With new technologies to better identify and study novel biomarkers in metabolomics and study interventions for modulating the microbiome, these fields are emerging areas of interest and show promise for ways to diagnose and treat sepsis.

REFERENCES

1. Shankar-Hari M, Phillips GS, Levy ML, et al. Developing a new definition and assessing new clinical criteria for septic shock: for the third international consensus definitions for sepsis and septic shock (Sepsis-3). Jama 2016;315:775–87.
2. Itenov TS, Murray DD, Jensen JUS. Sepsis: personalized medicine utilizing 'omic' technologies-a paradigm shift? Healthcare (Basel) 2018;6:1–9.
3. Beloborodova NV, Olenin AY, Pautova AK. Metabolomic findings in sepsis as a damage of host-microbial metabolism integration. J Crit Care 2018;43:246–55.
4. Ludwig KR, Hummon AB. Mass spectrometry for the discovery of biomarkers of sepsis. Mol Biosyst 2017;13:648–64.
5. Patti GJ, Yanes O, Siuzdak G. Innovation: metabolomics: the apogee of the omics trilogy. Nat Rev Mol Cell Biol 2012;13:263–9.
6. Liu X, Locasale JW. Metabolomics: a primer. Trends Biochem Sci 2017;42: 274–84.
7. Everett JR. Pharmacometabonomics in humans: a new tool for personalized medicine. Pharmacogenomics 2015;16:737–54.
8. Vincent JL, Brealey D, Libert N, et al. Rapid diagnosis of infection in the critically ill, a multicenter study of molecular detection in bloodstream infections, pneumonia, and sterile site infections. Crit Care Med 2015;43:2283–91.
9. Li B, He X, Jia W, et al. Novel applications of metabolomics in personalized medicine: a mini-review. Molecules 2017;22:2–10.
10. Clayton TA, Lindon JC, Cloarec O, et al. Pharmaco-metabonomic phenotyping and personalized drug treatment. Nature 2006;440:1073–7.
11. Levy MM, Fink MP, Marshall JC, et al. 2001 SCCM/ESICM/ACCP/ATS/SIS international sepsis definitions conference. Crit Care Med 2003;31:1250–6.
12. Su L, Huang Y, Zhu Y, et al. Discrimination of sepsis stage metabolic profiles with an LC/MS-MS-based metabolomics approach. BMJ Open Respir Res 2014;1: e000056.
13. Stringer KA, Serkova NJ, Karnovsky A, et al. Metabolic consequences of sepsis-induced acute lung injury revealed by plasma (1)H-nuclear magnetic resonance quantitative metabolomics and computational analysis. Am J Physiol Lung Cell Mol Physiol 2011;300:L4–l11.
14. Schmerler D, Neugebauer S, Ludewig K, et al. Targeted metabolomics for discrimination of systemic inflammatory disorders in critically ill patients. J Lipid Res 2012;53:1369–75.
15. Weinshilboum R, Wang L. Pharmacogenomics: bench to bedside. Nat Rev Drug Discov 2004;3:739–48.

16. Clayton TA, Baker D, Lindon JC, et al. Pharmacometabonomic identification of a significant host-microbiome metabolic interaction affecting human drug metabolism. Proc Natl Acad Sci U S A 2009;106:14728–33.
17. Dickson RP. The microbiome and critical illness. Lancet Respir Med 2016;4: 59–72.
18. Haak BW, Prescott HC, Wiersinga WJ. Therapeutic potential of the gut microbiota in the prevention and treatment of sepsis. Front Immunol 2018;9:2042.
19. Haak BW, Levi M, Wiersinga WJ. Microbiota-targeted therapies on the intensive care unit. Curr Opin Crit Care 2017;23:167–74.
20. Johanson WG, Pierce AK, Sanford JP. Changing pharyngeal bacterial flora of hospitalized patients. Emergence of gram-negative bacilli. N Engl J Med 1969; 281:1137–40.
21. Gunther A, Siebert C, Schmidt R, et al. Surfactant alterations in severe pneumonia, acute respiratory distress syndrome, and cardiogenic lung edema. Am J Respir Crit Care Med 1996;153:176–84.
22. Nakagawa NK, Franchini ML, Driusso P, et al. Mucociliary clearance is impaired in acutely ill patients. Chest 2005;128:2772–7.
23. Albenberg L, Esipova TV, Judge CP, et al. Correlation between intraluminal oxygen gradient and radial partitioning of intestinal microbiota. Gastroenterology 2014;147:1055–63.e8.
24. Manzanares W, Lemieux M, Langlois PL, et al. Probiotic and synbiotic therapy in critical illness: a systematic review and meta-analysis. Crit Care 2016;19:262.
25. Panigrahi P, Parida S, Nanda NC, et al. A randomized synbiotic trial to prevent sepsis among infants in rural India. Nature 2017;548:407–12.
26. Price R, MacLennan G, Glen J. Selective digestive or oropharyngeal decontamination and topical oropharyngeal chlorhexidine for prevention of death in general intensive care: systematic review and network meta-analysis. BMJ 2014;348: g2197.
27. Li Q, Wang C, Tang C, et al. Successful treatment of severe sepsis and diarrhea after vagotomy utilizing fecal microbiota transplantation: a case report. Crit Care 2015;19:37.

Lactate: Where Are We Now?

Jan Bakker, MD, PhD[a,b,c,d,]*, Radu Postelnicu, MD[a],
Vikramjit Mukherjee, MD[a]

KEYWORDS

• Sepsis • Shock • Tissue perfusion • Early goal directed therapy • Hemodynamics

KEY POINTS

• Lactate is a rapidly available variable that is closely linked to morbidity and mortality in almost every critically ill patient.

• A decrease in lactate levels during initial resuscitation of a patient with circulatory dysfunction is a universally good sign.

• Lactate clearance is a function of production and uptake of lactate, mostly by liver and kidney, followed by metabolism that results in a given serum lactate concentration. Lactate clearance in clinical practice refers to the changes in lactate over time.

• Using lactate levels as a marker of tissue hypoperfusion has limitations, especially in septic shock patients, and is likely to be limited to the initial hours of resuscitation.

• When initial therapy in the first 6 to 8 hours of septic shock resuscitation is aimed to decrease lactate levels guided by parameters of tissue perfusion this is likely to improve outcome of the patient.

INTRODUCTION

Following the definition of a biomarker lactate seems to be the ideal one in critically ill patients. Increased lactate levels are a universal sign of an abnormal condition. When using the correct treatment to correct the causing mechanism, lactate levels change quickly. A decrease in lactate levels following institution of treatment thus gives the clinician guidance on its adequacy and may serve to adjust treatment when needed. However, in contrast to what some guidelines suggest, lactate is not an easy to use parameter and an advice to measure it without a clinical direction on how to respond is not the way to go. Opinions on the clinical value of lactate levels still spur a lot of discussion[1–3] related to the many pitfalls of using lactate in critically ill.[4]

Disclosure Statement: The authors have nothing to disclose.
[a] Division of Pulmonary Critical Care, and Sleep Medicine, New York University School of Medicine, Bellevue Hospital, 462 First Avenue | NBV-10W18, New York, NY 10016, USA; [b] Department of Pulmonology and Critical Care, Columbia University Medical Center, New York, NY, USA; [c] Department Intensive Care Adults, Erasmus MC University Medical Center, Rotterdam, Netherlands; [d] Department of Intensive Care, Pontificia Universidad Católica de Chile, Santiago, Chile
* Corresponding author. Division of Pulmonary, Critical Care, and Sleep Medicine, New York University School of Medicine, Bellevue Hospital, 462 First Avenue | NBV-10W18, New York, NY 10016.
E-mail address: Jan.bakker@nyulangone.org

Crit Care Clin 36 (2020) 115–124
https://doi.org/10.1016/j.ccc.2019.08.009
0749-0704/20/© 2019 Elsevier Inc. All rights reserved.

criticalcare.theclinics.com

In clinical conditions we characterize circulatory dysfunction by a combination of abnormalities in different systems. Without a particular order of importance, it may consist of abnormal hemodynamic parameters like blood pressure and heart rate, abnormal tissue perfusion parameters like a cold, discolored sweaty skin, altered mental state and decreased urine production and abnormal metabolic parameters like lactate, arterial pH, and base excess. Under normal conditions, oxygen demand dictates oxygen delivery and is thus equal to oxygen consumption. Therefore, a decrease in oxygen consumption during unchanged oxygen demand denotes a state in which the delivery of oxygen to the tissues is inadequate to meet the demands for normal tissue function (tissue hypoxia) that will result in tissue damage and organ dysfunction. Invariably in both experimental and clinical conditions this situation is characterized by a sharp rise in lactate levels.[5,6] As increased lactate levels in critically ill patients have also been associated with this phenomenon[7,8] and increased lactate levels are related to the presence and severity of organ dysfunction,[9,10] increased lactate levels have been seen as a hallmark of circulatory dysfunction and tissue damage.

In this article, we review the current states on how to appropriately use lactate levels to that end and how they can be used to diagnose and treat circulatory dysfunction.

METABOLISM OF LACTATE

Under normal conditions, the metabolism of lactate produces a small amount of ATP in the presence or absence of a functional Krebs cycle. However, by accelerating the process of glucose metabolism, much more ATP can be generated.[11] Therefore, a clinical context associated with increased glucose metabolism might lead to increased lactate levels as the capacity of the Krebs cycle is limited. Many situations and treatments in critically ill patients lead to increased glucose metabolism. Increased sympathetic nervous system activation, prominently present in shock states, is only one of them.[12] In these conditions, lactate might even serve as a fuel being exchanged between tissues (liver, kidneys, muscles) and even cells (astrocytes, neurons) through lactate shuttles.[13,14] In contrast with the Cori cycle (hepatic and renal gluconeogenesis) requiring oxygen, the interorgan/cellular exchange does not make this an interesting energy transport mechanism.[15] Even exogenous lactate can be used as a fuel in this context.[13] Therefore, the old concept of lactate being an indicator of the presence of tissue hypoxia in shock states has been challenged and especially in sepsis, where lactate clearance is impaired, this relationship might be more problematic than suggested in guidelines[4,16]

LACTATE AND TISSUE HYPOPERFUSION

Oxygen delivery is a function of hemoglobin levels, arterial oxygen saturation, and cardiac output (and its distribution). In experimental conditions, decreasing any of these components of oxygen delivery will result in a decrease in oxygen consumption when a critical level is reached.[6,17] This state of oxygen delivery–dependent oxygen consumption is a hallmark of tissue hypoxia and further reductions in oxygen delivery will immediately result in sharp decreases in oxygen consumption (below the baseline level reflecting the demand for oxygen) and increases in lactate levels. Also, in clinical conditions, this supply dependent state is characterized by increased lactate levels.[7] The study by Ronco and colleagues[5] showed that this phenomenon also occurs when therapy is withdrawn during end-of-life care. In experimental conditions, reversing this state of supply dependency, corrects lactate levels to normal baseline levels.[18] Clinically, Friedman and colleagues[8] showed that supply dependency is present in the early phase of septic shock, whereas in the post resuscitation phase supply dependency was absent and lactate levels were normal. In addition, observational studies have associated increased morbidity and mortality to the presence of other markers of tissue hypoperfusion in patients with sepsis.

In the presence of normal oxygen delivery values, abnormal microcirculatory perfusion may still be present[19] and thus there will be limited cellular oxygen availability. Particularly in sepsis, microcirculatory derangement may lead to insufficient oxygen that is delivered to the cell, thereby increasing lactate levels.[17] This is indirectly illustrated by the observation that increased lactate levels have been associated with abnormal microcirculatory perfusion[20] and that improving capillary perfusion has been associated with a reduction in lactate levels in patients with septic shock, independent of changes in systemic hemodynamic variables.[21] In addition, normalization of tissue perfusion parameters has been associated with a sharp decrease in lactate levels.[22]

Nevertheless, given the abnormal metabolism in sepsis[23–25] and the decreased clearance of lactate[26–28] even restoration of microcirculatory perfusion in these conditions may still be associated with increased lactate levels.[29] This in contrast with low cardiac output forms of circulatory failure where correction of microcirculatory perfusion is associated with normalization of lactate levels.[29] Therefore, especially in septic shock conditions, the exclusive use of increased lactate levels to determine the presence of tissue hypoxia, following the initial period of resuscitation, is limited.[30] Additional parameters reflecting tissue perfusion and metabolism have been proposed to aid in the diagnosis.[22,31–33] Also, the lactate to pyruvate ratio has been proposed to aid in the diagnosis of hypoxia related tissue metabolism.[34–36] Although clinically available as a micro dialysate technique in brain tissue monitoring,[37] the interpretation in relation to tissue hypoxia is not straight forward but rather a complex parameter of metabolism.[38,39]

CLEARANCE OF LACTATE

As the blood lactate level is a result of the production and clearance, an impairment in the latter may thus result in increased lactate levels. Several conditions have been associated with impaired clearance. Liver dysfunction/failure, cardiac surgery, and sepsis have all been associated with decreased clearance capacity.[24,26,40,41] In clinical practice, lactate clearance has been used to describe the change in lactate levels over time. Although technically not correct,[4,42] the use of lactate clearance has been stimulated by studies linking the relative decrease of lactate levels over time to the patient's response to therapy and ultimately outcome.[43–48] In summary, almost in any context of critical illness, decreases in lactate levels following start of treatment are associated with improved outcome.[49] Meta-analysis of studies using decreases in lactate as a clinical endpoint showed improved survival both in hyperlactatemic patients as in patients with severe sepsis and septic shock.[50,51]

GOAL-DIRECTED THERAPY USING LACTATE LEVELS

Given the strong relationship among increased lactate levels tissue perfusion, organ failure, and ultimate outcome, this biomarker is frequently used in clinical practice to guide therapy. However, only a limited number of randomized studies have evaluated the value of this strategy.

Many studies evaluating the use of early goal-directed therapy (EGDT) aiming to optimize blood pressure, preload status, and tissue perfusion in patients with sepsis have shown minimal results in contrast to the first landmark study by Rivers and colleagues[52] using this concept. Three large randomized studies[53–55] randomizing more than 4000 patients in total did, not show a survival benefit when using the broad elements of EGDT. Although there might have been a survival benefit in patients with a high initial lactate level (>5.0 mmol/L),[53] lactate levels were not used to adjust therapy by protocol in these studies. Important to recognize here is that the landmark study by Rivers and colleagues[52] was started in native sepsis patients without any previous treatment, whereas the recent EGDT studies have all been done in patients who had already received some early treatment, in most cases fluid resuscitation or even already start of vasopressor therapy.[56]

In a study in patients with early sepsis by Jones and colleagues,[57] therapy aimed to normalize central venous oxygenation (ScvO$_2$) was compared with therapy aimed to decrease lactate levels by at least 10% in the 6-hour duration study protocol. In this study, fluid resuscitation in both groups was aimed to increase central venous pressure to 8 mm Hg or higher, vasopressors were used to maintain a mean arterial pressure (MAP) of 65 mm Hg or higher, and dobutamine and blood transfusions were used where needed to increase ScvO$_2$. In the lactate-guided group, the same interventions were used; however, ScvO$_2$ was not available in these patients and substituted with the lactate target of a 10% decrease in the first 2 hours or longer. The hospital mortality in the 2 groups, of each 150 patients, was lower in the lactate-guided group (17% vs 22%), although this difference was not statistically significant (difference 6; 95% CI −3% to 15%).

In a randomized trial in the Netherlands, Jansen and colleagues[58] studied 348 patients with a lactate level of more than 3.0 mmol/L irrespective of their diagnosis. Following the measurement of central venous oxygen saturation (ScvO$_2$), therapy was directed to optimize oxygen delivery and reduce oxygen demand in the lactate group. The aim of the protocol was to decrease lactate by at least 20% every 2 hours for the duration of the intervention period (first 8 hours of admission). The control group received standard treatment where lactate levels were not available. This combined use of ScvO$_2$ and lactate decreases resulted in an improvement in hospital survival when corrected for baseline imbalances (hazard ratio 0.61 [CI: 0.43–0.87]). When combining the patients with sepsis from this study with the study by Jones and colleagues[57] and two Chinese studies, using lactate to guide therapy in sepsis patients was shown to improve outcome.[50]

In a recent study in 424 patients with septic shock, Hernandez and colleagues[56] compared a strategy to decrease lactate levels similar to the study by Jansen and colleagues[58] with a strategy to normalize peripheral capillary refill time (CRT). In both groups, the protocol to reach the therapeutic goal was similar, with only a difference in the ultimate therapeutic goal: CRT of 3 seconds or less or a decrease in lactate by 20% every 2 hours for the duration of the 8-hour intervention period. In this study, there was improved survival in the group using CRT as the endpoint of resuscitation, although this was not statistically significant (34.9% vs 43.4% 28-day mortality, $P = .06$). However, the patients in the CRT-guided resuscitation had significantly less positive fluid balances during the intervention period and a faster recovery of organ failure when compared with the lactate-guided resuscitation.

HOW TO USE LACTATE IN CLINICAL PRACTICE

An increased lactate should always be a warning signal to the treatment team requiring immediate attention. The first line of assessment is very straightforward: the higher the lactate level, the higher the urgency. In the control group of the recent study by Jansen and colleagues,[58] in which patients with a suspected source of increased lactate levels other than circulatory were excluded, survival rapidly decreased with increasing initial lactate levels (**Fig. 1**). These data are compliant with older data in which increasing lactate levels were associated with rapidly decreasing survival.[59,60]

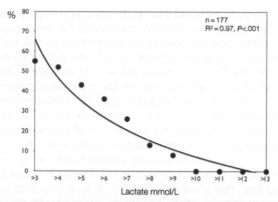

Fig. 1. Relationship between initial lactate level and survival in patients admitted with a lactate level of 3 mmol/L or more. Patients consist of the control group in the study by Jansen and colleagues.[58] (*From* Jansen TC, van Bommel J, Schoonderbeek FJ, et al. Early Lactate-Guided Therapy in Intensive Care Unit Patients A Multicenter, Open-Label, Randomized Controlled Trial. Am J Respir Crit Care Med 2010;182(6):752-761.)

The first line of action should then be to create context (**Fig. 2**). If the increased lactate is unlikely to be associated with decreased tissue perfusion but rather metabolic derangements or other causes,[12] this should be investigated and appropriate measures should be taken. In general, the urgency and line of actions in these contexts may be very different where generalized seizures, thiamine deficiency, and carbon monoxide or cyanide intoxication are extreme examples.[61–64]

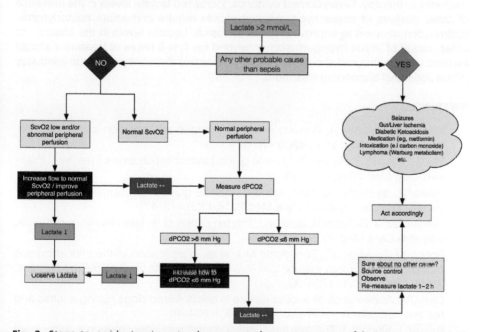

Fig. 2. Steps to guide treatment using repeated measurements of lactate using central venous oxygen saturation (ScvO$_2$) and central venous-to-arterial Pco$_2$ difference (dPCO2). (*From* Hernandez G, Bellomo R, Bakker J. The ten pitfalls of lactate clearance in sepsis. Intensive Care Med 2018;45(1):82-85; with permission.)

When there are signs of impaired tissue perfusion (eg, hypotension, tachycardia, abnormal peripheral perfusion, altered mentation), a measurement of $ScvO_2$ should be done. When normal, adding measurements of the delta-PCO_2 (difference between central venous and arterial P_{CO_2})[22] or a surrogate of the respiratory quotient (venous-arterial CO2 to arterial-venous O2 content difference ratio)[32] or the venous-arterial CO2 to arterial-venous O2 difference ratio[65] could help to diagnose tissue hypoperfusion that would require hemodynamic and microcirculatory perfusion improvements. Treatment should result in a rapid decrease or normalization of lactate levels and the parameters of tissue hypoperfusion.[30,43,66] Current evidence suggests to repeat measurements every 1 to 2 hours.[49] Given the available studies, targeting increased lactate levels by general optimization of perfusion to improve outcome is limited to the initial hours of admission. In the studies presented, this would be the first 6 to 8 hours of admission. Some guidelines suggest that the patient should be resuscitated to normalize lactate levels. Although this may be appropriate in the large community of patients, it does not fit an individualized approach where up to 50% of surviving patients with sepsis may still have increased lactate levels 24 hours after intensive care unit admission.[30] However, persistently increased lactate levels should urge the clinician to review diagnosis and adequacy of the treatment of the cause of increased lactate levels.

SUMMARY

When used correctly, lactate levels may aid in diagnosing and treating patients. Changes in lactate can provide an early and objective evaluation of the patient's response to therapy. Given current evidence, increased lactate levels in the presence of other markers of tissue hypoperfusion should require immediate hemodynamic optimization directed to improving tissue perfusion. Lactate levels in the absence of other marker of tissue hypoperfusion or beyond the first 8 hours of treatment should be used with caution and should warrant reassessment of diagnosis and the adequacy of the additional supporting treatment.

REFERENCES

1. Monnet X, Delaney A, Barnato A. Lactate-guided resuscitation saves lives: no. Intensive Care Med 2016;42(3):470–1.
2. Bloos F, Zhang Z, Boulain T. Lactate-guided resuscitation saves lives: yes. Intensive Care Med 2016;42(3):466–9.
3. Bakker J, de Backer D, Hernandez G. Lactate-guided resuscitation saves lives: we are not sure. Intensive Care Med 2016;42(3):472–4.
4. Hernandez G, Bellomo R, Bakker J. The ten pitfalls of lactate clearance in sepsis. Intensive Care Med 2018;45(1):82–5.
5. Ronco JJ, Fenwick JC, Tweeddale MG, et al. Identification of the critical oxygen delivery for anaerobic metabolism in critically ill septic and nonseptic humans. JAMA 1993;270(14):1724–30.
6. Cain SM. Appearance of excess lactate in anesthetized dogs during anemic and hypoxic hypoxia. Am J Physiol 1965;209(3):604–10.
7. Bakker J, Vincent J. The oxygen-supply dependency phenomenon is associated with increased blood lactate levels. J Crit Care 1991;6(3):152–9.
8. Friedman G, De Backer D, Shahla M, et al. Oxygen supply dependency can characterize septic shock. Intensive Care Med 1998;24(2):118–23.

9. Bakker J, Gris P, Coffernils M, et al. Serial blood lactate levels can predict the development of multiple organ failure following septic shock. Am J Surg 1996; 171(2):221–6.

10. Jansen TC, van Bommel J, Woodward R, et al. Association between blood lactate levels, Sequential Organ Failure Assessment subscores, and 28-day mortality during early and late intensive care unit stay: a retrospective observational study. Crit Care Med 2009;37(8):2369–74.

11. Bakker J, Nijsten MW, Jansen TC. Clinical use of lactate monitoring in critically ill patients. Ann Intensive Care 2013;3(1):12.

12. Jansen TC, van Bommel J, Bakker J. Blood lactate monitoring in critically ill patients: a systematic health technology assessment. Crit Care Med 2009;37(10): 2827–39.

13. Leverve XM. Energy metabolism in critically ill patients: lactate is a major oxidizable substrate. Curr Opin Clin Nutr Metab Care 1999;2(2):165–9.

14. Brooks GA. Lactate shuttles in nature. Biochem Soc Trans 2002;30(2):258–64.

15. Ferguson BS, Rogatzki MJ, Goodwin ML, et al. Lactate metabolism: historical context, prior misinterpretations, and current understanding. Eur J Appl Physiol 2018;118(4):691–728.

16. Garcia-Alvarez M, Marik P, Bellomo R. Sepsis-associated hyperlactatemia. Crit Care 2014;18(5):503.

17. Zhang H, Vincent JL. Oxygen extraction is altered by endotoxin during tamponade-induced stagnant hypoxia in the dog. Circ Shock 1993;40(3):168–76.

18. Zhang H, Spapen H, Benlabed M, et al. Systemic oxygen extraction can be improved during repeated episodes of cardiac tamponade. J Crit Care 1993; 8(2):93–9.

19. Ince C. Hemodynamic coherence and the rationale for monitoring the microcirculation. Crit Care 2015;19(Suppl 3):S8.

20. Hernandez G, Boerma EC, Dubin A, et al. Severe abnormalities in microvascular perfused vessel density are associated to organ dysfunctions and mortality and can be predicted by hyperlactatemia and norepinephrine requirements in septic shock patients. J Crit Care 2013;28(4):538.e9-14.

21. De Backer D, Creteur J, Dubois MJ, et al. The effects of dobutamine on microcirculatory alterations in patients with septic shock are independent of its systemic effects. Crit Care Med 2006;34(2):403–8.

22. Alegria L, Vera M, Dreyse J, et al. A hypoperfusion context may aid to interpret hyperlactatemia in sepsis-3 septic shock patients: a proof-of-concept study. Ann Intensive Care 2017;7(1):29.

23. Levy B. Lactate and shock state: the metabolic view. Curr Opin Crit Care 2006; 12(4):315–21.

24. Vary TC. Sepsis-induced alterations in pyruvate dehydrogenase complex activity in rat skeletal muscle: effects on plasma lactate. Shock 1996;6(2):89–94.

25. Levy B, Gibot S, Franck P, et al. Relation between muscle Na+K+ ATPase activity and raised lactate concentrations in septic shock: a prospective study. Lancet 2005;365(9462):871–5.

26. Tapia P, Soto D, Bruhn A, et al. Impairment of exogenous lactate clearance in experimental hyperdynamic septic shock is not related to total liver hypoperfusion. Crit Care 2015;19(1):188.

27. Levraut J, Ciebiera JP, Chave S, et al. Mild hyperlactatemia in stable septic patients is due to impaired lactate clearance rather than overproduction. Am J Respir Crit Care Med 1998;157(4):1021–6.

28. Levraut J, Ichai C, Petit I, et al. Low exogenous lactate clearance as an early predictor of mortality in normolactatemic critically ill septic patients. Crit Care Med 2003;31(3):705–10.

29. van Genderen ME, Klijn E, Lima A, et al. Microvascular perfusion as a target for fluid resuscitation in experimental circulatory shock. Crit Care Med 2014;42(2): E96–105.

30. Hernandez G, Luengo C, Bruhn A, et al. When to stop septic shock resuscitation: clues from a dynamic perfusion monitoring. Ann Intensive Care 2014;4:30.

31. Mekontso-Dessap A, Castelain V, Anguel N, et al. Combination of venoarterial PCO2 difference with arteriovenous O2 content difference to detect anaerobic metabolism in patients. Intensive Care Med 2002;28(3):272–7.

32. Ospina-Tascon GA, Umana M, Bermudez WF, et al. Can venous-to-arterial carbon dioxide differences reflect microcirculatory alterations in patients with septic shock? Intensive Care Med 2016;42(2):211–21.

33. Ospina-Tascon GA, Umana M, Bermudez W, et al. Combination of arterial lactate levels and venous-arterial CO2 to arterial-venous O2 content difference ratio as markers of resuscitation in patients with septic shock. Intensive Care Med 2015;41(5):796–805.

34. Leverve XM. From tissue perfusion to metabolic marker: assessing organ competition and co-operation in critically ill patients? Intensive Care Med 1999;25(9): 890–2.

35. Levy B, Sadoune LO, Gelot AM, et al. Evolution of lactate/pyruvate and arterial ketone body ratios in the early course of catecholamine-treated septic shock. Crit Care Med 2000;28(1):114–9.

36. Levy B, Bollaert PE, Charpentier C, et al. Comparison of norepinephrine and dobutamine to epinephrine for hemodynamics, lactate metabolism, and gastric tonometric variables in septic shock: a prospective, randomized study. Intensive Care Med 1997;23(3):282–7.

37. Lazaridis C, Andrews CM. Brain tissue oxygenation, lactate-pyruvate ratio, and cerebrovascular pressure reactivity monitoring in severe traumatic brain injury: systematic review and viewpoint. Neurocrit Care 2014;21(2):345–55.

38. Haitsma IK, Maas AI. Advanced monitoring in the intensive care unit: brain tissue oxygen tension. Curr Opin Crit Care 2002;8(2):115–20.

39. Nortje J, Gupta AK. The role of tissue oxygen monitoring in patients with acute brain injury. Br J Anaesth 2006;97(1):95–106.

40. Almenoff PL, Leavy J, Weil MH, et al. Prolongation of the half-life of lactate after maximal exercise in patients with hepatic dysfunction. Crit Care Med 1989; 17(9):870–3.

41. Mustafa I, Roth H, Hanafiah A, et al. Effect of cardiopulmonary bypass on lactate metabolism. Intensive Care Med 2003;29(8):1279–85.

42. Vincent JL. Serial blood lactate levels reflect both lactate production and clearance. Crit Care Med 2015;43(6):e209.

43. Vincent JL, Dufaye P, Berre J, et al. Serial lactate determinations during circulatory shock. Crit Care Med 1983;11(6):449–51.

44. Nichol A, Bailey M, Egi M, et al. Dynamic lactate indices as predictors of outcome in critically ill patients. Crit Care 2011;15(5):R242.

45. Donnino MW, Andersen LW, Giberson T, et al. Initial lactate and lactate change in post-cardiac arrest: a multicenter validation study*. Crit Care Med 2014;42(8): 1804–11.

46. During J, Dankiewicz J, Cronberg T, et al. Lactate, lactate clearance and outcome after cardiac arrest: a post-hoc analysis of the TTM-trial. Acta Anaesthesiol Scand 2018;62(10):1436–42.

47. Zhang Z, Xu X. Lactate clearance is a useful biomarker for the prediction of all-cause mortality in critically ill patients: a systematic review and meta-analysis*. Crit Care Med 2014;42(9):2118–25.

48. Li S, Peng K, Liu F, et al. Changes in blood lactate levels after major elective abdominal surgery and the association with outcomes: a prospective observational study. J Surg Res 2013;184(2):1059–69.

49. Vincent JL, Quintairos ESA, Couto L Jr, et al. The value of blood lactate kinetics in critically ill patients: a systematic review. Crit Care 2016;20(1):257.

50. Gu WJ, Zhang Z, Bakker J. Early lactate clearance-guided therapy in patients with sepsis: a meta-analysis with trial sequential analysis of randomized controlled trials. Intensive Care Med 2015;41(10):1862–3.

51. Ding XF, Yang ZY, Xu ZT, et al. Early goal-directed and lactate-guided therapy in adult patients with severe sepsis and septic shock: a meta-analysis of randomized controlled trials. J Transl Med 2018;16(1):331.

52. Rivers E, Nguyen B, Havstad S, et al. Early goal-directed therapy in the treatment of severe sepsis and septic shock. N Engl J Med 2001;345(19):1368–77.

53. Investigators P, Yealy DM, Kellum JA, et al. A randomized trial of protocol-based care for early septic shock. N Engl J Med 2014;370(18):1683–93.

54. Investigators A, Group ACT, Peake SL, et al. Goal-directed resuscitation for patients with early septic shock. N Engl J Med 2014;371(16):1496–506.

55. Investigators PT, Mouncey PR, Osborn TM, et al. Trial of early, goal-directed resuscitation for septic shock. N Engl J Med 2015;372(14):1301–11.

56. Hernandez G, Ospina-Tascon GA, Damiani LP, et al. Effect of a resuscitation strategy targeting peripheral perfusion status vs serum lactate levels on 28-day mortality among patients with septic shock: the ANDROMEDA-SHOCK randomized clinical trial. JAMA 2019;321(7):654–64.

57. Jones AE, Shapiro NI, Trzeciak S, et al. Lactate clearance vs central venous oxygen saturation as goals of early sepsis therapy: a randomized clinical trial. JAMA 2010;303(8):739–46.

58. Jansen TC, van Bommel J, Schoonderbeek FJ, et al. Early lactate-guided therapy in intensive care unit patients a multicenter, open-label, randomized controlled trial. Am J Respir Crit Care Med 2010;182(6):752–61.

59. Weil MH, Afifi AA. Experimental and clinical studies on lactate and pyruvate as indicators of the severity of acute circulatory failure (shock). Circulation 1970; 41(6):989–1001.

60. Peretz DI, Scott HM, Duff J, et al. The significance of lacticacidemia in the shock syndrome. Ann N Y Acad Sci 1965;119(3):1133–41.

61. Moskowitz A, Graver A, Giberson T, et al. The relationship between lactate and thiamine levels in patients with diabetic ketoacidosis. J Crit Care 2014;29(1); 182.e5–8.

62. Orringer CE, Eustace JC, Wunsch CD, et al. Natural history of lactic acidosis after grand-mal seizures. A model for the study of an anion-gap acidosis not associated with hyperkalemia. N Engl J Med 1977;297(15):796–9.

63. Sokal JA, Kralkowska E. The relationship between exposure duration, carboxyhemoglobin, blood glucose, pyruvate and lactate and the severity of intoxication in 39 cases of acute carbon monoxide poisoning in man. Arch Toxicol 1985;57(3): 196–9.

64. Baud FJ, Haidar MK, Jouffroy R, et al. Determinants of lactic acidosis in acute cyanide poisonings. Crit Care Med 2018;46(6):e523–9.
65. Monnet X, Julien F, Ait-Hamou N, et al. Lactate and venoarterial carbon dioxide difference/arterial-venous oxygen difference ratio, but not central venous oxygen saturation, predict increase in oxygen consumption in fluid responders. Crit Care Med 2013;41(6):1412–20.
66. Lara B, Enberg L, Ortega M, et al. Capillary refill time during fluid resuscitation in patients with sepsis-related hyperlactatemia at the emergency department is related to mortality. PLoS One 2017;12(11):e0188548.

The Role of Biomarkers in Acute Kidney Injury

Nattachai Srisawat, MD, PhD[a,b,c,d,e,f], John A. Kellum, MD[b,*]

KEYWORDS

- NGAL • TIMP-2 • IGFBP7 • KIM-1 • IL-18

KEY POINTS

- Indicators of kidney function, including serum creatinine and urine output, are insufficient for timely detection of acute kidney injury.
- Several acute kidney injury biomarkers have been discovered and validated, often in large clinical studies and in experimental models.
- Anatomic sources within the nephron and new mechanistic insights have been discovered for these markers.
- Implementation trials have been slow to emerge but are becoming available for newer tests such as those measuring tissue inhibitor of metalloproteinases-2 and insulin-like growth factor-binding protein 7 ([TIMP2]•[IGFBP7]).

INTRODUCTION

In the past 50 years, the diagnosis of acute kidney injury (AKI) has been mainly based on serum creatinine.[1] It is well known that an increase in serum creatinine level occurs after a significant reduction in glomerular filtration rate (GFR). However, for most forms of AKI, the renal tubular epithelium, not glomeruli, is the primary locus of injury, and a decreased GFR is a late and insensitive indicator. Thus, reliance solely on changes in

Disclosures: N. Srisawat discloses grant support from Baxter. J.A. Kellum discloses grant support and consulting fees from Astute Medical, bioMerieux, and Bioporto.
[a] Division of Nephrology, Faculty of Medicine, Chulalongkorn University, Bangkok, Thailand; 3rd floor, Anantamahidol Building, Henri Dunant Road, Pathumwan, Bangkok 10330, Thailand; [b] Department of Critical Care Medicine, Center for Critical Care Nephrology, The CRISMA Center, University of Pittsburgh School of Medicine, 3347 Forbes Avenue, Suite 220, Pittsburgh, PA 15213, USA; [c] Excellence Center for Critical Care Nephrology, King Chulalongkorn Memorial Hospital, 1873 Rama IV Road, Khwaeng Pathum Wan, Khet Pathum Wan, Krung Thep Maha Nakhon 10330, Thailand; [d] Critical Care Nephrology Research Unit, Chulalongkorn University, 3rd floor, Anantamahidol Building, Henri Dunant Road, Pathumwan, Bangkok 10330, Thailand; [e] Academic of Science, Royal Society of Thailand, 197 Rama 5 Road Khwaeng Dusit, Khet Dusit, Bangkok 10300, Thailand; [f] Tropical Medicine Cluster, Chulalongkorn University, 3rd floor, Anantamahidol Building, Henri Dunant Road, Pathumwan, Bangkok 10330, Thailand
* Corresponding author.
E-mail address: kellum@pitt.edu

Table 1
The origin of biomarkers based on biological properties

Biology	Biomarkers
Filtered-impaired tubular reabsorption	Albumin, Cystatin C, Beta 2 microglobulin, L-FABP
Upregulation	NGAL, KIM-1, Clusterin, IL-18, Netrin-1
Downregulation	TFF3
Preformed	ALP, GGT, GST, NAG, L-FABP, TIMP-2, IGFBP7

Abbreviations: ALP, alkaline phosphatase; GGT, gamma glutaryl transferase; GST, glutathione S-transferase; IGFBP7, insulinlike growth factor–binding protein 7; IL, interleukin; KIM-1, kidney injury molecule-1; L-FABP, liver-type fatty acid–binding protein; NAG, *N*-acetyl-beta-D-glucosaminidase; NGAL, neutrophil gelatinase associated lipocalin; TIMP-2, tissue inhibitor of mettaloproteinase-2; TFF3, trefoil factor 3.

serum creatinine level might result in a delay in AKI management and lead to unfavorable outcomes. Over the past 10 years, many efforts have been made to find specific biomarkers that can detect acute damage in the renal tubular epithelium. This idea is similar to the concept of markers for myocyte injury (eg, troponin), which are specific markers in the diagnosis of myocardial infarction.[2,3]

However, unlike myocardial ischemia, in which acute coronary syndrome is the dominant cause, AKI can be caused by many different conditions. Furthermore, injury to renal epithelial cells may not manifest in subsequent functional change and, thus, specificity may be difficult to confirm. Most studies have aimed to discover biomarkers through high-throughput techniques and validate them in large cohorts of patients. Very few studies have examined clinical implementation of AKI biomarkers to improve AKI care and patient outcomes.

Biomarkers can be detected in both blood and urine. However, urine biomarkers have been most extensively studied because urine is a more proximal fluid to the location of injury and because blood is a more complex substrate for biomarker discovery work. The pathway for biomarker research in general is shown in **Fig. 1**.

LIMITATIONS OF SERUM CREATININE IN THE DIAGNOSIS OF ACUTE KIDNEY INJURY

Serum creatinine has been used to detect changes in kidney function for more than 50 years. The half-life of serum creatinine is about 4 hours. At the point of a 50%

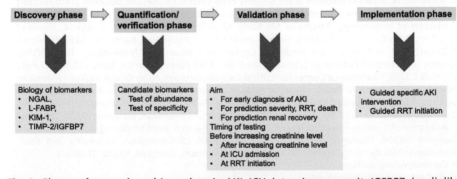

Fig. 1. Phases of research on biomarkers in AKI. ICU, intensive care unit; IGFBP7, insulinlike growth factor–binding protein 7; KIM-1, kidney injury molecule-1; L-FABP, liver-type fatty acid–binding protein; NGAL, neutrophil gelatinase associated lipocalin; RRT, renal replacement therapy; TIMP-2, tissue inhibitor of metalloproteinases-2.

reduction in creatinine clearance, the half-life of serum creatinine is about 8 hours and it takes another 3 to 5 half-lives before reaching its peak or reaching a steady state (ie, it takes 24 to 40 hours). This limitation makes serum creatinine a delayed marker of AKI even when GFR has decreased by half.

In certain situations, an increase in serum creatinine level overestimates the change in GFR (eg, rhabdomyolysis, exposure to certain medications such as cephalosporins and sulfa). In other conditions, serum creatinine level may underestimate changes in GFR (eg, cirrhosis, hyperbilirubinemia, fluid overload, elderly patients, and others with an acute loss in muscle mass). Thus, serum creatinine level is limited by lack of specificity, sensitivity, and timeliness.

Urine output may provide more timely information about AKI because anuric patients have a GFR of zero. Even less severe alterations in renal function may manifest as oliguria long before serum creatinine level increases. However, urine output also lacks sensitivity and nonoliguric AKI may also occur. Specificity is also limited.

PHASES OF ACUTE KIDNEY INJURY BIOMARKER DEVELOPMENT

There are several discrete phases to biomarker discovery. At each stage the number of candidates decreases and complexity of studies increases. Only a small number of AKI biomarkers have progressed across most of these stages and only 1 has gone all the way.

Discovery Phase

In this phase, so-called proximal fluids (eg, urine), cell culture supernatants, and tissues from animal models are used. Gold-standard samples are used (both cases and controls) to reduce biological variation. The goal is to find candidates that can be tested in the next phases. Technologies such as proteomic analysis are applied to differentiate protein expression in samples from cases (patients, animals, cells) with and without AKI. The first-generation AKI biomarkers, such as neutrophil gelatinase–associated lipocalin (NGAL), were initially identified by such techniques.

Quantification/Verification Phase

In this phase, candidates are first confirmed to have differential abundance (quantification) in samples from humans with disease (gold standards: low variation) and then verification is performed in population-derived samples (normal background variation). Verification is aimed primarily at understanding specificity so the number of samples tested must be large enough to confidently include potential sources of false-positivity (typically a few hundred). In this phase, multiple candidates are still often compared.

Validation Phase

In addition, candidates that survive these first 2 phases are then subjected to a more rigorous validation, typically using a clinical assay (high throughput) and sensitivity and specificity are established. Most often a single candidate marker or maker panel is subjected to a validation phase. Larger sample sizes are required (typically several hundred patients) to ensure adequate representation of clinical heterogeneity. Moreover, if a multicenter study is performed, the results will be more convincing and its acceptance will be higher. For example, the Sapphire study,[4] which was a study of 2 biomarkers, insulinlike growth factor–binding protein 7 (IGFBP7) and tissue inhibitor of metalloproteinases-2 (TIMP-2), revealed that the combination of IGFBP7 and TIMP-2 was significantly superior to all other existing biomarkers for detection of AKI manifesting in the next 12 hours, with an area under the receiver operating curve (AUC) of 0.80. A test incorporating this combination (Nephrocheck, Astute Medical, San Diego, CA) was subsequently approved by the US Food and Drug Administration (FDA) for clinical use after an additional validation study[4] was performed.

Implementation Phase

In this phase, biomarkers are applied in clinical use in many ways, and patient-centered outcomes are measured. The challenge for new biomarkers is that effective treatments need to be paired with the test in order to show benefit. For AKI, 2 single-center studies have shown benefit associated with the use of [TIMP-2]•[IGFBP7] in patients after surgery.[5,6] In the first study,[5] biomarker-positive patients were randomized to receive a care bundle that included a hemodynamic management algorithm based on mean arterial pressure and stroke volume variation. AKI was significantly reduced with the intervention compared with controls (55.1 vs 71.7%; absolute risk reduction (ARR) 16.6% [95 confidence interval [CI], 5.5%–27.9%]; $P = .004$). Rates of moderate to severe AKI were also significantly reduced by the intervention compared with controls (41 out of 138 [29.7%] vs 62 out of 138 [44.9%]; $P = .009$; odds ratio [OR], 0.518 [95% CI, 0.316–0.851]; ARR, 15.2% [95% CI, 4.0%–26.5%]). The intervention resulted in significantly improved hemodynamics ($P<.05$) as well as less hyperglycemia ($P<.001$) and use of angiotensin-converting enzyme inhibitors/angiotensin receptor blockers ($P<.001$) compared with controls. The total administered volume was not different between the two groups, but the distribution of fluid was different, with patients in the intervention group receiving significantly less volume during the last 3 hours of the intervention period ($P = .024$). However, there were no differences in rates of renal replacement therapy between intervention and control, whether within 72 hours (7.2% vs 5.1%, $P = .45$), during hospitalization (10.1% vs 6.5%, $P = .28$), or at 30 days (3.1% vs 2.3%. $P = .72$). Neither were there differences in mortality or persistent renal dysfunction at 30, 60, or 90 days.

In the second study,[6] a similar care bundle, including early optimization of fluids and maintenance of perfusion pressure, was applied to noncardiac major surgery patients after testing positive for the biomarker. Overall AKI rates were not statistically different between groups (19 out of 60 [31.7%] in the intervention group vs. 29 out of 61 [47.5%] in the standard care group; $P = .076$). However, rates of moderate and severe AKI, a secondary end point, were reduced with the intervention (4 out of 60 [6.7%] vs 12 out of 61 [19.7%; $P = .04$), as were lengths of intensive care unit (ICU) stay (median difference, 1 day; $P = .035$) and hospital stay (median difference, 5 days; $P = .04$). There were no significant differences regarding renal replacement therapy, in-hospital mortality, or major kidney events at hospital discharge.

ORIGIN OF URINARY BIOMARKERS

There are 3 broad categories of urinary biomarkers. The first group includes biomarkers that have low molecular weight and are freely filtered at the glomerulus. Under normal circumstances, these biomarkers are reabsorbed by the process of proximal tubule endocytosis. For example, low-molecular-weight proteins (eg, β2-microglobulin, lysozyme, α1-microglobulin, light chains, and cystatin C) are filtered by the glomerulus and reabsorbed completely by proximal tubular epithelial cells so that only following epithelial cell injury can these biomarkers be detected in the urine.[7–11]

A second group of biomarkers are upregulated in renal cells in response to kidney injury. These molecules include NGAL and kidney injury molecule-1 (KIM-1), which are expressed mainly in distal and proximal tubular epithelial cells respectively. Some bio-markers are also upregulated in interstitial cells in response to kidney injury, such as hepatocyte growth factor (HGF).[12–14] A third group of biomarkers are constitutively expressed by tubular epithelial cells and then released into the urine in response to AKI. Examples of this group include the lysosomal enzyme N-acetyl-b-D-glucosami-nidase (NAG),[15] the cytosolic protein lactate dehydrogenase,[16] and the brush border. protein gp130.[17] The recently discovered biomarkers TIMP-2 and IGFBP7 seem to also be constitutively produced but are released rapidly in response to injurious (or even non injurious) noxious stimuli.[18] In addition, biomarkers such as interleukin (IL)-18 are released by inflammatory cells such as macrophages or neutrophils entering the kidneys during AKI. The origins of the urinary biomarkers are summarized in **Fig. 2** and **Table 1**.

CURRENT ACUTE KIDNEY INJURY BIOMARKERS

The following biomarkers have been extensively studied and widely used as diag-nostic tests of AKI. **Table 2** compares the characteristic of AKI biomarkers and avail-able clinical studies.

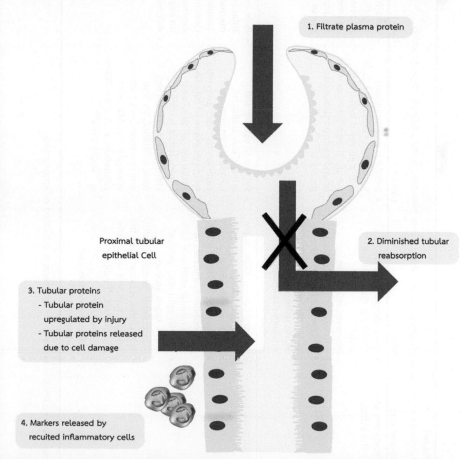

Fig. 2. The origin of biomarkers in urine.

Table 2
Comparison of characteristics of acute kidney injury biomarkers and available clinical studies

Biomarkers	NGAL	L-FABP	KIM-1	TIMP-2/IGFBP7
Producing sites in the kidney	• Thick ascending limb, collecting duct tubular cells[19] • However, NGAL can be detected at the proximal tubular epithelium because of the failure of filtered NGAL reabsorption in a megalin-dependent manner.[20–22]	• L-FABP is predominantly found in the proximal tubule and is excreted into the tubular lumen together with bound toxic peroxisomal products[52–54]	• Data from ischemia/reperfusion injury models and nephrotoxic induced AKI models indicated that the proximal tubule is the site of KIM-1 production[62,63]	• Although various parts of the nephron can produce both markers, the main source of TIMP-2 is the distal tubule and, for IGFBP7, the proximal tubule[18,76]
Functional role in the kidney	• Iron-trafficking: NGAL is an important transport protein in the process of iron transport by binding to iron-siderophore complexes in renal tubular epithelial cells • Tubular epithelial genesis: NGAL forms an iron-siderophore complex (Holo-NGAL) that is secreted by the ureteric bud and can induce the genesis of tubular epithelium[23] • Antiinflammatory and antiapoptotic[20]	• Fatty acid uptake and intracellular transport: L-FABP might help to mobilize the lipid peroxides from cytoplasm of tubular epithelial cell to tubular lumen, hence preventing kidney damage from this toxic substance. Various proteins/conditions that can upregulate L-FABP gene expression, such as the PPAR-α,[56] hypoxemia[54,57]	• Role in renal recovery and tubular regeneration: the mechanism related to apoptotic body clearance,[65,66] peak expression of KIM-1 occurs on day 2–3 after injury[64] • Antiinflammation effect[63]	• Cell-cycle arrest: both TIMP-2 and IGFBP7 are cell-cycle regulators and can induce cell-cycle arrest, thought to be a protective mechanism[68]

Abbreviation: PPAR-α, peroxisome proliferator activated receptor-alpha.

Neutrophil Gelatinase–Associated Lipocalin

NGAL is the most studied AKI biomarker. This 25-kDa protein was first discovered in the granules of neutrophils. NGAL plays a role in innate immunity via a bacteriostatic effect in which NGAL can block iron uptake by bacteria. Later it was found in many organs, such as kidney (proximal/distal tubular epithelial cells), lung, and large intestine. Increase of plasma NGAL level can also be seen as result of hepatic production. The origin of urinary NGAL was debated for many years until Paragas and colleagues[19] showed that the thick ascending limb and the intercalated cells of the collecting duct were the main intrarenal production site, and NGAL can also be detected at the proximal tubular epithelium because of the failure of filtered NGAL reabsorption in a megalin-dependent manner.[20–22] **Fig. 3** shows the site of NGAL in the nephron and the role of NGAL in the functioning of renal tubule cells.[23–25]

Clinical studies of neutrophil gelatinase–associated lipocalin in acute kidney injury

At present, NGAL is the most widely studied AKI biomarker. An important caveat is that age, gender (female), urinary tract infection, and impaired renal function (chronic kidney disease) may increase levels of urine NGAL.[26–30]

- To predict/diagnosis AKI

  NGAL has been found to be most useful following cardiac surgery (especially in children), in kidney transplant, and in the critically ill.[25,31–36] Two recent meta-analyses, by Hasse and colleagues[37] and Ho and colleagues,[38] included 19 studies with 2538 patients and 16 studies with 2906 patients, respectively, and found the AUC for urine NGAL to predict AKI was 0.82 and 0.72, respectively.

- To prediction persistent AKI

  The distinction between transient and persistent AKI is clinically important because the treatment of these conditions can be different. For example, the use of renal replacement therapy (RRT) is typically reserved for

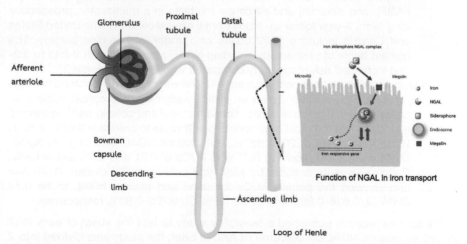

Fig. 3. The site of NGAL production in the nephron; intercalated cells of collecting tubule, and the role of NGAL in renal tubule cells. NGAL is involved in the iron transport and binds siderophore to form iron-siderophore complex, which enters renal tubule cells via megalin. Iron-siderophore NGAL complex in renal tubule cells is stored in endosome and then iron is released, which directly results in the function of iron-responsive gene.

persistent AKI. In 2 studies the predictive ability for NGAL for this indication was low, with an AUC of only 0.5.[39,40]Singer and colleagues[41] used urine NGAL to distinguish so-called prerenal AKI from intrinsic AKI from the clinical course and response to therapy. Although roughly a quarter of patients could not be classified, urine NGAL was able to distinguish remaining patients between the two conditions with 87% accuracy. If urine NGAL level was greater than 104 ng/mL, it is likely to be intrinsic AKI (likelihood ratio, 5.97), and, if urine NGAL level is less than 47 ng/mL, it is less likely to be intrinsic AKI.

- To predict short-term outcome and renal recovery

   Urine NGAL and KIM-1 may predict the composite outcome of death and dialysis.[41,42] Prediction of recovery of renal function after AKI is clinically important. In addition to renal prognosis, it helps in quickly making decisions for some treatments, such as RRT. The authors tested the role of plasma NGAL in predicting recovery of kidney function in patients with severe AKI (stage 3) and found an AUC of 0.74. Patients with renal recovery had lower plasma NGAL levels compared with patients with no renal recovery.[43] In another study, the authors tested biomarkers of NGAL, cystatin C, HGF, matrix metalloproteinase (MMP)-9, and IL-18 in the urine.[26] These biomarkers were measured during the first 2 weeks after starting RRT. None of the available markers could predict the recovery of renal function on their own, but models that included multiple markers along with clinical variables could perform reasonably well (AUC, 0.78) even on day 1.[42]

- To predict long-term outcomes

   Only a few studies of NGAL, or other AKI biomarkers, have focused on long-term outcomes. Ralib and colleagues[44] explored the predictability role of urine NGAL, IL-18, and KIM-1 in the critical care setting for 1-year mortality and found modest discrimination, with an AUC of 0.60. Coca and colleagues[45] studied the association between 5 urinary kidney injury biomarkers (NGAL, IL-18, KIM-1, liver-type fatty acid–binding protein [L-FABP], and albumin) and all-cause mortality in a multicenter, prospective long-term, 3-year follow-up study from 6 clinical centers in the United States and Canada including 1199 adults who underwent cardiac surgery. The highest tertile of biomarkers including NGAL associated with 2-fold to 3.2-fold increased risk of mortality compared with the lowest tertile.[46]

- Decision making on treatment such as RRT and withdrawal of nephrotoxic drugs

   At present, RRT initiation relies on clinical judgment, and considerable variability in clinical practice exists. Tiranathanagul and colleagues[47] performed a study to find the most appropriate cutoff value to predict initiation of RRT. Urine NGAL level of 2000 ng/mL and plasma NGAL level of 1000 ng/mL could predict AKI requiring RRT with AUCs of 0.81 and 0.81, respectively. Recently, a meta-analysis by Klein and colleagues[48] included 41 studies and showed the pooled AUCs for urine and plasma NGAL to be 0.72 (95% CI, 0.638–0.803) and 0.755 (95% CI, 0.706–0.803), respectively.

The authors recently published a feasibility study to test the effect of early RRT guided by plasma NGAL on outcome of AKI. In brief, the study was divided into 2 phases, triage and interventional phase, running subsequently. As a guide for triage to RRT, the authors measured plasma NGAL (pNGAL) at enrollment. Forty patients with plasma NGAL level greater than or equal to 400 ng/mL (high pNGAL group) were randomized to the early or standard group. Patients with plasma

NGAL level less than 400 ng/mL (n = 20) were defined as the low pNGAL group. Plasma NGAL selected patients with AKI with more severity of illness and worse clinical outcome. However, in the high pNGAL group, early RRT did not result in different 28-day mortality from the standard group. However, the median number of days free from mechanical ventilation were significantly higher in the early RRT group.[49]

In summary, of the available AKI biomarkers, NGAL has been most widely investigated. Different investigators analyzed diverse patient populations and determined the performance of NGAL for different indications. It is clear that NGAL is expressed in a severity-dependent fashion in AKI and is activated at the time of patient presentation; for example, in the after contrast exposure, after cardiac surgery, and after kidney transplant. It is also clear that dehydration alone does not trigger NGAL expression, whereas kidney damage does. However, NGAL expression lacks specificity for AKI, and the diversity of test kits on the market means that cutoffs are unclear.

Liver-type Fatty Acid–Binding Protein

This biomarker has a molecular weight of 14 kDa and is member of a superfamily of lipid-binding proteins, consisting of 9 members named for the organs in which they were first identified: liver (L), intestine (I), muscle (M), heart (H), adipocyte (A), epidermal (E), ileum (IL), brain (B), testis (T), and myelin (MY). L-FABP is critical for fatty acid uptake and facilitates the transfer of fatty acids between extracellular and intracellular membranes.

L-FABP is not only found in the liver but also in many organs, such as intestine, stomach, lung, and kidney. L-FABP can be detected in urine and but there is no standard cutoff point for the diagnosis of AKI. Recently, urinary L-FABP was approved as an AKI biomarker in Japan. **Fig. 4** shows the production sites in the kidney, and the functional role of L-FABP is described in **Table 2**.[50–55] Recently, 249 critically ill patients were studied to analyze the distinct clinical characteristics of NGAL and L-FABP. NGAL showed linear correlations with inflammatory markers (white blood cell count and C-reactive protein), whereas L-FABP showed linear correlations with

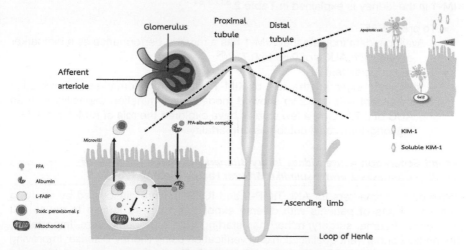

Fig. 4. The role of L-FABP in transport of free fatty acid (FFA) into renal tubule cells and elimination of toxic peroxisomal products from renal tubule cells. Also shown is the role of KIM-1 in removal of apoptotic bodies during kidney injury.

hypoperfusion and hepatic injury markers (lactate, liver transaminases, and bilirubin). This finding is compatible with the basic mechanism of L-FABP, which is thought to be a marker of renal hypoxia (see **Fig. 4**).

- To predict/diagnosis AKI

    Ho and colleagues[38] analyzed the role of L-FABP to predict AKI after cardiac surgery by included 6 major studies and showed AUCs between 0.52 and 0.85 with a composite AUC of 0.72. In critically ill patients, Noiri and colleagues[55] showed the superiority of L-FABP in predicting AKI compared with other biomarkers, including NGAL, IL-18, NAG, and albumin, with an AUC of 0.75. In the setting of contrast-associated AKI, Nakamura and colleagues[56] explored the utility of urine L-FABP in patients undergoing nonemergency cardiac catheterization and found a significant increase of urine L-FABP level in patients developing AKI, whereas there was no change in those patients not developing AKI.

- To prediction persistent AKI

    Recently, Matsuura and colleagues,[57] summarized 3 prospective studies conducted in Japan and Thailand to evaluate the accuracy of renal angina index (RAI) and L-FABP. At a cutoff of 6, the RAI showed a good performance, with an AUC of 0.73. When combined with L-FABP, the predictive performance for predicting persistent AKI increased to an AUC of 0.79. Few studies have explored the role of L-FABP in predicting short-term or long-term renal outcomes or mortality.

Kidney Injury Molecule-1

KIM-1 is a 38.7-kDa protein. It is a type 1 transmembrane glycoprotein. After ischemic/reperfusion injury and nephrotoxic exposure, KIM-1 is markedly upregulated in the injured proximal tubular epithelium. In response to injury, the extracellular component of KIM-1 is shed from the cell membrane into the tubular lumen in an MMP-dependent manner.[58,59]

Fig. 4 shows the sites of production of KIM-1 in the kidney, and the functional role of KIM-1 in the kidney is explained in **Table 2**.[58,60–64]

- To predict AKI

    Available data indicate that KIM-1 has a modest performance as a biomarker of AKI, with AUCs of 0.69 to 0.7.[65,66]

- To predict persistent AKI

    Nickolas[67] explored the role of KIM-1 with other biomarkers in predicting persistent AKI and also showed modest discrimination capability with an AUC of 0.7.[40] Only a few studies have explored the role of KIM-1 in predicting long-term renal outcomes or mortality.

Second-Generation Acute Kidney Injury Biomarkers: Tissue Inhibitor of Metalloproteinases-2 and Insulinlike Growth Factor–Binding Protein 7

Unlike other biomarkers for AKI, TIMP-2 and IGFBP7 were discovered by studying multiple cohorts of patients with diverse exposures that are known to cause AKI (eg, sepsis, trauma, surgery) rather than starting from a model system. Importantly, the markers underwent qualification and verification using Kidney Disease: Improving Global Outcomes (KDIGO) criteria for AKI (stage 2–3), which were not available when other biomarkers were discovered. Thus, TIMP-2 and IGFP7 are the first second-generation AKI biomarkers (**Fig. 5**).

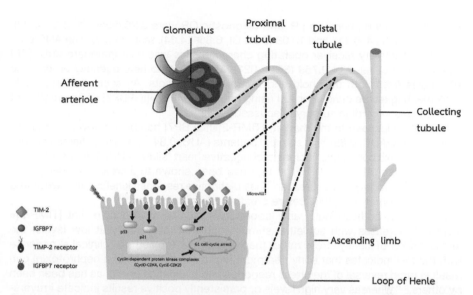

Fig. 5. The mechanisms that occur within renal tubule cells during AKI. TIMP-2 and IGFBP7 increase and activate p53, p21, and p27, which results in the inhibition of the function of cyclin-dependent protein kinase (CDK) complexes and cell-cycle arrest in renal tubule cells.

The first report of TIMP-2 and IGFBP7 as markers of AKI came from Kashani and colleagues.[68] This study included adult patients in ICUs in 35 centers across North America and Europe. In the discovery phase, 522 patients were enrolled in 3 distinct cohorts, including patients with sepsis, shock, major surgery, and trauma, and were examined for 300 markers. In the validation phase, the final analysis cohort was a heterogeneous sample of 728 critically ill patients. The primary end point was moderate to severe AKI (KDIGO stage 2–3) within 12 hours of sample collection, which occurred in 14% of subjects. Urinary [TIMP-2]•[IGFBP7] showed an AUC of 0.80 and was significantly superior to all existing markers of AKI ($P<.002$), none of which achieved an AUC greater than 0.72. In sensitivity analyses, [TIMP-2]•[IGFBP7] remained significant and superior to all other markers regardless of changes in reference creatinine method.

A second large multicenter study was conducted for FDA registration and this study took the additional step of requiring that the end point be subject to confirmation by a clinical adjudication committee who were blinded to the biomarker results.[4] This study enrolled 420 critically ill patients, and urinary TIMP-2 and IGFBP7 were measured using a clinical immunoassay platform. The primary end point (stage 2–3 AKI confirmed by clinical adjudication) was reached in 17% of patients. For a single urinary [TIMP-2]•[IGFBP7] test, sensitivity at the prespecified high-sensitivity cutoff of 0.3 $(ng/mL)^2/1000$ was 92% (95% CI, 85%–98%), with a negative likelihood ratio of 0.18 (95% CI, 0.06–0.33). Critically ill patients with urinary [TIMP-2]•[IGFBP7] greater than 0.3 had 7 times the risk for AKI (95% CI, 4–22) compared with critically ill patients with a test result less than 0.3. Thus, urinary [TIMP-2]•[IGFBP7] greater than 0.3 $(ng/mL)^2/1000$ identifies patients at risk for imminent AKI.

Several subsequent studies have confirmed the initial results in various cohorts; however, cardiac surgery remains the most common.[69] In this area, a total of 10 studies have enrolled 747 patients. Pooled sensitivity and specificity were 0.77 (95% CI, 0.70–0.83) and 0.76 (95% CI, 0.72–0.79), respectively. Pooled positive likelihood ratio (LR), negative LR, and diagnostic OR were 3.26 (95% CI, 2.51–4.23), 0.32 (95% CI, 0.24–0.41), and 10.08 (95% CI, 6.85–14.84), respectively. The AUC estimated by summary receiver operating characteristics was 0.83 (standard error [SE] 0.023) with a Q value of 0.759 (SE, 0.021). There was no heterogeneity among the 10 studies from both threshold and nonthreshold effects. As such, the first study implementing a care bundle for AKI using urinary [TIMP-2]•[IGFBP7] as an enrollment criterion was in cardiac surgery (discussed earlier).[5]

Since its release onto the market, [TIMP-2]•[IGFBP7] has been shown to perform well in sepsis (AUC, 0.85)[70]; in surgical patients (AUC, 0.84)[71]; and in patients with underlying chronic conditions, including congestive heart failure (AUC, 0.89) and chronic kidney disease (AUC, 0.91).[72] The test has been shown to increase rapidly (within 4 hours) after various exposures, and has distinctive response kinetics after exposure to various nephrotoxins, well before creatinine level increases.[73]

Importantly, both clinical[74] and laboratory[18] studies have shown that [TIMP-2]•[IGFBP7] increases with sublethal stimuli such that (particularly at low levels) the test is marker of kidney stress rather than damage.[75] The authors' clinical experience with the test indicates that early treatment (eg, discontinuation of a nephrotoxin) can result in rapid reversal of the stress response and avoidance of AKI, as has been seen by others,[5,6] whereas very high levels or persistently positive results indicate irreversible AKI.

SUMMARY

Although AKI has trailed other areas in the development of biomarkers, there are now multiple tests available in various parts of the world. Both [TIMP-2]•[IGFBP7] and KIM-1 have FDA approval, for clinical risk assessment and nephrotoxicity respectively. The recent studies showing clinical application are still small and single centered but will likely be starting points for large multicenter trials. In addition, new questions concerning the evaluation of the cause of AKI, and prediction of outcomes, including recovery and need for RRT, are being asked and new biomarkers are being evaluated. The future will likely bring many more tests.

REFERENCES

1. Kidney Disease: Improving Global Outcomes (KDIGO) Acute Kidney Injury Work Group. KDIGO clinical practice guideline for acute kidney injury. Kidney Int Suppl 2012;2:1–138.
2. Schrezenmeier EV, Barasch J, Budde K, et al. Biomarkers in acute kidney injury - pathophysiological basis and clinical performance. Acta Physiol (Oxf) 2017; 219(3):554–72.
3. Alge JL, Arthur JM. Biomarkers of AKI: a review of mechanistic relevance and potential therapeutic implications. Clin J Am Soc Nephrol 2015;10(1):147–55.
4. Bihorac A, ChawlaL S, Shaw AD, et al. Validation of cell-cycle arrest biomarkers for acute kidney injury using clinical adjudication. Am J Respir Crit Care Med 2014;189(8):932–9.
5. Meersch M, Schmidt C, Hoffmeier A, et al. Prevention of cardiac surgery-associated AKI by implementing the KDIGO guidelines in high risk patients identified by biomarkers: the PrevAKI randomized controlled trial. Intensive Care Med 2017;43(11):1551–61.
6. Gocze I, Jauch D, Götz M, et al. Biomarker-guided intervention to prevent acute kidney injury after major surgery: the prospective randomized BigpAK study. Ann Surg 2017;267(6):1013–20.

7. Argyropoulos CP, Chen SS, Ng YH, et al. Rediscovering beta-2 microglobulin as a biomarker across the spectrum of kidney diseases. Front Med (Lausanne) 2017;4:73.
8. Tataranni G, Logallo G, Gilli P, et al. Functional recovery phase of acute renal insufficiency. Behavior and significance of urinary excretion of alpha-glucosidase, gamma-glutamyl transferase, lysozyme and beta 2 microglobulin. Minerva Nefrol 1980;27:625–9 [in Italian].
9. Zager RA, Johnson AC, Frostad K, et al. An evaluation of the antioxidant protein a1-microglobulin as a renal tubular cytoprotectant. Am J Physiol Renal Physiol 2016;311:640–51.
10. Zhang R, Li M, Chouhan KK, et al. Urine free light chains as a novel biomarker of acute kidney allograft injury. Clin Transplant 2013;27:953–60.
11. Lagos-Arevalo P, Palijan A, Vertullo L, et al. Cystatin C in acute kidney injury diagnosis: early biomarker or alternative to serum creatinine? Pediatr Nephrol 2015; 30(4):665–76.
12. Zager RA, Vijayan A, Johnson AC. Proximal tubule haptoglobin gene activation is an integral component of the acute kidney injury "stress response". Am J Physiol Renal Physiol 2012;303(1):139–48.
13. Zager RA, Johnson AC, Becker K. Plasma and urinary heme oxygenase-1 in AKI. J Am Soc Nephrol 2012;23:1048–57.
14. Ware LB, Johnson AC, Zager RA. Renal cortical albumin gene induction and urinary albumin excretion in response to acute kidney injury. Am J Physiol Renal Physiol 2011;300:628–38.
15. Cheng B, Jin Y, Liu G, et al. Urinary N-acetyl-beta-D-glucosaminidase as an early marker for acute kidney injury in full-term newborns with neonatal hyperbilirubinemia. Dis Markers 2014;315843:201.
16. Zager RA, Johnson AC, Becker K. Renal cortical lactate dehydrogenase: a useful, accurate, quantitative marker of in vivo tubular injury and acute renal failure. PLoS One 2013;8(6):e66776.
17. Zager RA, Carpenter CB. Radioimmunoassay for urinary renal tubular antigen: a potential marker of tubular injury. Kidney Int 1978;13(6):505–12.
18. Emlet DR, Pastor-Soler N, Marciszyn A, et al. Insulin-like growth factor binding protein 7 and tissue inhibitor of metalloproteinases-2: differential expression and secretion in human kidney tubule cells. Am J Physiol Renal Physiol 2017; 312(2):284–96.
19. Paragas N, Qiu A, Zhang Q, et al. The Ngal reporter mouse detects the response of the kidney to injury in real time. Nat Med 2011;17(2):216–22.
20. Mori K, Lee HT, Rapoport D, et al. Endocytic delivery of lipocalin-siderophore-iron complex rescues the kidney from ischemia-reperfusion injury. J Clin Invest 2005; 115:610–21.
21. Schmidt-Ott KM, Mori K, Kalandadze A, et al. Neutrophil gelatinase-associated lipocalin-mediated iron traffic in kidney epithelia. Curr Opin Nephrol Hypertens 2006;15(4):442–9.
22. Hvidberg V, Jacobsen C, Strong RK, et al. The endocytic receptor megalin binds the iron transporting neutrophil-gelatinase-associated lipocalin with high affinity and mediates its cellular uptake. FEBS Lett 2005;579:773–7.
23. Li JY, Ram G, Gast K, et al. Detection of intracellular iron by its regulatory effect. Am J Physiol Cell Physiol 2004;287(6):1547–59.
24. Mishra J, Dent C, Tarabishi R, et al. Neutrophil gelatinase-associated lipocalin (NGAL) as a biomarker for acute renal injury after cardiac surgery. Lancet 2005;365(9466):1231–8.

25. Parikh CR, Coca SG, Thiessen-Philbrook H, et al. Postoperative biomarkers predict acute kidney injury and poor outcomes after adult cardiac surgery. J Am Soc Nephrol 2011;22(9):1748–57.
26. Ronco C, Bellomo R, Kellum JA. Emerging biomarkers of acute kidney injury. Contrib Nephrol 2007;156:203–12.
27. Schmidt-Ott KM. Neutrophil gelatinase-associated lipocalin as a biomarker of acute kidney injury–where do we stand today? Nephrol Dial Transplant 2011; 26(3):762–4.
28. McIlroy DR, Wagener G, Lee HT. Neutrophil gelatinase-associated lipocalin and acute kidney injury after cardiac surgery: the effect of baseline renal function on diagnostic performance. Clin J Am Soc Nephrol 2010;5(2):211–9.
29. Cullen MR, Murray PT, Fitzgibbon MC. Establishment of a reference interval for urinary neutrophil gelatinase-associated lipocalin. Ann Clin Biochem 2012; 49(2):190–3.
30. Pennemans V, Rigo JM, Faes C, et al. Establishment of reference values for novel urinary biomarkers for renal damage in the healthy population: are age and gender an issue? Clin Chem Lab Med 2013;51(9):1795–802.
31. Dent CL, Ma Q, Dastrala S, et al. Plasma neutrophil gelatinase-associated lipocalin predicts acute kidney injury, morbidity and mortality after pediatric cardiac surgery: a prospective uncontrolled cohort study. Crit Care 2007;11(6):127.
32. Prowle JR, Calzavacca P, Licari E, et al. Combination of biomarkers for diagnosis of acute kidney injury after cardiopulmonary bypass. Ren Fail 2015;37(3):408–16.
33. Pajek J, Škoberne A, Šosterič K, et al. Non-inferiority of creatinine excretion rate to urinary L-FABP and NGAL as predictors of early renal allograft function. BMC Nephrol 2014;15:117.
34. Pianta TJ, Peake PW, Pickering JW, et al. Clusterin in kidney transplantation: novel biomarkers versus serum creatinine for early prediction of delayed graft function. Transplantation 2015;99(1):171–9.
35. De Geus HR, Bakker J, Lesaffre EM, et al. Neutrophil gelatinase-associated lipocalin at ICU admission predicts for acute kidney injury in adult patients. Am J Respir Crit Care Med 2011;183(7):907–14.
36. Bennett M, Dent CL, Ma Q, et al. Urine NGAL predicts severity of acute kidney injury after cardiac surgery: a prospective study. Clin J Am Soc Nephrol 2008; 3(3):665–73.
37. Haase M, Bellomo R, Devarajan P, et al. Accuracy of neutrophil gelatinase-associated lipocalin (NGAL) in diagnosis and prognosis in acute kidney injury: a systematic review and meta-analysis. Am J Kidney Dis 2009;54(6):1012–24.
38. Ho J, Tangri N, Komenda P, et al. Urinary, plasma, and serum biomarkers' utility for predicting acute kidney injury associated with cardiac surgery in adults: a meta-analysis. Am J Kidney Dis 2015;66(6):993–1005.
39. Pons B, Lautrette A, Oziel J, et al. Diagnostic accuracy of early urinary index changes in differentiating transient from persistent acute kidney injury in critically ill patients: multicenter cohort study. Crit Care 2013;17(2):56.
40. Darmon M, Vincent F, Dellamonica J, et al. Diagnostic performance of fractional excretion of urea in the evaluation of critically ill patients with acute kidney injury: a multicenter cohort study. Crit Care 2011;15(4):178.
41. Singer E, Elger A, Elitok S, et al. Urinary neutrophil gelatinase-associated lipocalin distinguishes pre-renal from intrinsic renal failure and predicts outcomes. Kidney Int 2011;80(4):405–14.
42. Srisawat N, Wen X, Lee M, et al. Urinary biomarkers and renal recovery in critically ill patients with renal support. Clin J Am Soc Nephrol 2011;6(8):1815–23.

43. Choy E, Hornicek F, MacConaill L, et al. High-throughput genotyping in osteosarcoma identifies multiple mutations in phosphoinositide-3-kinase and other oncogenes. Cancer 2011;118(11):2905–14.
44. Ralib AM, Pickering JW, Shaw GM, et al. Test characteristics of urinary biomarkers depend on quantitation method in acute kidney injury. J Am Soc Nephrol 2012;23(2):322–33.
45. Coca SG, Garg AX, Thiessen-Philbrook H, et al. TRIBE-AKI Consortium. Urinary biomarkers of AKI and mortality 3 years after cardiac surgery. J Am Soc Nephrol 2014;25(5):1063–71.
46. Zachar RM, Skjødt K, Marcussen N, et al. The epithelial sodium channel γ-subunit is processed proteolytically in human kidney. J Am Soc Nephrol 2014;26(1): 95–106.
47. Tiranathanagul K, Amornsuntorn S, Avihingsanon Y, et al. Potential role of neutrophil gelatinase-associated lipocalin in identifying critically ill patients with acute kidney injury stage 2-3 who subsequently require renal replacement therapy. Ther Apher Dial 2013;17(3):332–8.
48. Klein SJ, Brandtner AK, Lehner GF, et al. Biomarkers for prediction of renal replacement therapy in acute kidney injury: a systematic review and meta-analysis. Intensive Care Med 2018;44(3):323–36.
49. Srisawat N, Laoveeravat P, Limphunudom P, et al. The effect of early renal replacement therapy guided by plasma neutrophil gelatinase associated lipocalin on outcome of acute kidney injury: a feasibility study. J Crit Care 2018;43: 36–41.
50. Maatman RG, Van Kuppevelt TH, Veerkamp JH. Two types of fatty acid-binding protein in human kidney. Isolation, characterization and localization. Biochem J 1991;273:759–66.
51. Maatman RG, van deWesterlo EM, van Kuppevelt TH, et al. Molecular identification of the liver- and the heart-type fatty acid-binding proteins in human and rat kidney. Use of the reverse transcriptase polymerase chain reaction. Biochem J 1992;288:285–90.
52. Yamamoto T, Noiri E, Ono Y, et al. Renal L-type fatty acid–binding protein in acute ischemic injury. J Am Soc Nephrol 2007;18:2894–902.
53. Kamijo-Ikemori A, Sugaya T, Matsui K, et al. Roles of human liver type fatty acid binding protein in kidney disease clarified using hL-FABP chromosomal transgenic mice. Nephrology 2011;16(6):539–44.
54. Landrier JF, Thomas C, Grober J, et al. Statin induction of liver fatty acid-binding protein (L-FABP) gene expression is peroxisome proliferator-activated receptor-alpha-dependent. J Biol Chem 2004;279(44):45512–8.
55. Noiri E, Doi K, Negishi K, et al. Urinary fatty acid-binding protein 1: an early predictive biomarker of kidney injury. Am J Physiol Renal Physiol 2009;296:669–79.
56. Nakamura T, Sugaya T, Node K, et al. Urinary excretion of liver-type fatty acid-binding protein in contrast medium-induced nephropathy. Am J Kidney Dis 2006;47(3):439–44.
57. Matsuura R, Srisawat N, Claure-Del Granado R, et al. Use of the renal angina index in determining acute kidney injury. Kidney Int Rep 2018;3(3):677–83.
58. Ichimura T, Bonventre JV, Bailly V, et al. Kidney injury molecule-1 (KIM-1), a putative epithelial cell adhesion molecule containing a novel immunoglobulin domain, is up-regulated in renal cells after injury. J Biol Chem 1998;273(7): 4135–42.
59. Amin RP, Vickers AE, Sistare F, et al. Identification of putative gene based markers of renal toxicity. Environ Health Perspect 2004;112(4):465–79.

60. Ichimura T, Hung CC, Yang SA, et al. Kidney injury molecule-1: a tissue and urinary biomarker for nephrotoxicant-induced renal injury. Am J Physiol Renal Physiol 2004;286(3):552–63.
61. Han WK, Bailly V, Abichandani R, et al. Kidney Injury Molecule-1 (KIM-1): a novel biomarker for human renal proximal tubule injury. Kidney Int 2002;62(1):237–44.
62. Yang QH, Liu DW, Long Y, et al. Acute renal failure during sepsis: potential role of cell cycle regulation. J Infect 2009;58(6):459–64.
63. Ichimura T, Asseldonk EJ, Humphreys BD, et al. Kidney injury molecule-1 is a phosphatidylserine receptor that confers a phagocytic phenotype on epithelial cells. J Clin Invest 2008;118(5):1657–68.
64. Ismail OZ, Zhang X, Wei J, et al. Kidney injury molecule-1 protects against Gα12 activation and tissue damage in renal ischemia-reperfusion injury. Am J Pathol 2015;185(5):1207–15.
65. Jay L, Vishal S, Michael R, et al. Urinary biomarkers in the clinical prognosis and early detection of acute kidney injury. Clin J Am Soc Nephrol 2010;5(12):2154–65.
66. Parikh CR, Thiessen-Philbrook H, Garg AX, et al. Performance of kidney injury molecule-1 and liver fatty acid-binding protein and combined biomarkers of AKI after cardiac surgery. Clin J Am Soc Nephrol 2013;8(7):1079–88.
67. Nickolas TL, Schmidt-Ott KM, Canetta P, et al. Diagnostic and prognostic stratification in the emergency department using urinary biomarkers of nephron damage: a multicenter prospective cohort study. J Am Coll Cardiol 2012;59(3):246–55.
68. Kashani K, Al-Khafaji A, Ardiles T, et al. Discovery and validation of cell cycle arrest biomarkers in human acute kidney injury. Crit Care 2013;17(1):25.
69. Su LJ, Li YM, Kellum JA, et al. Predictive value of cell cycle arrest biomarkers for cardiac surgery-associated acute kidney injury: a meta-analysis. Br J Anaesth 2018;121(2):350–7.
70. Honore PM, Nguyen HB, Gong M, et al. Urinary tissue inhibitor of metalloproteinase-2 and insulin-like growth factor-binding protein 7 for risk stratification of acute kidney injury in patients with sepsis. Crit Care Med 2016;44(10):1851–60.
71. Gunnerson KJ, Shaw AD, Chawla LS, et al. TIMP2•IGFBP7 biomarker panel accurately predicts acute kidney injury in high-risk surgical patients. J Trauma Acute Care Surg 2016;80(2):243–9.
72. Heung M, Ortega LM, Chawla LS, et al. Common chronic conditions do not affect performance of cell cycle arrest biomarkers for risk stratification of acute kidney injury. Nephrol Dial Transplant 2016;31(10):1633–40.
73. Ostermann M, McCullough PA, Forni LG, et al. Kinetics of urinary cell cycle arrest markers for acute kidney injury following exposure to potential renal insults. Crit Care Med 2018;46(3):375–83.
74. Zarbock A, Schmidt C, Van AH, et al. Effect of remote ischemic preconditioning on kidney injury among high-risk patients undergoing cardiac surgery: a randomized clinical trial. JAMA 2015;313(21):2133–41.
75. Kellum JA, Chawla LS. Cell-cycle arrest and acute kidney injury: the light and the dark sides. Nephrol Dial Transplant 2016;31(1):16–22.
76. Wen X, Cui L, Morrisroe S, et al. A zebrafish model of infection-associated acute kidney injury. Am J Physiol Renal Physiol 2018;315(2):F291–9.

Biomarkers and Right Ventricular Dysfunction

Natasha M. Pradhan, MBBS[a], Christopher Mullin, MD, MHS[b], Hooman D. Poor, MD[a],*

KEYWORDS

- Right ventricular dysfunction • Biomarkers • Pulmonary embolism
- Pulmonary hypertension • Troponin • Brain natriuretic peptide

KEY POINTS

- Right ventricular failure is commonly encountered in critically ill patients, most often due to pulmonary embolism or pulmonary hypertension, and is associated with poor prognosis and outcomes.
- Laboratory biomarkers such as troponin and brain natriuretic peptide are sensitive, but not specific, indicators of right ventricular dysfunction and aide in the risk stratification, prognosis, and management of right ventricular failure in various critical illnesses.
- Cardiac biomarkers are most widely studied and clinically used to risk stratify patients with acute pulmonary embolism.
- Novel biomarkers such as heart-type fatty acid–binding protein, growth differentiation factor 15, and neutrophil gelatinase–associated lipocalin have been shown to predict mortality in acute pulmonary embolism but are not currently used in routine clinical practice.
- Although awareness of the possibility of right ventricular dysfunction in common critical illnesses such as acute respiratory distress syndrome and sepsis is imperative, biomarkers are not standardly used to assess right ventricular function.

INTRODUCTION

Right ventricular failure is defined as the inability of the right ventricle (RV) to maintain adequate cardiac output in the presence of sufficient preload.[1] RV dysfunction may result from increased RV afterload, decreased RV contractility, or a combination of both. RV failure is common in critically ill patients, as it frequently results from pulmonary embolism (PE) or pulmonary arterial hypertension (PAH), and it often

None of the authors have any financial disclosures.
[a] Division of Pulmonary, Critical Care, and Sleep Medicine, Icahn School of Medicine at Mount Sinai Hospital, 1 Gustave L. Levy Place, New York, NY 10029-5674, USA; [b] Division of Pulmonary, Critical Care, and Sleep Medicine, Warren Alpert Medical School of Brown University, 593 Eddy Street, Providence, RI 02903, USA
* Correspondence: Division of Pulmonary, Critical Care, and Sleep Medicine, Icahn School of Medicine at Mount Sinai Hospital, 1 Gustave L. Levy Place, New York, NY 10029-5674.
E-mail address: hooman.poor@mountsinai.org

complicates common critical illnesses such as the acute respiratory distress syndrome (ARDS) and sepsis. Acute PE increases RV afterload and is a common cause of RV dysfunction, estimated to affect up to 900,000 people and resulting in more than 60,000 deaths per year in the United States.[2] PAH, although rare in comparison, can result in devastating RV failure, cardiogenic shock, and death. In both acute PE and PAH, RV function is the most important determinant of survival.[2,3] Hypoxemic respiratory failure, particularly ARDS, can result in pulmonary hypertension (PH) and RV dysfunction. Echocardiographic evidence of RV dysfunction can be seen in 22% to 50% of patients with moderate ARDS and is associated with increased mortality.[4,5] Increased circulating cytokines in sepsis may cause myocardial depression and increased pulmonary vascular resistance (PVR), resulting in RV dysfunction, which is ultimately associated with increased mortality.[6–8] RV ischemia, cardiomyopathy, or myocarditis can result in decreased RV contractility and primary RV failure, often in the presence of normal pulmonary vascular impedance. Although this is less commonly encountered, it is important to diagnose because there are critical differences in management between RV failure resulting from increased RV afterload and decreased RV contractility.[1]

Given the poor outcomes and challenges with managing RV dysfunction, the intensivist must be equipped to recognize RV dysfunction, identify the underlying pathophysiology, and intervene appropriately. Echocardiography, advanced cardiac imaging such as cardiac MRI, and invasive hemodynamic measurements are often used in the diagnosis and management of RV dysfunction; however, they are costly, time consuming, challenging to obtain in the intensive care unit (ICU), and may require specialized skill for performance and interpretation. Laboratory biomarkers are rapid, noninvasive, accurate, inexpensive, and widely available and thus are attractive for use in the recognition and management of RV dysfunction in critically ill patients. Understanding the role of biomarkers in RV dysfunction requires insight into normal and abnormal RV function.

NORMAL RIGHT VENTRICULAR FUNCTION

The RV consists of the interventricular septum and a free wall that embraces the left ventricle (LV). The RV is efficient because it matches the same cardiac output as the LV with one-fifth of the energy expenditure. Its ability to do so stems from unique structural and functional adaptations to the low-resistance, high-capacitance pulmonary circulation.[9] The RV free wall is thinner than that of the LV and lacks the middle circumferential layer of constrictor fibers of the LV that provides the contractility against higher systemic pressures.[9,10] Instead, the RV relies on longitudinal shortening for systolic ejection, bringing the apex toward the tricuspid annulus, along with flattening of the free wall, producing a bellows movement.[9,11] Its high compliance allows for a greater surface area to volume ratio, enabling the RV to eject a large volume of blood with minimal changes in wall stretch.[12] In addition, the lower RV cavity pressures allow for myocardial perfusion throughout both diastole and systole, in contrast to the LV, where perfusion occurs only when cavity pressures are lower than aortic root pressures during diastole.[13] These mechanisms allow the RV to function efficiently under physiologic conditions.

PATHOPHYSIOLOGY OF RIGHT VENTRICULAR FAILURE

A significant increase in RV afterload or a significant decrease in RV contractility, often compounded by excessive RV preload, can set into motion a downward spiral of RV failure. Although the normal RV is capable of accommodating increases in preload, it is not tolerant of significant increases in RV afterload, particularly when the increase occurs acutely.[12] When subjected to acute pressure overload, the RV dilates and maintains its stroke volume by the Frank-Starling mechanism.[14] Once this compensatory capacity is exceeded, maladaptive dilation results in further worsening of RV performance and a precipitous drop in RV cardiac output.[15] Because the RV and LV are arranged in series, a drop in RV cardiac output reduces LV preload and subsequently LV cardiac output. Dilation of the RV chamber extends to the tricuspid annulus, producing functional tricuspid regurgitation, increasing preload, and furthering RV stretch.

The progressively rising RV end-diastolic pressure and volume cause thinning of the RV myocardium and increase RV wall stress.[16,17] The higher wall stress increases myocardial oxygen demand and also reduces RV myocardial perfusion as the myocardium becomes perfused only during diastole.[18,19] This mismatch between RV myocardial oxygen demand and supply leads to RV ischemia, myocyte necrosis, and impaired RV contractility.

Because constraint from the pericardium prevents the RV free wall from dilating outwards, progressive RV dilation displaces the interventricular septum, leading to decreased LV cavity size in diastole and LV deformation during systole.[20] Decreased LV cavity size during diastole reduces LV preload and LV deformation during systole impairs LV contractility, both of which lead to decreased LV cardiac output[20–23] (**Fig. 1**).

BIOMARKERS IN RIGHT VENTRICULAR DYSFUNCTION

Biomarkers are disease-associated molecular changes in body tissues and fluids[24] that can serve as standardized, reproducible, noninvasive, and objective measures to assist in the diagnosis, assess prognosis, and monitor response to therapy in specific disease states. Laboratory biomarkers serve as sensitive, but not specific, indicators of RV dysfunction and aide in risk stratification, prognosis, and management in various critical illnesses. These biomarkers are often used in combination with clinical assessment, risk scores, and imaging modalities such as echocardiography and computed tomography. Many of the biomarkers are linked to the underlying pathophysiologic changes that occur during RV failure.

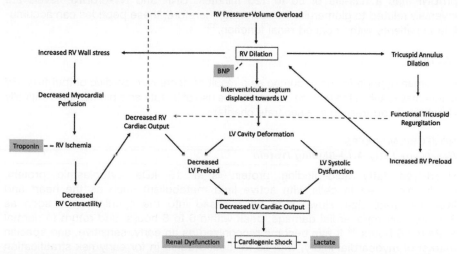

Fig. 1. Pathophysiology of RV failure.

TROPONIN

Troponin is most commonly used for detection of myocardial ischemia and infarction because it relates to the LV.[25,26] However, troponin I and T are also released into the systemic circulation from myocardial injury due to RV ischemia. Troponin I and T are largely structurally bound to myofilaments, with a small soluble unbound cytoplasmic pool of 3% and 6%, respectively.[18] This cytoplasmic pool is thought to be released due to myocardial injury from RV ischemia and may explain the distinct pattern of troponin release seen in PE compared with non-ST-elevation myocardial infarction (MI).[27] In MI, extensive myocardial necrosis causes troponin T to appear as early as 3 hours after onset of symptoms, peak at 24 hours, and remain detectable for up to 10 to 14 days. In PE, however, troponin peaks at 10 hours after presentation and remains detectable for only 40 hours. The peak is lower than that of MI, and remains detectable for a shorter period of time.[28] In patients presenting greater than 72 hours after symptom onset, troponin is undetectable despite the presence of RV dysfunction on echocardiogram.[29] Understanding the kinetics of troponin release is essential to determine optimal timing of blood sampling for accurate risk stratification.

BRAIN NATRIURETIC PEPTIDE

Secretion of brain natriuretic peptide (BNP) is stimulated by an increase in wall stress from pressure overload in the failing RV. Ventricular cardiomyocytes secrete the inactive prohormone pro-BNP, which is split into biologically active BNP hormone and inactive N-terminal pro-BNP (NT-proBNP). Both hormones are measurable in plasma and serve as biomarkers of RV dysfunction.[30] Timing of measurement, mechanism of secretion, half-life, and clearance all affect plasma levels and are important considerations in the interpretation of BNP and NT-proBNP levels. In contrast to troponin, which is a normal constituent of the cardiomyocyte, only small amounts of BNP and NT-proBNP are stored in the cell under physiologic conditions. Instead, BNP and Nt-proBNP secretion is stimulated by a constitutive mechanism in response to stretch and may take several hours before it appears in circulation.[30–32] BNP has a half-life of 20 minutes, whereas NT-proBNP has a half-life of 60 to 120 minutes. BNP and NT-proBNP levels are inversely related to glomerular filtration rate; therefore, these peptides can accumulate in patients with impaired renal function.[33]

LACTATE

End-organ hypoperfusion occurring as a result of decreased cardiac output from RV failure may result in the release of lactate. The use of lactate as a biomarker in critically ill patients is addressed in a separate chapter.

NOVEL BIOMARKERS
Heart-type Fatty Acid–Binding Protein

Heart-type fatty acid–binding protein is a 15 kDa cytoplasmic protein, highly expressed in cells with active lipid metabolism such as the heart and liver. Its small size allows it to be released into the circulation as soon as 2 hours after myocardial damage, peak within 6 to 8 hours, and return to normal at 24 to 36 hours.[34] It has become recognized as an early, sensitive, and specific marker of myocardial injury, with so far best studied in for early risk stratification of PE.[35]

Other Novel Biomarkers

Several novel biomarkers have been investigated in the diagnostic and prognostic assessment of PE. Growth differentiation factor 15 (GDF-15) is a cytokine that is produced in cardiomyocytes in the setting of ischemia or pressure overload. Elevated GDF-15 is an independent predictor of complicated 30-day outcome in acute PE.[36] Elevated levels of copeptin, a stable precursor protein of vasopressin, were also associated with increased risk of 30-day adverse outcome in normotensive patients with PE.[37,38] Various markers of impaired renal function have prognostic value in acute PE. In normotensive patients with acute PE, a GFR less than 35 mL/min was an independent predictor of 30-day mortality and improved troponin-based risk stratification.[39] Neutrophil gelatinase–associated lipocalin (N-GAL) is produced by the kidney and has been shown to rapidly accumulate in acute kidney injury.[40] Likewise, cystatin C is also a marker of renal dysfunction that has been used to diagnose acute kidney injury in critically ill patients 24 to 48 hours before increase in creatinine level.[41] Elevated levels of N-GAL and cystatin C have been shown to predict 30-day all-cause mortality in acute PE.[42]

APPLICATIONS
Biomarkers for Right Ventricular Dysfunction in Acute Pulmonary Embolism

Acute PE is one of the most common causes of RV dysfunction in the emergency room and ICU. Several biomarkers are well established as predictors of mortality and morbidity in acute PE and as such play an important role in prognostication and risk stratification in patients with acute PE.

Troponin is released into the systemic circulation in response to RV myocardial ischemia in acute PE. In a subgroup of normotensive patients with acute PE, elevated levels of troponin (greater than 99th percentile of healthy subjects) measured on admission and/or up to 24 hours after admission were associated with a higher risk of in-hospital or 30-day mortality (odds ratio [OR] 5.90, 95% confidence interval [CI] 2.68–12.95) and need for cardiopulmonary resuscitation, vasopressors, mechanical ventilation, and thrombolysis. Although a greater proportion of patients with a positive troponin had RV dysfunction on echocardiography, both troponin and echocardiographic RV dysfunction had independent, additive prognostic value without significant interaction.[43,44] The prognostic value of troponin has been supported with subsequent meta-analyses.[45,46]

High-sensitivity troponin (Hs-TnT) also has predictive value in acute PE and may be more accurate than troponin T. In one study, an Hs-TNT greater than 14 pg/mL in normotensive patients with acute PE predicted 30-day mortality and adverse outcomes with better accuracy than troponin T. Unlike troponin T, which has not been shown to correlate with long-term prognosis, patients with acute PE with Hs-TnT greater than 14 pg/mL had a reduced probability of long-term survival over a median period of 965 days.[45,46] Although this is a promising option to optimize risk stratification in acute PE, the number of studies is small and widespread application of Hs-TnT is still limited.

BNP is released as a result of increased myocardial wall stress in the setting of RV dysfunction due to PE. As would be expected, increased levels of BNP or NT-proBNP in patients with acute PE have been shown to be associated with RV dysfunction.[47] In a meta-analysis of 1132 patients with acute PE, elevated BNP and NT-pro BNP were associated with an increased risk of 30-day mortality (OR 6.5; 95% CI 2–21) and in-hospital adverse clinical outcomes, including death, cardiopulmonary resuscitation, mechanical ventilation, use of vasopressors, thrombolysis, thrombosuction, surgical embolectomy, or admission to the ICU (OR 8.7; 95% CI 2.8–27).[48] This meta-analysis, however, also included hemodynamically unstable patients, in whom RV dysfunction is likely clinically apparent and in whom risk stratification with biomarkers may be unnecessary. In another study that included only normotensive patients with acute PE, BNP and NT-proBNP levels similarly predicted short-term mortality.[45] Because their values can be elevated in other conditions such as LV dysfunction, renal impairment, chronic respiratory illness, and advanced age, elevation of BNP and NT-proBNP are nonspecific and have a low positive predictive value for RV dysfunction.[49]

Heart-type fatty acid–binding protein (hFABP) is an early marker of myocardial damage, and because it is both sensitive and specific, it has been used for early identification of low-risk patients with acute PE.[35,45] In a study of 126 normotensive patients with acute PE, hFABP greater than 6 ng/mL predicted death or complications at 30 days with a sensitivity of 0.89 and specificity of 0.82.[50] All patients who developed complications had an elevated hFABP level, whereas troponin T and NT-proBNP levels did not significantly differ,[50] which suggests that hFABP may be a more useful biomarker in acute PE; however, more studies of this biomarker are necessary.

RISK STRATIFICATION IN ACUTE PULMONARY EMBOLISM

Once the diagnosis of PE has been confirmed by computed tomography pulmonary angiography (CTPA), ventilation-perfusion scan, or pulmonary angiography, prompt risk stratification using validated predictive models is used to estimate early mortality risk and help guide management decisions. The European Society of Cardiology 2014 guidelines recommend stratifying patients into low-, intermediate-, and high-risk groups,[51] using biomarkers to differentiate between low- and intermediate-risk groups. Assessment of hemodynamic status is the first step in risk stratification for a patient with confirmed or suspected PE. Shock or sustained hypotension (defined as systolic blood pressure less than 90 mm Hg or drop of >40 mm Hg for 15 minutes or longer) classifies patients as high risk, with an estimated 90-day mortality as high as 58% (**Fig. 2**).[52] Patients without sustained hypotension or shock are further classified into low and intermediate risk. These 2 groups are distinguished from each other with the evaluation of the pulmonary embolism severity index (PESI), imaging assessment (eg, echocardiography, CTPA) of the RV, and biomarkers. Specifically, patients with low-risk PE demonstrate no imaging signs of RV dysfunction, do not have elevations in cardiac biomarkers, and do not have elevated PESI risk score. Intermediate-risk PE, on the other hand, requires only the presence of one of those listed abnormalities. Intermediate-risk patients are further stratified into intermediate-high or intermediate-low risk. Patients with imaging evidence of RV dysfunction *and* positive biomarkers (especially troponin) are classified as intermediate-high risk, whereas those with only one abnormality (RV dysfunction *or* positive biomarkers) are deemed intermediate-low risk. This distinction is important to make because it enables the identification of a group of normotensive patients with more significant RV dysfunction who are at increased risk of the short-term mortality and may benefit from ICU monitoring and the consideration of reperfusion therapy.[53]

Negative biomarkers when measured at the appropriate time can help identify patients with PE at low risk of death or complications and allow for shorter duration of hospital stay or early discharge from the emergency department. NT pro-BNP of less than 500 ng/L to less than 1000 ng/L measured on admission predicts a benign clinical outcome in patients with PE with a negative predictive value between 97% and 100%.[46,54] Admission BNP values of less than 50 pg/mL have better negative

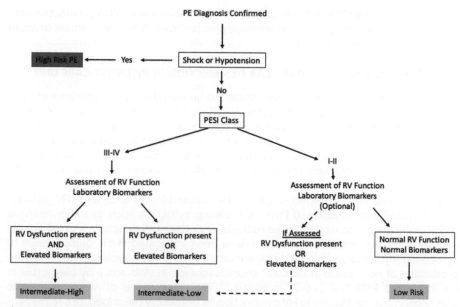

Fig. 2. Risk stratification of pulmonary embolism.

predictive value for short-term adverse events than the more widely used cut-off less than 90 pg/L.[55] However, with a negative likelihood ratio (NLR) of 0.33 for all-cause mortality and NLR of 0.41 for short-term adverse events, BNP does not accurately identify low-risk patients.[45] Hs-TnT of less than 14 pg/mL was 100% sensitive in identifying patients who would not experience short-term adverse events.[46] A meta-analysis also confirmed NLR of 0.21 for all-cause mortality, making it a useful marker for early risk stratification. Low hFABP measured on admission is a sensitive, early marker with excellent negative predictive value for short-term adverse events.[50]

BIOMARKERS FOR RIGHT VENTRICULAR DYSFUNCTION IN PULMONARY HYPERTENSION

PH is a pathophysiologic disorder, defined by a mean pulmonary artery pressure of more than 20 mm Hg at rest, measured via right heart catheterization.[56] PAH, a type of PH, is a chronic, progressive pulmonary arterial vasculopathy, characterized by medial hypertrophy, intimal fibrosis, and in situ thrombosis of the pulmonary arterioles that causes an increase in PVR.[57] PAH can result in progressive RV failure, multi-organ dysfunction, and ultimately death.[58] RV failure is a leading cause of death in PAH,[59] and patients with PAH admitted to the ICU have high mortality rates.[17] Cardiac biomarkers are frequently used in both the chronic management of patients with PAH as well as in the intensive care setting. BNP and NT-proBNP are the most commonly used biomarkers in PH, as they correlate with functional and hemodynamic measures[60–62] and are independent predictors of mortality.[63,64] In addition, changes in hemodynamics correlate with changes in BNP, making BNP a useful tool to noninvasively assess response to therapy.[61] Troponin is used less frequently but has been identified as an independent marker of mortality in patients with precapillary PH.[65] There is less data for the use of biomarkers in the patients with PAH with RV failure. One study of 46 patients with PAH or inoperable chronic thromboembolic pulmonary hypertension with acute RV failure in the ICU found BNP to be an independent predictor of mortality.[66] Practically speaking, biomarkers are used in conjunction with other clinical, laboratory, and echocardiographic parameters in management of acute RV failure in patients with PAH.[17]

BIOMARKERS FOR RIGHT VENTRICULAR DYSFUNCTION IN INTENSIVE CARE UNIT

RV dilation and dysfunction has been shown to be an independent predictor of mortality in patients with moderate to severe ARDS.[67,68] A myriad of factors contribute to the elevated PVR in ARDS that leads to RV dysfunction, including hypoxic pulmonary vasoconstriction, elevated $Paco_2$, acidemia, endothelial dysfunction, imbalance between vasoconstrictors and vasodilators, microthrombosis, and pulmonary vascular remodeling.[69–72] Biomarkers specific to acute RV dysfunction in ARDS have yet to be investigated.

RV dysfunction during sepsis stems from a combination of decreased RV myocardial contractility and increased PVR.[6] Circulating cytokines such as tumor necrosis factor alpha increased oxidative free radicals, endothelial dysfunction, and toll-like receptors activation that occur in sepsis have been implicated in the pathogenesis of myocardial dysfunction.[73,74] Bacterial endotoxins have been shown to decrease the production of nitric oxide in vascular endothelial cells in vitro and may play a role in the increased PVR that occurs in sepsis.[75] The coexistence of ARDS in patients with sepsis also contributes to RV dysfunction as previously described. In a retrospective cohort study that evaluated 100 patients with sepsis or septic shock with RV dysfunction, isolated RV dysfunction was independently associated with worse 1-year survival (hazard ratio 1.6, 95% CI 1.2–2.1, $P = .001$) when adjusted for age, comorbidities, illness severity, septic shock, and the use of mechanical ventilation.[8]

RV dysfunction due to decreased myocardial contractility may occur due to several reasons, namely RV MI, myocarditis, and pericarditis. Clinically significant RV infarction usually occurs in conjunction with left-sided acute inferior-posterior MI and is due to occlusion of the proximal right coronary artery.[76–78] The hemodynamic compromise in RV MI may be compounded by bradycardia that is frequently seen in conjunction with inferior MI and left atrial ischemia due to proximal right coronary artery occlusion, which leads to loss of left atrial augmentation to preload.[79–81] Cardiac biomarkers used to aide the diagnosis of RV MI are similar to those used in LV MI, such as troponin T, troponin I, and creatine kinase-MB.[82]

SUMMARY

RV dysfunction is an important prognostic marker in the wide array of cardiopulmonary diseases that frequently cause or contribute to critical illness. Assessment of RV function is vital in the intensive care setting for management of acute PE, pulmonary hypertension, ARDS, and sepsis. Biomarkers used to assess RV dysfunction are primarily cardiac in origin, being released into circulation as a result of RV stretch and ischemia that are central in the pathophysiology of RV dysfunction. These biomarkers, namely troponin and brain natriuretic peptides, have several applications in RV dysfunction, most notably in acute PE, where they play an important role in risk stratification and assessment of prognosis.

REFERENCES

1. Konstam MA, Kiernan MS, Bernstein D, et al. Evaluation and management of right-sided heart failure: a scientific statement from the American Heart Association. Circulation 2018;137(20):e578–622.

2. Beckman MG, Hooper WC, Critchley SE, et al. Venous thromboembolism: a public health concern. Am J Prev Med 2010;38(4):S495–501.
3. Noordegraaf AV, Chin KM, Haddad F, et al. Pathophysiology of the right ventricle and of the pulmonary circulation in pulmonary hypertension: an update. Eur Respir J 2019;53(1):1801900.
4. Zochios V, Parhar K, Tunnicliffe W, et al. The right ventricle in ARDS. Chest 2017; 152(1):181–93.
5. Zapol WM, Snider MT. Pulmonary hypertension in severe acute respiratory failure. N Engl J Med 1977;296(9):476–80.
6. Chan CM, Klinger JR. The right ventricle in sepsis. Clin Chest Med 2008;29(4): 661–76.
7. Furian T, Aguiar C, Prado K, et al. Ventricular dysfunction and dilation in severe sepsis and septic shock: relation to endothelial function and mortality. J Crit Care 2012;27(3):319. e9–e15.
8. Vallabhajosyula S, Kumar M, Pandompatam G, et al. Prognostic impact of isolated right ventricular dysfunction in sepsis and septic shock: an 8-year historical cohort study. Ann Intensive Care 2017;7(1):94.
9. Sheehan F, Redington A. The right ventricle: anatomy, physiology and clinical imaging. Heart 2008;94(11):1510–5.
10. James TN. Anatomy of the crista supraventricularis: its importance for understanding right ventricular function, right ventricular infarction and related conditions. J Am Coll Cardiol 1985;6(5):1083–95.
11. Buckberg G, Hoffman JI. Right ventricular architecture responsible for mechanical performance: unifying role of ventricular septum. J Thorac Cardiovasc Surg 2014;148(6):3166–71.e1-4.
12. Greyson CR. Pathophysiology of right ventricular failure. Crit Care Med 2008; 36(1):S57–65.
13. Greyson CR. The right ventricle and pulmonary circulation: basic concepts. Rev Esp Cardiol 2010;63(1):81–95.
14. Hon J, Steendijk P, Khan H, et al. Acute effects of pulmonary artery banding in sheep on right ventricle pressure-volume relations: relevance to the arterial switch operation. Acta Physiol Scand 2001;172(2):97–106.
15. Guyton AC, Lindsey AW, Gilluly JJ. The limits of right ventricular compensation following acute increase in pulmonary circulatory resistance. Circ Res 1954; 2(4):326–32.
16. Kerbaul F, Rondelet B, Motte S, et al. Effects of norepinephrine and dobutamine on pressure load-induced right ventricular failure. Crit Care Med 2004;32(4): 1035–40.
17. Poor HD, Ventetuolo CE. Pulmonary hypertension in the intensive care unit. Prog Cardiovasc Dis 2012;55(2):187–98.
18. Katus HA, Remppis A, Scheffold T, et al. Intracellular compartmentation of cardiac troponin T and its release kinetics in patients with reperfused and nonreperfused myocardial infarction. Am J Cardiol 1991;67(16):1360–7.
19. Kroeker CAG, Adeeb SM, Shrive NG, et al. Compression induced by RV pressure overload decreases regional coronary blood flow in anesthetized dogs. Am J Physiol Heart Circ Physiol 2006;290(6):H2432–8.
20. Gan C, Lankhaar JW, Marcus JT, et al. Impaired left ventricular filling due to right-to-left ventricular interaction in patients with pulmonary arterial hypertension. Am J Physiol Heart Circ Physiol 2006;290(4):H1528–33.

21. Weyman AE, Wann S, Feigenbaum H, et al. Mechanism of abnormal septal motion in patients with right ventricular volume overload: a cross-sectional echocardiographic study. Circulation 1976;54(2):179–86.
22. Mahmud E, Raisinghani A, Hassankhani A, et al. Correlation of left ventricular diastolic filling characteristics with right ventricular overload and pulmonary artery pressure in chronic thromboembolic pulmonary hypertension. J Am Coll Cardiol 2002;40(2):318–24.
23. Brookes C, Ravn H, White P, et al. Acute right ventricular dilatation in response to ischemia significantly impairs left ventricular systolic performance. Circulation 1999;100(7):761–7.
24. Poste G. Bring on the biomarkers. Nature 2011;469(7329):156.
25. Antman E, Bassand J-P, Klein W, et al. Myocardial infarction redefined—a consensus document of the Joint European Society of Cardiology/American College of Cardiology committee for the redefinition of myocardial infarction: the Joint European Society of Cardiology/American College of Cardiology Committee. J Am Coll Cardiol 2000;36(3):959–69.
26. Hallén J, Jensen JK, Fagerland MW, et al. Cardiac troponin I for the prediction of functional recovery and left ventricular remodelling following primary percutaneous coronary intervention for ST-elevation myocardial infarction. Heart 2010; 96(23):1892–7.
27. Coma-Canella I, Gamallo C, Onsurbe PM, et al. Acute right ventricular infarction secondary to massive pulmonary embolism. Eur Heart J 1988;9(5):534–40.
28. Müller-Bardorff M, Weidtmann B, Giannitsis E, et al. Release kinetics of cardiac troponin T in survivors of confirmed severe pulmonary embolism. Clin Chem 2002;48(4):673–5.
29. Punukollu G, Khan IA, Gowda RM, et al. Cardiac troponin I release in acute pulmonary embolism in relation to the duration of symptoms. Int J Cardiol 2005; 99(2):207–11.
30. Hall C. Essential biochemistry and physiology of (NT-pro)BNP. Eur J Heart Fail 2004;6(3):257–60.
31. Mäntymaa P, Vuolteenaho O, Marttila M, et al. Atrial stretch induces rapid increase in brain natriuretic peptide but not in atrial natriuretic peptide gene expression in vitro. Endocrinology 1993;133(3):1470–3.
32. Hama N, Itoh H, Shirakami G, et al. Rapid ventricular induction of brain natriuretic peptide gene expression in experimental acute myocardial infarction. Circulation 1995;92(6):1558–64.
33. Van Kimmenade RR, Januzzi JL, Bakker JA, et al. Renal clearance of B-type natriuretic peptide and amino terminal pro-B-type natriuretic peptide a mechanistic study in hypertensive subjects. J Am Coll Cardiol 2009;53(10):884–90.
34. Pelsers MM, Hermens WT, Glatz JF. Fatty acid-binding proteins as plasma markers of tissue injury. Clin Chim Acta 2005;352(1–2):15–35.
35. Kaczyñska A, Pelsers MM, Bochowicz A, et al. Plasma heart-type fatty acid binding protein is superior to troponin and myoglobin for rapid risk stratification in acute pulmonary embolism. Clin Chim Acta 2006;371(1–2):117–23.
36. Lankeit M, Kempf T, Dellas C, et al. Growth differentiation factor-15 for prognostic assessment of patients with acute pulmonary embolism. Am J Respir Crit Care Med 2008;177(9):1018–25.
37. Bolignano D, Cabassi A, Fiaccadori E, et al. Copeptin (CTproAVP), a new tool for understanding the role of vasopressin in pathophysiology. Clin Chem Lab Med 2014;52(10):1447–56.

38. Hellenkamp K, Schwung J, Rossmann H, et al. Risk stratification of normotensive pulmonary embolism: prognostic impact of copeptin. Eur Respir J 2015;46(6): 1701–10.
39. Kostrubiec M, Łabyk A, Pedowska-Włoszek J, et al. Assessment of renal dysfunction improves troponin-based short-term prognosis in patients with acute symptomatic pulmonary embolism. J Thromb Haemost 2010;8(4):651–8.
40. Mishra J, Ma Q, Prada A, et al. Identification of neutrophil gelatinase-associated lipocalin as a novel early urinary biomarker for ischemic renal injury. J Am Soc Nephrol 2003;14(10):2534–43.
41. Coca S, Yalavarthy R, Concato J, et al. Biomarkers for the diagnosis and risk stratification of acute kidney injury: a systematic review. Kidney Int 2008;73(9): 1008–16.
42. Kostrubiec M, Łabyk A, Pedowska-Włoszek J, et al. Neutrophil gelatinase-associated lipocalin, cystatin C and eGFR indicate acute kidney injury and predict prognosis of patients with acute pulmonary embolism. Heart 2012;98(16):1221–8.
43. Becattini C, Vedovati MC, Agnelli G. Prognostic value of troponins in acute pulmonary embolism: a meta-analysis. Circulation 2007;116(4):427–33.
44. Choi HS, Kim KH, Yoon HJ, et al. Usefulness of cardiac biomarkers in the prediction of right ventricular dysfunction before echocardiography in acute pulmonary embolism. J Cardiol 2012;60(6):508–13.
45. Bajaj A, Rathor P, Sehgal V, et al. Prognostic value of biomarkers in acute non-massive pulmonary embolism: a systematic review and meta-analysis. Lung 2015;193(5):639–51.
46. Lankeit M, Friesen D, Aschoff J, et al. Highly sensitive troponin T assay in normotensive patients with acute pulmonary embolism. Eur Heart J 2010;31(15): 1836–44.
47. Krüger S, Graf J, Merx MW, et al. Brain natriuretic peptide predicts right heart failure in patients with acute pulmonary embolism. Am Heart J 2004;147(1):60 5.
48. Klok FA, Mos IC, Huisman MV, et al. Brain-type natriuretic peptide levels in the prediction of adverse outcome in patients with pulmonary embolism: a systematic review and meta-analysis. Am J Respir Crit Care Med 2008;178(4):425–30.
49. de Lemos JA, McGuire DK, Drazner MH. B-type natriuretic peptide in cardiovascular disease. Lancet 2003;362(9380):316–22.
50. Dellas C, Puls M, Lankeit M, et al. Elevated heart-type fatty acid-binding protein levels on admission predict an adverse outcome in normotensive patients with acute pulmonary embolism. J Am Coll Cardiol 2010;55(19):2150–7.
51. Konstantinides SV, Torbicki A, Agnelli G, et al. Task force for the diagnosis and management of acute pulmonary embolism of the European Society of Cardiology (ESC). 2014 ESC guidelines on the diagnosis and management of acute pulmonary embolism. Eur Heart J 2014;35(43):3033–73.
52. Goldhaber SZ, Visani L, De Rosa M. Acute pulmonary embolism: clinical outcomes in the International Cooperative Pulmonary Embolism Registry (ICOPER). Lancet 1999;353(9162):1386–9.
53. Becattini C, Agnelli G, Lankeit M, et al. Acute pulmonary embolism: mortality prediction by the 2014 European Society of Cardiology risk stratification model. Eur Respir J 2016;48(3):780–6.
54. Kucher N, Printzen G, Doernhoefer T, et al. Low pro-brain natriuretic peptide levels predict benign clinical outcome in acute pulmonary embolism. Circulation 2003;107(12):1576–8.
55. Kucher N, Printzen G, Goldhaber SZ. Prognostic role of brain natriuretic peptide in acute pulmonary embolism. Circulation 2003;107(20):2545–7.

56. Galiè N, Humbert M, Vachiery JL, et al. 2015 ESC/ERS guidelines for the diagnosis and treatment of pulmonary hypertension: the joint task force for the diagnosis and treatment of pulmonary hypertension of the European Society of Cardiology (ESC) and the European Respiratory Society (ERS): endorsed by: Association for European Paediatric and Congenital Cardiology (AEPC), International Society for Heart and Lung Transplantation (ISHLT). Eur Respir J 2016; 37(1):67–119.

57. Humbert M, Guignabert C, Bonnet S, et al. Pathology and pathobiology of pulmonary hypertension: state of the art and research perspectives. Eur Respir J 2019; 53(1):1801887.

58. Thenappan T, Shah SJ, Gomberg-Maitland M, et al. Clinical characteristics of pulmonary hypertension in patients with heart failure and preserved ejection fraction. Circ Heart Fail 2011;4(3):257–65.

59. Tonelli AR, Arelli V, Minai OA, et al. Causes and circumstances of death in pulmonary arterial hypertension. Am J Respir Crit Care Med 2013;188(3):365–9.

60. Nagaya N, Nishikimi T, Okano Y, et al. Plasma brain natriuretic peptide levels increase in proportion to the extent of right ventricular dysfunction in pulmonary hypertension. J Am Coll Cardiol 1998;31(1):202–8.

61. Leuchte HH, Holzapfel M, Baumgartner RA, et al. Characterization of brain natriuretic peptide in long-term follow-up of pulmonary arterial hypertension. Chest 2005;128(4):2368–74.

62. Leuchte HH, Holzapfel M, Baumgartner RA, et al. Clinical significance of brain natriuretic peptide in primary pulmonary hypertension. J Am Coll Cardiol 2004; 43(5):764–70.

63. Al-Naamani N, Palevsky HI, Lederer DJ, et al. Prognostic significance of biomarkers in pulmonary arterial hypertension. Ann Am Thorac Soc 2016;13(1): 25–30.

64. Benza RL, Miller DP, Gomberg-Maitland M, et al. Predicting survival in pulmonary arterial hypertension: insights from the Registry to Evaluate Early and Long-Term Pulmonary Arterial Hypertension Disease Management (REVEAL). Circulation 2010;122(2):164–72.

65. Torbicki A, Kurzyna M, Kuca P, et al. Detectable serum cardiac troponin T as a marker of poor prognosis among patients with chronic precapillary pulmonary hypertension. Circulation 2003;108(7):844–8.

66. Sztrymf B, Souza R, Bertoletti L, et al. Prognostic factors of acute heart failure in patients with pulmonary arterial hypertension. Eur Respir J 2010;35(6):1286–93.

67. Dessap AM, Boissier F, Charron C, et al. Acute cor pulmonale during protective ventilation for acute respiratory distress syndrome: prevalence, predictors, and clinical impact. Intensive Care Med 2016;42(5):862–70.

68. Boissier F, Katsahian S, Razazi K, et al. Prevalence and prognosis of cor pulmonale during protective ventilation for acute respiratory distress syndrome. Intensive Care Med 2013;39(10):1725–33.

69. Price LC, Wort SJ, Finney SJ, et al. Pulmonary vascular and right ventricular dysfunction in adult critical care: current and emerging options for management: a systematic literature review. Crit Care 2010;14(5):R169.

70. Snow RL, Davies P, Pontoppidan H, et al. Pulmonary vascular remodeling in adult respiratory distress syndrome. Am Rev Respir Dis 1982;126(5):887–92.

71. Zapol WM, Kobayashi K, Snider MT, et al. Vascular obstruction causes pulmonary hypertension in severe acute respiratory failure. Chest 1977;71(2):306–7.

72. Wort SJ, W Evans T. The role of the endothelium in modulating vascular control in sepsis and related conditions. Br Med Bull 1999;55(1):30–48.

73. Batista Lorigados C, Garcia Soriano F, Szabo C. Pathomechanisms of myocardial dysfunction in sepsis. Endocrine, metabolic & immune disorders-drug targets (formerly current drug targets-immune, endocrine & metabolic disorders) 2010;10(3):274–84.
74. Carlson DL, Willis MS, White DJ, et al. Tumor necrosis factor-α-induced caspase activation mediates endotoxin-related cardiac dysfunction. Crit Care Med 2005; 33(5):1021–8.
75. Myers PR, Wright TF, Tanner MA, et al. EDRF and nitric oxide production in cultured endothelial cells: direct inhibition by E. coli endotoxin. Am J Physiol 1992;262(3):H710–8.
76. Goldstein JA. Pathophysiology and management of right heart ischemia. J Am Coll Cardiol 2002;40(5):841–53.
77. Isner JM, Roberts WC. Right ventricular infarction complicating left ventricular infarction secondary to coronary heart disease. Frequency, location, associated findings and significance from analysis of 236 necropsy patients with acute or healed myocardial infarction. Am J Cardiol 1978;42(6):885–94.
78. Andersn HR, Falk E, Nielsen D. Right ventricular infarction: frequency, size and topography in coronary heart disease: a prospective study comprising 107 consecutive autopsies from a coronary care unit. J Am Coll Cardiol 1987;10(6): 1223–32.
79. Goldstein JA, Tweddell JS, Barzilai B, et al. Right atrial ischemia exacerbates hemodynamic compromise associated with experimental right ventricular dysfunction. J Am Coll Cardiol 1991;18(6):1564–72.
80. Goldstein JA, Harada A, Yagi Y, et al. Hemodynamic importance of systolic ventricular interaction, augmented right atrial contractility and atrioventricular synchrony in acute right ventricular dysfunction. J Am Coll Cardiol 1990;16(1):181–9.
81. Adgey AA, Geddes JS, Mulholland HC, et al. Incidence, significance, and management of early bradyarrhythmia complicating acute myocardial infarction. Lancet 1968;2(7578):1097–101.
82. Mythili S, Malathi N. Diagnostic markers of acute myocardial infarction. Biomed Rep 2015;3(6):743–8.

Biomarkers and Precision Medicine: State of the Art

Aartik Sarma, MD[a], Carolyn S. Calfee, MD, MAS[a,b,c],
Lorraine B. Ware, MD[d,e,f],*

KEYWORDS

- Biomarkers • Precision medicine • Prognostic enrichment • Predictive enrichment
- ARDS • Sepsis

KEY POINTS

- Biomarkers can identify clinically distinct molecular phenotypes in heterogenous populations of critically ill patients, including patients with acute respiratory distress syndrome (ARDS) and sepsis.
- Advances in computational and molecular methods have found genomic, transcriptomic, and metabolomic biomarkers that identify potential pathways involved in the biology of these complex syndromes.
- Molecular phenotypes predict differential response to therapies in retrospective analyses of clinical trials in ARDS and sepsis; these findings need to be validated in prospective studies.
- Future clinical trials should use biomarkers for prognostic and predictive enrichment to improve power to identify effective treatments.

Disclosure Statement: A. Sarma: No disclosures. C.S. Calfee: Grant funding from Bayer (current) and GlaxoSmithKline (United Kingdom) (past) (in addition to the National Institutes of Health [NIH]); consulting for Bayer, Roche-Genentech, Prometric, CSL Behring (Germany), Quark. L.B. Ware: Grant funding from NIH (United States) and DOD (United States) (current); research contract with Boehringer Ingelheim (Germany) (past), Global Blood Therapeutics (past), CSL Behring (current); consulting for Bayer (Germany), CSL Behring, Quark.
a Department of Medicine, University of California, San Francisco, 505 Parnassus Avenue, Box 0111, San Francisco, CA 94143-0111, USA; b Department of Anesthesia, University of California, San Francisco, 505 Parnassus Avenue, Box 0111, San Francisco, CA 94143-0111, USA; c Cardiovascular Research Institute, University of California, San Francisco, 505 Parnassus Avenue, Box 0111, San Francisco, CA 94143-0111, USA; d Department of Medicine, Vanderbilt University School of Medicine, T1218 MCN, 1161 21st Avenue South, Nashville, TN 37232-2650, USA; e Department of Pathology, Microbiology, and Immunology, Vanderbilt University School of Medicine, Nashville, TN, USA; f Allergy, Pulmonary and Critical Care Medicine, Vanderbilt University Medical Center, T1218 MCN, 1161 21st Avenue South, Nashville, TN 37232-2650, USA
* Corresponding author. Allergy, Pulmonary and Critical Care Medicine, Vanderbilt University Medical Center, T1218 MCN, 1161 21st Avenue South, Nashville, TN 37232-2650.
E-mail address: lorraine.ware@vanderbilt.edu

Crit Care Clin 36 (2020) 155–165
https://doi.org/10.1016/j.ccc.2019.08.012
0749-0704/20/© 2019 Elsevier Inc. All rights reserved.

INTRODUCTION

In this article, we discuss the important role of biomarkers in bringing precision medicine to the intensive care unit (ICU), particularly for patients with 2 prototypical critical illness syndromes, sepsis, and the acute respiratory distress syndrome (ARDS). Precision medicine uses the available clinical, biological, and environmental data about patients to identify subgroups of patients with common clinical and biological features that can guide diagnostic and therapeutic decisions.[1,2]

This approach stands in contrast to a decades-long effort in critical care to create broad definitions of syndromes, including ARDS[3] and sepsis,[4] based on clinically available criteria. These definitions allow early recognition and treatment of critical illness and include criteria for basic prognostication. Shared definitions have also been essential to forming multicenter clinical trial groups to study these conditions. One notable success of these efforts was the National Heart Lung and Blood Institute ARDS Clinical Trials Network trial demonstrating decreased mortality with low tidal volume ventilation in ARDS.[5]

Notwithstanding these successes, there is a growing recognition that a new paradigm is required for future clinical trials in critical care. There is still no targeted pharmacologic therapy available to treat ARDS or sepsis despite decades of large randomized controlled trials and robust preclinical models. The current definitions of these syndromes incorporate vast clinical heterogeneity without an underlying unifying mechanism, which may limit the power to identify new treatments in clinical trials. Preliminary studies in carefully selected homogeneous cohorts may not be generalizable to the heterogeneous patients enrolled in phase II/III clinical trials of therapies for these syndromes. Biomarker-driven precision medicine offers potential solutions to address these barriers to bringing new therapies into clinical practice.

BIOMARKERS ENABLE PRECISION MEDICINE IN CLINICAL RESEARCH AND PRACTICE

Clinicians use biomarkers to make diagnoses, prognosticate, and monitor treatment. Researchers also can use biomarkers to understand the pathobiology of a disease. In the context of precision medicine, biomarkers enable 2 forms of "enrichment"[6] to more efficiently recruit patients for future clinical trials in critical care (**Fig. 1**):

1. Prognostic enrichment: identifying patients at increased risk of an outcome of interest, which improves the statistical power to detect a relative risk reduction.
2. Predictive enrichment: identifying subgroups of patients who are more likely to respond to a specific treatment based on their specific clinical and/or biological phenotype.

This approach has been used in other specialties. Oncologists, for example, are using increasingly sophisticated molecular biomarkers to identify subgroups of malignancies with distinct biology and for development of targeted therapies. The history of human epidermal growth factor receptor 2 (HER-2) in breast cancer therapy demonstrates the many roles of biomarkers in precision medicine. Early oncogene studies demonstrated HER-2 overexpression on tumor cells predicted increased risk of relapse and worse overall survival in patients with breast cancer.[7] This biomarker provided key insights to the biology of the HER-2–positive subgroup of breast cancer, and motivated the development of trastuzumab, a monoclonal antibody targeting HER-2.[8] HER-2 was then used as a prognostic and predictive biomarker for clinical trials of trastuzumab. These trials demonstrated a marked decrease in mortality in the HER-2–positive subgroup; due to these targeted treatments, HER-2 is now a favorable prognostic biomarker.[9] These early successes have driven further research into

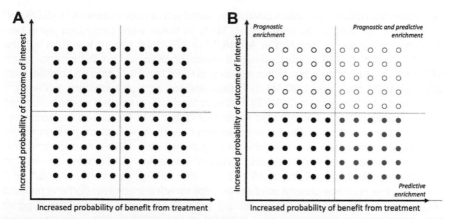

Fig. 1. Biomarkers enable design of enriched clinical trials. (*A*) Without biomarkers, clinical trials will enroll patients with a wide range of outcomes and likelihood of responding to treatment. (*B*) Biomarkers that identify patients at higher risk of the outcome of interest (*empty circles*), or improved response to treatment (*blue circles*) can be used to enrich clinical trials.

identifying targetable mutations. As of 2018, the Food and Drug Administration (FDA) had approved 31 drugs to treat specific mutations in cancers.[10]

There is considerable interest in applying a similar approach to patients in the ICU, but this comes with additional challenges. Critical illnesses frequently present in patients with many comorbidities. They also have rapidly evolving physiology that requires urgent intervention. Finally, in contrast to cancers, critical illnesses can involve multiple organ systems and the optimal site for biomarker sampling is not always apparent. Despite this, progress has been made in identifying predictive and prognostic biomarkers in critical care that are used in clinical research and may soon be implemented in clinical practice. For the remainder of this review, we discuss the role of biomarkers in prognostic and predictive enrichment in ARDS and sepsis, with a focus on novel computational and genomic approaches that identify subgroups of patients with distinct biology.

BIOMARKERS AND PRECISION MEDICINE IN ACUTE RESPIRATORY DISTRESS SYNDROME

There have been many attempts to identify clinical, physiologic, and laboratory biomarkers that define relevant subgroups of ARDS. The best described of these clinical biomarkers is the Pao_2/Fio_2 (PF) ratio, which is included in the 2012 Berlin Definition of ARDS and has been used for prognostic and predictive enrichment in clinical trials. In the derivation cohort for the Berlin Definition, patients were stratified into mild (200 < PF ≤300), moderate (100 < PF ≤200), and severe ARDS (PF ≤100), which were associated with 27%, 32%, and 45% mortality, respectively. Many ARDS trials have restricted enrollment to patients with lower PF ratios for prognostic enrichment, including the Proning Severe ARDS patients (PROSEVA) trial, which demonstrated a mortality benefit for prone positioning in patients with a PF ratio less than 150.[11] Although physiologic markers such as PF are useful for prognostic enrichment, they do not explain underlying mechanisms of disease, and there is considerable interest in identifying additional molecular biomarkers in ARDS.

Several protein biomarkers have been associated with a poor outcome in ARDS and could be used for prognostic enrichment. Many of these were described using biospecimens from patients enrolled in ARMA,[5] the ARDSNet trial of low tidal volume ventilation. In the ARMA cohort, elevated levels of plasma von Willebrand factor (VWF),[12] soluble tumor necrosis factor receptor (sTNFr) I and II,[13] plasma soluble intercellular adhesion molecule-1 (ICAM-1),[14] plasminogen activator inhibitor-1 (PAI-1),[15] and plasma surfactant protein D (SP-D)[16] all independently predicted worse outcomes in ARDS. Lower protein C levels also were associated with increased mortality and fewer ventilator-free days.[15] Similar associations of outcomes with single biomarkers have been demonstrated in other cohorts of patients with ARDS. Kovach and colleagues[17] observed that higher plasma levels of interleukin (IL)-2R were associated with increased 28-day mortality in 48 patients with ARDS. In a meta-analysis of 8 studies, a higher baseline plasma soluble receptor for advanced glycation end product (sRAGE) was associated with higher 90-day mortality.[18] These biomarkers suggest dysregulated immune responses, lung epithelial and endothelial injury, and alterations in coagulation and fibrinolysis play a key role in the pathophysiology of ARDS, but the sensitivity and specificity of individual biomarkers is limited and most are not available for clinical use.

Models combining clinical variables and multiple biomarkers can improve prognostication. In subjects enrolled in the ARDS Network ALVEOLI trial of 2 different levels of positive end-expiratory pressure,[19] a model combining 6 clinical variables and 8 biomarkers (area under the curve [AUC] = 0.850) was superior to a model using only clinical variables (AUC = 0.815) or only biomarkers (AUC = 0.756) for predicting mortality.[20] A simplified version of this model that included 2 clinical variables (APACHE III and age) and 2 biomarkers (SP-D, IL-8) also performed well in this cohort (AUC = 0.834), and was subsequently validated in 2 additional clinical trials and an observational cohort.[21] These studies demonstrate the potential to combine multiple biomarkers both for prognostication in complex critical illness syndromes and to investigate the biology of these heterogeneous diseases.

Advanced computational methods offer new opportunities to further investigate combinations of biomarkers and develop signatures of clinically distinct groups. Calfee and colleagues applied latent class analysis, a mixture modeling method that can be used to determine whether there are distinct subgroups of patients within a cohort, to patients in the ARMA[5] and ALVEOLI[19] trials. The modeling identified a "hyperinflammatory" molecular phenotype with elevated serum inflammatory markers in approximately one-third of the patients and a "hypoinflammatory" phenotype in approximately two-thirds of the patients.[22] Mortality was significantly higher in this hyperinflammatory group (44% vs 23% in ARMA and 51% vs 19% in ALVEOLI, $P<.001$). These molecular phenotypes were found in independent analyses of 3 additional clinical trials, and, in each trial, the hyperinflammatory phenotype had increased mortality.[23–25] These molecular phenotypes can be identified by a parsimonious 3 biomarker model that includes IL-8, sTNFr, and serum bicarbonate.[23] Using a Ward cluster analysis, Bos and colleagues[26] had a similar finding, identifying "reactive" and "uninflamed" molecular phenotypes of patients with ARDS that could be distinguished by IL-6, interferon-gamma, angiopoietin-1/2, and plasminogen activator inhibitor-1. A subsequent analysis of the same cohort identified genes that were differentially expressed in peripheral blood between the reactive and uninflamed groups and identified upregulation of pathways associated with oxidative phosphorylation and mitochondrial dysfunction in the reactive group,[27] further supporting the hypothesis that these 2 groups have distinct underlying biology.

The hyperinflammatory molecular phenotype also predicts differential responses to treatment in retrospective analyses of clinical trials in ARDS. In the original ALVEOLI[19] trial, there was no difference between a high positive end-expiratory pressure (PEEP) and low PEEP strategy in patients with ARDS. In contrast, for the hyperinflammatory patients, mortality at 90 days was 51% in the low PEEP group versus 42% in the high PEEP group (P = .049 for interaction). For the hypoinflammatory patients, mortality at 90 days was 16% in the low PEEP group versus 24% in the high PEEP group. In FACTT,[28] the hyperinflammatory molecular phenotype had a lower mortality with a liberal fluid strategy in ARDS, whereas the original trial reported more ventilator-free days with a conservative fluid strategy and no effect of fluid strategy on mortality.[23] A similar effect was observed for simvastatin in HARP-2,[29] which found no benefit to simvastatin compared with placebo in patients with ARDS. Patients with the hyperinflammatory phenotype had improved survival in the simvastatin arm compared with the placebo arm, whereas no difference was observed in the hypoinflammatory group.[24] Notably, in SAILS,[30] which compared rosuvastatin to placebo in patients with sepsis-associated ARDS, there was no interaction between hyperinflammatory molecular phenotype and rosuvastatin. Although these analyses provide compelling evidence that there are at least 2 distinct molecular phenotypes in ARDS with distinct physiology and responses to treatment, their findings will have to be validated in prospective studies.

BIOMARKERS AND PRECISION MEDICINE IN SEPSIS

As with ARDS, there has been a longstanding interest in identifying prognostic and predictive biomarkers in sepsis. Three biomarkers of particular interest in sepsis, lactate, procalcitonin, and soluble triggering receptor expressed on myeloid cells-1, are described in greater detail in separate reviews in this volume. Other biomarkers that prognosticate increased mortality in sepsis include plasma cell-free hemoglobin,[31] IL-6,[32] IL-8,[33] angiopoietin-1 and angiopoietin-2,[34] and cell-free host DNA.[35] Significant clinical and biological heterogeneity in sepsis has motivated further research into biomarkers that can identify molecular phenotypes of sepsis with distinct biology and clinical features.

As of 2019, multiple groups have identified distinct subgroups of patients with sepsis based on transcriptomic profiles. Wong and colleagues[36] developed a gene expression score that can identify 2 septic shock molecular phenotypes, called endotype A and endotype B. These groups are distinguished by an increased expression of genes associated with adaptive immunity and glucocorticoid receptor signaling in endotype B. Using a similar approach in adults, Davenport and colleagues[37] identified 2 distinct transcriptional signatures that were present at the time of ICU admission in patients with community-acquired pneumonia (CAP) and septic shock as part of the UK Genomic Advances in Sepsis (GAinS) study. These expression profiles were identified as Sepsis Response Signature (SRS) 1 and 2. SRS1 was associated with higher 14-day mortality (22% vs 10%). The differentially expressed pathways included genes that regulate hypoxia inducible factor alpha (HIF-alpha) and mammalian target of rapamycin (mTOR), and components of immune response. Interestingly, there was no significant difference in infectious pathogen or the expression of proinflammatory cytokine genes, including *TNF*, *IL6*, and *IL1B* between the 2 groups. In a subsequent study of patients from the GAinS cohort with fecal peritonitis, an unsupervised clustering approach again identified 2 subgroups of patients with differentially expressed genes that correlated well with the differentially expressed genes in SRS1 and SRS2 observed in CAP.[38]

Although these initial analyses identified 2 molecular phenotypes within sepsis, Sweeney and colleagues[39] used unsupervised clustering on transcriptomic samples from a multinational cohort of 700 patients in 14 datasets and identified 3 molecular phenotypes, which they described as "adaptive, inflammopathic, and coagulopathic" molecular phenotypes. The adaptive subgroup was associated with lower mortality compared with the inflammopathic and coagulopathic groups (18.5%, vs 29.3% and 31.%, respectively, $P = .01$). Finally, an analysis of patients in the Molecular Diagnosis and Risk Stratification of Sepsis (MARS) project identified 4 molecular phenotypes (Mars1–Mars4) using a 140-gene signature, which was then validated in 3 separate cohorts.[40] All 4 molecular phenotypes shared common changes in gene expression relative to healthy patients. The Mars1 molecular phenotype was associated with increased mortality. Further research is required to understand the shared and distinct features of these different molecular phenotypes, but these studies suggest that gene signatures are a potentially effective tool to identify patients at high risk of sepsis mortality in future clinical trials.

Finally, gene signatures may predict response to corticosteroids. Despite multiple large randomized controlled trials (RCTs) since the 1970s, data remain inconclusive on the benefit of steroids in septic shock.[41,42] Recent studies suggest that molecular phenotyping using the gene expression signatures described previously could be used for predictive enrichment to identify patients who may benefit from steroids. The Vasopressin versus Norepinephrine as Initial Therapy in Septic Shock (VANISH) trial was a 2×2 factorial prospective, double-blind RCT of vasopressin versus norepinephrine and hydrocortisone versus placebo in patients with septic shock.[43] In the original trial, there was no significant difference in mortality or acute kidney injury between the hydrocortisone and placebo arms, nor was there any difference between the pressor arms. Antcliffe and colleagues[44] used the previously described SRS1 and SRS2 scores for a post hoc stratification of patients in this trial. Patients with the SRS2 signature who were treated with hydrocortisone had higher mortality than those treated with placebo, and there was no benefit of hydrocortisone identified in the SRS1 group. The 28-day mortality in this study was markedly lower than in prior studies of septic shock, so it is unclear if these results are generalizable. A separate association between gene signatures and corticosteroids was reported with endotypes A and B in pediatric septic shock. In a subgroup of patients with endotype B with septic shock who were at intermediate to high risk of mortality based on serum protein biomarker score, patients had a lower relative risk of a complicated ICU course (defined as persistence of 2 or more organ failures at 7 days or death at 28 days) when treated with steroids at the discretion of the treating physician.[36] As there are many differences between pediatric and adult physiology in sepsis, it is similarly unclear if these results can be applied to adults. Further research is required to identify gene signatures that may be used for predictive enrichment in sepsis clinical trials.

Several protein biomarkers also identify patients who may benefit from targeted anti-inflammatory therapies. IL-6 is upregulated in response to TNF and is a key proinflammatory signal in sepsis.[32] In the MONARCS trial, patients were prospectively stratified into IL-6 high and IL-6 low groups and then were randomly assigned to receive afelimomab, a monoclonal antibody fragment that targets TNF versus placebo for 3 days.[45] Treatment with afelimomab was associated with a lower absolute risk of mortality (adjusted reduction in risk of death 5.8%) in patients with elevated serum IL-6 levels before randomization, but not in the patients with low serum IL-6, consistent with the hypothesis that IL-6 predicted increased TNF activity that would respond to treatment with an inhibitor.

Cell-free hemoglobin (CFH) contains iron protoporphyrin radicals that may cause oxidative injury to lipid membranes and is associated with increased mortality in sepsis.[31] Acetaminophen reduces iron protoporphyrin radicals found in hemoglobin[46] and could therefore be a targeted treatment in sepsis. A phase II RCT randomized 40 patients with severe sepsis and a detectable level of CFH to treatment with enteral acetaminophen versus placebo.[47] The primary outcome of this trial, a reduction of plasma levels of F2-isoprostanes, a marker of lipid peroxidation, on day 3 of ICU admission was negative; however, F2-isoprostanes were significantly reduced on study day 2, and creatinine on study day 3 was significantly lower in the acetamino-phen group. CFH is therefore a potential easily measured biomarker for prognostic and predictive enrichment in clinical trials.

IL-1 receptor antagonist (IL1RA) is an anti-inflammatory cytokine that may play a role in regulating inflammation in sepsis and predicted response to treatment with re-combinant human IL1RA (rhIL1RA) in the Sepsis Syndrome Study. In this multicenter RCT of rhIL1RA in patients with sepsis and hypotension, patients were randomized to rhIL1RA versus placebo for 72 hours,[48] and the initial trial showed no benefit compared with placebo. In a retrospective subgroup analysis, Meyer and colleagues[49] observed significant heterogeneity in the effect of rhIL1RA depending on the plasma IL1RA concentration. Contrary to the hypothesis motivating the original study, patients with higher IL-1RA had higher mortality in both the placebo and treatment arms, but in these patients, treatment with rhIL1RA was associated with decreased mortality (45.4% vs 34.3%, $P = .044$), whereas there was no significant treatment effect in pa-tients with lower IL1RA levels ($P = .028$ for interaction). This counterintuitive finding highlights our limited understanding of the complex biology of clinical sepsis.

SUMMARY

Advances in molecular and computational methods have opened new biomarker-based approaches to precision medicine in critically ill patients, but several challenges remain. Critically ill patients often have comorbid and overlapping conditions. Because these syndromes are dynamic, biomarkers can have temporal variability. Any clinically relevant test must have a short processing time to be used to manage critically ill patients. The biomarkers used in the previously described studies were pri-marily analyzed in research laboratories after trials had concluded and are not avail-able for use to quickly inform clinical decisions or assignment to treatment in the heterogeneous critically ill population. However, development of rapidly available as-says for molecular phenotyping of patients is not infeasible. One recent advance was the FDA approval of SeptiCyte LAB, a 4-gene signature of host immune response that distinguishes between sepsis and noninfectious systemic inflammatory response syn-drome.[50,51] This test was compared with diagnosis by 3 expert physicians in a cohort of 249 patients from the United States and validated in 198 additional patients from the MARS cohort (AUC = 0.85).

Once biomarker measurements are available rapidly at the bedside, their utility will have to be validated in prospective trials. One notable early attempt to use clinical phenotypes for prognostic and predictive enrichment in critical care was the PROWESS-SHOCK trial.[52] The original PROWESS trial was an RCT of recombinant activated protein C (drotrecogin alfa) in patients with severe sepsis.[53] In this trial, a 96-hour infusion of the study drug was associated with a significant reduction in mor-tality (30.8% vs 24.7%). Secondary analyses suggested this benefit was largely in pa-tients with higher APACHE scores or organ dysfunction, and regulatory bodies eventually required a follow-up trial, PROWESS-SHOCK, which was limited to patients with septic shock. However, despite this predictive enrichment strategy, this trial showed no mortality benefit at 28 or 90 days, and the drug was withdrawn from the market, highlighting the importance of prospective validation.

Enriched clinical trials also introduce new challenges in developing and testing new therapies; these trials, by definition, are less generalizable than the current generation of clinical trials. In oncology, for example, genome-targeted therapies, such as trastuzumab, are available for only 8.3% of patients with advanced or metastatic cancer in the United States, despite rapid growth of precision oncology.[10] The more narrowly tailored indications will also spread the fixed costs of drug development over a smaller population, potentially increasing the price of new therapies. These costs must be weighed against the potential benefit of reductions in the high morbidity, mortality, and financial costs of caring for critically ill patients.

Biomarkers are useful tools to understand the biology of ARDS and sepsis and may in the future be able to guide clinical care via identification of distinct molecular phenotypes of critical illness. Further studies are required to identify biomarkers that can be translated to the bedside for precision therapy and to improve on the clinically available criteria that are currently used for patient management.

ACKNOWLEDGMENTS

The authors thank Dr Stephanie Christenson for her many helpful comments and suggestions on our article.

REFERENCES

1. Collins FS, Varmus H. A new initiative on precision medicine. N Engl J Med 2015; 372:793–5.
2. Seymour CW, Gomez H, Chang C-CH, et al. Precision medicine for all? Challenges and opportunities for a precision medicine approach to critical illness. Crit Care 2017;21:257.
3. ARDS Definition Task Force. Acute respiratory distress syndrome: the Berlin definition. JAMA 2012;307(23):2526–33.
4. Singer M, Deutschman CS, Seymour CW, et al. The Third International Consensus definitions for sepsis and septic shock (Sepsis-3). JAMA 2016;315:801–10.
5. The Acute Respiratory Distress Syndrome Network, Brower RG, Matthay MA, Morris A, et al. Ventilation with lower tidal volumes as compared with traditional tidal volumes for acute lung injury and the acute respiratory distress syndrome. N Engl J Med 2000;342:1301–8.
6. US Food and Drug Administration. Enrichment strategies for clinical trials to support determination of effectiveness of human drugs and biological products guidance for industry. 2019. Available at: https://www.fda.gov/downloads/drugs/guidancecomplianceregulatoryinformation/guidances/ucm332181.pdf. Accessed April 21, 2019.
7. Slamon D, Clark G, Wong S, et al. Human breast cancer: correlation of relapse and survival with amplification of the HER-2/neu oncogene. Science 1987;235: 177–82.
8. Harries M, Smith I. The development and clinical use of trastuzumab (Herceptin). Endocr Relat Cancer 2002;9:75–85.
9. Waks AG, Winer EP. Breast cancer treatment. JAMA 2019;321:288–300.
10. Marquart J, Chen EY, Prasad V. Estimation of the percentage of us patients with cancer who benefit from genome-driven oncology. JAMA Oncol 2018. https://doi.org/10.1001/jamaoncol.2018.1660.

11. Guérin C, Reignier J, Richard J-C, et al. Prone positioning in severe acute respiratory distress syndrome. N Engl J Med 2013;368:2159–68.

12. Ware LB, Eisner MD, Thompson BT, et al. Significance of von Willebrand factor in septic and nonseptic patients with acute lung injury. Am J Respir Crit Care Med 2004;170:766–72.

13. Parsons PE, Matthay MA, Ware LB, et al, National Heart, Lung, Blood Institute Acute Respiratory Distress Syndrome Clinical Trials Network. Elevated plasma levels of soluble TNF receptors are associated with morbidity and mortality in patients with acute lung injury. Am J Physiol Lung Cell Mol Physiol 2004;288: L426–31.

14. Calfee CS, Eisner MD, Parsons PE, et al. Soluble intercellular adhesion molecule-1 and clinical outcomes in patients with acute lung injury. Intensive Care Med 2009;35:248–57.

15. Ware LB, Matthay MA, Parsons PE, et al. Pathogenetic and prognostic significance of altered coagulation and fibrinolysis in acute lung injury/acute respiratory distress syndrome. Crit Care Med 2007;35:1821–8.

16. Eisner MD, Parsons P, Matthay MA, et al. Acute Respiratory Distress Syndrome Network. Plasma surfactant protein levels and clinical outcomes in patients with acute lung injury. Thorax 2003;58:983–8.

17. Kovach MA, Stringer KA, Bunting R, et al. Microarray analysis identifies IL-1 receptor type 2 as a novel candidate biomarker in patients with acute respiratory distress syndrome. Respir Res 2015;16:29.

18. Jabaudon M, Blondonnet R, Pereira B, et al. Plasma sRAGE is independently associated with increased mortality in ARDS: a meta-analysis of individual patient data. Intensive Care Med 2018;44:1388–99.

19. Brower RG, Lanken PN, MacIntyre N, et al. Higher versus lower positive end-expiratory pressures in patients with the acute respiratory distress syndrome. N Engl J Med 2004;351:327–36.

20. Ware LB, Koyama T, Billheimer DD, et al. Prognostic and pathogenetic value of combining clinical and biochemical indices in patients with acute lung injury. Chest 2010;137:288–96.

21. Zhao Z, Wickersham N, Kangelaris KN, et al. External validation of a biomarker and clinical prediction model for hospital mortality in acute respiratory distress syndrome. Intensive Care Med 2017;43:1123–31.

22. Calfee CS, Delucchi K, Parsons PE, et al. Subphenotypes in acute respiratory distress syndrome: latent class analysis of data from two randomised controlled trials. Lancet Respir Med 2014;2:611–20.

23. Famous KR, Delucchi K, Ware LB, et al. Acute respiratory distress syndrome subphenotypes respond differently to randomized fluid management strategy. Am J Respir Crit Care Med 2017;195:331–8.

24. Calfee CS, Delucchi KL, Sinha P, et al. Acute respiratory distress syndrome subphenotypes and differential response to simvastatin: secondary analysis of a randomised controlled trial. Lancet Respir Med 2018;6:691–8.

25. Sinha P, Delucchi KL, Thompson BT, et al. Latent class analysis of ARDS subphenotypes: a secondary analysis of the statins for acutely injured lungs from sepsis (SAILS) study. Intensive Care Med 2018;44:1859–69.

26. Bos LD, Schouten LR, van Vught LA, et al. Identification and validation of distinct biological phenotypes in patients with acute respiratory distress syndrome by cluster analysis. Thorax 2017;72:876.

27. Bos LD, Scicluna BP, Ong DY, et al. Understanding heterogeneity in biological phenotypes of ARDS by leukocyte expression profiles. Am J Respir Crit Care Med 2019. https://doi.org/10.1164/rccm.201809-1808oc.
28. National Heart, Lung, and Blood Institute Acute Respiratory Distress Syndrome (ARDS) Clinical Trials Network, Wiedemann HP, Wheeler AP, Bernard GR, et al. Comparison of two fluid-management strategies in acute lung injury. N Engl J Med 2006;354:2564–75.
29. McAuley DF, Laffey JG, O'Kane CM, et al. Simvastatin in the acute respiratory distress syndrome. N Engl J Med 2014;371:1695–703.
30. National Heart, Lung, Blood Institute ARDS Clinical Trials Network, Douglas IS, Bernard GR, Steingrub J, et al. Rosuvastatin for sepsis-associated acute respiratory distress syndrome. N Engl J Med 2014;370:2191–200.
31. Janz DR, Bastarache JA, Peterson JF, et al. Association between cell-free hemoglobin, acetaminophen, and mortality in patients with sepsis. Crit Care Med 2013; 41:784–90.
32. Casey LC, Balk RA, Bone RC. Plasma cytokine and endotoxin levels correlate with survival in patients with the sepsis syndrome. Ann Intern Med 1993;119: 771–8.
33. Wong HR, Cvijanovich N, Wheeler DS, et al. Interleukin-8 as a stratification tool for interventional trials involving pediatric septic shock. Am J Respir Crit Care Med 2008;178:276–82.
34. Ricciuto DR, dos Santos CC, Hawkes M, et al. Angiopoietin-1 and angiopoietin-2 as clinically informative prognostic biomarkers of morbidity and mortality in severe sepsis*. Crit Care Med 2011;39:702–10.
35. Dwivedi DJ, Toltl LJ, Swystun LL, et al. Prognostic utility and characterization of cell-free DNA in patients with severe sepsis. Crit Care 2012;16:R151.
36. Wong HR, Atkinson SJ, Cvijanovich NZ, et al. Combining prognostic and predictive enrichment strategies to identify children with septic shock responsive to corticosteroids. Crit Care Med 2016;44:e1000–3.
37. Davenport EE, Burnham KL, Radhakrishnan J, et al. Genomic landscape of the individual host response and outcomes in sepsis: a prospective cohort study. Lancet Respir Med 2016;4:259–71.
38. Burnham KL, Davenport EE, Radhakrishnan J, et al. Shared and distinct aspects of the sepsis transcriptomic response to fecal peritonitis and pneumonia. Am J Respir Crit Care Med 2017;196:328–39.
39. Sweeney TE, Azad TD, Donato M, et al. Unsupervised analysis of transcriptomics in bacterial sepsis across multiple datasets reveals three robust clusters. Crit Care Med 2018;46:915–25.
40. Scicluna BP, van Vught LA, Zwinderman AH, et al. Classification of patients with sepsis according to blood genomic endotype: a prospective cohort study. Lancet Respir Med 2017;5.
41. Annane D, Renault A, Brun-Buisson C, et al. Hydrocortisone plus fludrocortisone for adults with septic shock. N Engl J Med 2018;378:809–18.
42. Venkatesh B, Finfer S, Cohen J, et al. Adjunctive glucocorticoid therapy in patients with septic shock. N Engl J Med 2018;378:797–808.
43. Gordon AC, Mason AJ, Thirunavukkarasu N, et al. Effect of early vasopressin vs norepinephrine on kidney failure in patients with septic shock: the VANISH randomized clinical trial. JAMA 2016;316:509–18.
44. Antcliffe DB, Burnham KL, Al-Beidh F, et al. Transcriptomic signatures in sepsis and a differential response to steroids: from the VANISH randomized trial. Am J Respir Crit Care Med 2018. https://doi.org/10.1164/rccm.201807-1419oc.

45. Panacek EA, Marshall JC, Albertson TE, et al. Efficacy and safety of the monoclonal anti-tumor necrosis factor antibody F(ab′)2 fragment afelimomab in patients with severe sepsis and elevated interleukin-6 levels. Crit Care Med 2004; 32:2173–82.

46. Boutaud O, Moore KP, Reeder BJ, et al. Acetaminophen inhibits hemoprotein-catalyzed lipid peroxidation and attenuates rhabdomyolysis-induced renal failure. Proc Natl Acad Sci U S A 2010;107(6):2699–704.

47. Janz DR, Bastarache JA, Rice TW, et al. Randomized, placebo-controlled trial of acetaminophen for the reduction of oxidative injury in severe sepsis. Crit Care Med 2015;43:534–41.

48. Fisher CJ, Slotman GJ, Opal SM, et al. Initial evaluation of human recombinant interleukin-1 receptor antagonist in the treatment of sepsis syndrome: a randomized, open-label, placebo-controlled multicenter trial. Crit Care Med 1994;22: 12–21.

49. Meyer NJ, Reilly JP, Anderson BJ, et al. Mortality benefit of recombinant human interleukin-1 receptor antagonist for sepsis varies by initial interleukin-1 receptor antagonist plasma concentration. Crit Care Med 2018;46:21–8.

50. Miller RR III, Lopansri BK, Burke JP, et al. Validation of a host response assay, SeptiCyte LAB, for discriminating sepsis from systemic inflammatory response syndrome in the ICU. Am J Respir Crit Care Med 2018;198:903–13.

51. McHugh L, Seldon TA, Brandon RA, et al. A molecular host response assay to discriminate between sepsis and infection-negative systemic inflammation in critically ill patients: discovery and validation in independent cohorts. PLoS Med 2015;12:e1001916.

52. Ranieri VM, Thompson BT, Barie PS, et al. Drotrecogin alfa (activated) in adults with septic shock. N Engl J Med 2012;366:2055–64.

53. Bernard GR, Vincent J-L, Laterre P-F, et al. Efficacy and safety of recombinant human activated protein C for severe sepsis. N Engl J Med 2001;344:699–709.

Biomarkers of Immunosuppression

Abinav K. Misra, MD, Mitchell M. Levy, MD, MCCM, Nicholas S. Ward, MD, FCCM*

KEYWORDS

- Sepsis • Immunosuppression • Biomarkers • IL-10 • HLA-DR

KEY POINTS

- Sepsis can no longer be described as a primarily proinflammatory response. There is a complimentary anti-inflammatory response, the timing, duration, and intensity of which is as variable as the proinflammatory response.
- The combination of proinflammatory and anti-inflammatory activation, along with patient-specific variables, such as genetics and health status, can lead to tremendous heterogeneity of immunologic states in patients with sepsis at any given stage of sepsis.
- There is renewed focus on biomarkers that can identify patients at different stages of the immune response to facilitate precision medicine and therapeutics.
- The immunosuppressive response has a distinct set of cytokines and cellular responses, and may have a powerful influence on clinical outcomes in sepsis.
- Despite promising data, the use of HLA expression as clinical biomarker in practice is not likely to be common for some time.

INTRODUCTION

In recent decades, two important concepts have emerged in sepsis research. The first is that the damaging response to infection can no longer be described as primarily proinflammatory in nature. It is now known that accompanying an inflammatory phase there is a complimentary anti-inflammatory response, the timing, duration, and intensity of which is as variable as the proinflammatory response. The second important concept is that the combination of proinflammatory and anti-inflammatory activation, along with patient-specific variables, such as genetics and health status, can lead to tremendous heterogeneity of immunologic states in patients with sepsis at any given stage. Moreover, this immunologic response changes almost continuously. The result of this new understanding of the complexity of the sepsis syndrome is that there has been a major shift in creating new antisepsis therapies. After many years spent trying

Division of Pulmonary, Critical Care, and Sleep Medicine, Alpert Medical School of Brown University, Physicians Office Building, Suite 224, 110 Lockwood street, Providence, RI 02903, USA
* Corresponding author.
E-mail address: nicholas_ward@brown.edu

Crit Care Clin 36 (2020) 167–176
https://doi.org/10.1016/j.ccc.2019.08.013
0749-0704/20/© 2019 Elsevier Inc. All rights reserved.

to find agents that would suppress the proinflammatory response and use them in a "one size fits all" manner, researchers are now also looking at agents meant to enhance or stimulate the immune system. Furthermore, given the question of optimal timing for administration of these agents, there is renewed focus on biomarkers that can identify patients at different stages of the immune response to facilitate precision medicine and therapeutics.

BACKGROUND AND HISTORY

In 1996, a paper by Bone[1] described an immunologic phenomenon that was increasingly noticed to occur in sepsis. Like the systemic inflammatory response syndrome (SIRS), this immunosuppressed state he called the compensatory anti-inflammatory response syndrome is a complex and incompletely defined pattern of immunologic responses to severe infection. The difference was that whereas SIRS was a proinflammatory state aimed at eliminating infectious organisms through activation of the immune system, compensatory anti-inflammatory response syndrome was a deactivation of the immune system tasked with restoring homeostasis from an inflammatory state. Since then understanding of the immunosuppression of sepsis has grown. It has become apparent that this response is not merely to counterbalance the proinflammatory response and furthermore, that the anti-inflammatory response does not necessarily "follow" the proinflammatory phase of sepsis. Instead, this immunosuppressive response has a distinct set of cytokines and cellular responses, and may have a powerful influence on clinical outcomes in sepsis.

Since Bone's paper there has been an ongoing evolution in understanding of sepsis immunosuppression. The work of Hotchkiss and others has shown that the spleens of patients who succumb to sepsis are seen to have an abundance of dying/apoptotic lymphocytes, and macrophages harvested from patients with sepsis are blunted in their ability to secrete proinflammatory cytokines (reviewed in Refs.[2,3]). Perhaps the most significant data, however, comes from the fact that a decade's worth of clinical trials on agents meant to suppress the immune system have not been shown to have a positive effect on sepsis outcomes and in some instances proved harmful. Later, studies began to show that using these markers of immunosuppression as individual biomarkers might be able to help predict outcomes in patients with sepsis. More recently, however, these data are now being used to determine patient selection for clinical trials and the timing of administration.

MARKERS OF SEPSIS IMMUNOSUPPRESSION
Lymphocyte Death and Deactivation

Lymphocytes play a key role in initiating and maintaining the sepsis response. Their importance relates to their capacity to interact with the innate and adaptive immune responses and their ability to coordinate, amplify, and attenuate the inflammatory response. Lymphocyte anergy has long been demonstrated in patients following major surgery, blunt trauma, and thermal injury.[4–6] In 2009, Hotchkiss and colleagues,[7] showed that spleens harvested from newly deceased patients with sepsis demonstrated copious apoptotic cell death of lymphocytes. Further studies using animal and human in vitro models helped better characterize these lymphocyte alterations.

Loss of lymphocytes or their dysfunction can significantly impair the immune system. Although loss of CD4$^+$ effector T cells has been shown repeatedly in patients with sepsis, the loss of CD8$^+$ cells was historically more debatable. In 2001 Hotchkiss and colleagues[8] showed caspase-9 mediated deletion of CD4$^+$ and B cells but not of CD8[+] T cells and natural killer cells in sepsis. Conversely, in 2002, Le Tulzo and colleagues[9] demonstrated lymphopenia in patients with sepsis that affected CD4[+] and CD8[+] subsets of T cells. This was also demonstrated, in postmortem studies, in patients dying with sepsis as apoptosis induced loss of cells of innate and adaptive immune system including CD4 and CD8 T cells, B cells, and dendritic cells.[7] In 2015, Roger and colleagues[10] also showed enhanced apoptosis in CD4[+] and CD8[+] T cells during early phase of human sepsis. In their study Le Tulzo and colleagues[9] showed that lymphocyte apoptosis was increased five-fold in patients with septic shock and two-fold in other critically ill patients when compared with control subjects. Severe lymphopenia occurred in 25% to 63% of patients with septic shock.[11] Drewry and colleagues,[12] among others, revealed persistent prolonged lymphopenia to be linked to decreased survival in an observational human study.[7]

Given the crucial role of lymphocytes in the immune response, it might be possible to reverse immunosuppression by restoring their function. Currently, the best available test to assess lymphocyte functionality remains ex vivo measurement of proliferation in response to recall antigens or mitogen stimulation.[13] However, as flow cytometry and enzyme-linked immunosorbent assays become available, these provide alternative routes for testing T-cell functionality.

T-Lymphocyte Anergy

Another feature of sepsis-induced immunosuppression is T-lymphocyte anergy.[14,15] This is characterized by decreased proliferation; decreased effector T-cell variability; decreased production of proinflammatory cytokines; and increased levels of anti-inflammatory cytokines, such as interleukin (IL)-10. Changes on cell surface receptors, such as reduced coactivating receptors (CD28) and increased coinhibitory receptors (PD-1, CTLA-4), also occur.[16-18] This shift in cell surface receptors leads to impaired responsiveness to stimuli. T-cell exhaustion usually occurs in the setting of persistent exposure to antigens, infection-mediated inflammation, or high antigen load, all of which are seen in patients with sepsis.[19,20] In 2012 Boomer and colleagues[21] conducted a prospective study looking at changing phenotypes of T cells as acute sepsis progressed and demonstrated increased expression of coinhibitory receptors and decreased IL-7R expression and γ-interferon secretion. They also saw increased expression of PD-L1 on dendritic cells, which can lead to cell death. This complex interplay is also affected by various other host/patient factors, such as age, comorbidities, overall health and functional status, and by the virulence and pathogenicity of the microbe.

The ability to diagnose T-cell exhaustion and apoptosis in real time would enable the use of several factors known to stimulate the immune system by preventing these phenomena, such as IL-7. IL-7 is a potent antiapoptotic cytokine produced in multiple organs, such as thymus gland, liver, peripheral lymphoid organs, and in a small amount by dendritic cells. IL-7 is essential for lymphocyte survival, development, and expansion.[22-24] Unsinger and colleagues[25] were able to show IL-7 decreased sepsis-induced apoptosis, reversed sepsis-induced depression of γ-interferon, and increased survival in murine polymicrobial sepsis model. In humans, IL-7 has been shown to increase CD4[+] and CD8[+] T cells and has been safely used in patients without significant side effects.[26-28] In 2018, the first phase II multicenter trial was conducted with immunoadjuvant therapy looking to reverse sepsis-induced defects in adaptive immunity. IL-7 was given to patients with sepsis and lymphopenia significantly raising lymphocyte counts with this effect persisting even after the experimental drug was stopped.[29]

HLA-DR

The expression of the HLA-DR receptor has been an important story in developing a biomarker of sepsis immunosuppression. HLA-DR receptor is expressed on monocytes, macrophages, and other immune cells that are key to activating the adaptive immune system.[30] These cells digest foreign proteins and express a receptor/protein complex on their surface for cobinding with T-cell receptors. Customarily, high levels of expression of this receptor correspond to an activated immune system. In many patients with sepsis, however, there is seen a deactivation of monocytes characterized by a downregulation of their HLA-DR receptors. Furthermore, this downregulation correlates with other markers of immunosuppression.

Several studies have focused on monocytes downregulation of HLA receptors as a biomarker.[31–36] In 1995 Asadullah and colleagues[31] studied 57 neurosurgical patients and found that HLA-DR expression was lower in 14 patients who developed infection, compared with patients with an uncomplicated postoperative course. Out of 10 patients with less than 30% HLA-DR-positive monocytes, 9 developed infection. They hypothesized that the mechanism of this downregulation was high levels of endogenous cortisol because the effect coincided with high adrenocorticotrophic hormone and cortisol concentrations and similar downregulation was seen in other patients who received high doses of exogenous corticosteroids. Subsequent studies supported the theory that the magnitude of HLA-DR receptor downregulation predicted a variety of other poor outcomes, such as sepsis in liver transplant patients[34]; however, that study was confounded by exogenous steroids in some patients.[33] Allen and colleagues[37] found HLA levels predicted sepsis in pediatric cardiac surgery patients. In a small study of adults with sepsis, Su and colleagues[38] found that levels of HLA-DR-positive monocytes less than 30% were more predictive of mortality than Acute Physiology, Age, Chronic Health Evaluation II scores.

More recent studies looking at the predictive power of HLA receptor have yielded mixed results. In 2003, three papers were published that yielded similar findings. Hynninen and colleagues[39] evaluated the HLA-DR expression of 61 patients with sepsis at admission and showed no predictive power of HLA expression for survival. Another study of 70 patients with sepsis also found no correlation between HLA expression and infectious or mortality outcomes.[40] This study showed that if patients' monocytes were stimulated with granulocyte colony–stimulating factor ex vivo, their HLA expression increased. The third study looked at 85 cardiac surgery patients. HLA expression was measured at presurgery, immediately after, and 1 day later. Their data showed that although all patients' HLA levels declined after surgery, the magnitude of the response did not correlate with sepsis/SIRS, or other infectious complications.[41] In one of the largest studies to date, Gomez and colleagues[42] did a complete immunologic assessment on 148 patients with sepsis, looking at a variety of proinflammatory and anti-inflammatory markers. They were unable to find a good correlation between HLA downregulation or lymphocyte apoptosis and mortality when adjusted for confounders, such as steroid use. Reasons for the different results are still being investigated but may be the result of small sample sizes, timing, or well-described variation caused by the different laboratory techniques used. In one study, the same samples were analyzed in two different laboratories and differed by 20%.[40]

In 2013, Venet and colleagues[13] published a comprehensive review of the use of HLA levels with outcomes. They looked at 13 studies done in the preceding 10 years and analyzed them for methodology and result. They analyzed a virtual cohort of patients using real data from the prior studies and concluded that analysis of immunosuppression by HLA at Day 4 of sepsis could be used to predict a group of patients with higher mortality. The authors go on to advocate for the use of such biomarker in any future studies looking at immunostimulators.

Several studies have examined the use of HLA expression as a marker for the use of γ-interferon, which has been shown in vivo to reverse monocyte deactivation.[43–45] Two small trials were done on human subjects with sepsis. In both studies, subjects with sepsis and monocyte HLA-DR expression of 30% or less were given γ-interferon. Both groups reported increases in HLA-DR expression, usually after just one dose. One of the studies also examined the monocytes ex vivo and showed that interferon improved monocyte cytokine production.[44] Another human trial was different in that it sought to study the effects of γ-interferon regionally.[46] In this study, the authors selected 21 patients with severe trauma and alveolar macrophage dysfunction as determined by a bronchoalveolar lavage sample showing macrophage HLA-DR expression of 30% or less. γ-Interferon was administered via inhalation. They found about 50% of the subjects had an increase in their alveolar macrophage HLA-DR expression. These patients had a lower incidence of pneumonia but no other differences in outcomes. The small numbers and lack of a control population in all three of these studies limits the conclusions that can be drawn, especially because HLA-DR expression is known to increase as patients recover.

Despite these promising data, the use of HLA expression as clinical biomarker in practice is not likely to be common for some time. Technical difficulties are a major concern. There are three assays that can be used and all are expensive, slow, not commonly available, and fraught with potential error.[47] The most common assay is to use some version of flow cytometry, either showing mean fluorescence intensity or percentage of cells expressing HLA. The first technique suffers from differing levels of calibration among laboratories. The second method suffers from lack of agreement as to what constitutes "low levels" of expression and "normal" levels of expression. Quantitative polymerase chain reaction can also be done to look for downregulation of the genes for HLA. This method is also complicated and expensive and suffers from the need to carefully isolate the monocytes from other cells.

Interleukin-10

IL-10 is another important cytokine in sepsis immunosupression. IL-10 was first characterized around 1990 and was shown to regulate T-cell population.[48] It has now been established that IL-10 has multiple immunosuppressive roles (reviewed in Ref.[49]) with its most important being the downregulation of tumor necrosis factor (TNF). In animal models of sepsis, the administration of IL-10 has been shown to have positive[50–52] and negative[53,54] effects on outcome, which likely are dependent on the time of administration and the severity of the infection. In one carefully done animal model, Ashare and colleagues[55] followed levels of proinflammatory cytokines and anti-inflammatory cytokines throughout the whole course of sepsis in mice. They found that bacterial levels in tissue correlated with IL-10 levels and that if the complementary proinflammatory response was blocked by pretreatment with IL-10 receptor antagonist, bacterial levels were higher as was mortality. Similarly, Song and colleagues[56] showed that blocking IL-10 activity early had no effect on mortality, and blocking it late (12 hours) after sepsis improved mortality. The totality of these studies helps to show the complex role of IL-10, because it helps to maintain a careful balance of the immune system in inflammation. Thus, manipulation of IL-10 leads to negative or positive consequences depending on the underlying state of the patient with sepsis.

IL-10 has been evaluated as a marker of sepsis outcomes. Most of these studies have been on human patients and showed mixed results. These data likely reflect the varied magnitudes and time courses of proinflammatory and anti-inflammatory cytokine expression in real patients. In 1998, Doughty and colleagues[57] sampled 53 pediatric intensive care unit patients and found that high IL-10 levels correlated with three or more organ dysfunction and mortality. Ahlstrom and coworkers[58] found no predictive value in IL-10 levels in patients with SIRS, but Simmons and colleagues[59] found that IL-10 levels did correlate with mortality in a sample of 93 critically ill patients with acute renal failure. Perhaps the most interesting data comes from two studies that looked at the ratio of IL-10 to TNF. In a large study of more than 400 patients admitted to the hospital for fever, van Dissel and colleagues[60] showed that a higher IL-10 to TNF ratio was predictive of mortality. A similar study by Gogos and colleagues[61] in a population of patients with mixed sepsis showed the same results.

More recently two large human studies were conducted in which IL-10 was evaluated for utility in predicting outcomes. Frencken and colleagues[62] analyzed the blood of more than 700 patients admitted for sepsis. They specifically looked for the ratio of IL-10 to IL-6 levels seeking patients with an immunosuppression imbalance. Although they did find correlations between high IL-10 and IL-6 with mortality, the ratio of the two seemed to have no predictive utility. In 2016 one of the largest ever evaluations of serum cytokine levels with outcomes was published by van Vught and colleagues.[63] In this study of 1719 admissions, clinical and biologic risk factors were analyzed as predictors of outcomes. Although the presence of a secondary infection had an impact on mortality, the levels of IL-10 production as measured by gene expression in leukocytes did not.

GENOMICS

The use of genomics as biomarkers of sepsis immunosuppression is a newer field of study that has yet to provide any major breakthroughs for clinicians. Genomic analysis is limited by the difficulty of isolating the cells of interest and the large number of genes that could be assayed. Further complicating the analysis is the imperfect correlation between gene expression and protein expression. Some progress is being made, however. In 2014, Fairfax and colleagues[64] showed that leukocytes with different genomic variants had different gene expression in response to inflammatory stimuli, such as endotoxin.

In a more clinical-based study from 2016, Davenport and colleagues[65] did gene expression analysis on leukocytes extracted from a cohort of 265 patients with sepsis from pneumonia and organ failure. Their analysis identified two distinct response signatures they labeled SRS1 and SRS2. The SRS1 signature identified individuals with an immunosuppressed phenotype characterized by endotoxin tolerance, T-cell exhaustion, and downregulation of monocyte HLA receptors. The SRS1 signature was also associated with a higher 14-day mortality rate. They then found that a set of just seven genes could predict if a patient falls into this group. Of note, this signature was only present in 41% of the patients studied, which lends further weight to the concept that future sepsis therapies, especially those used to boost the immune system, be used in conjunction with some biomarker. The only other recent clinical trial to look at genomics was a large study done by van Vught and colleagues,[63] in 2016, in which genomic analysis was done on a subset of patients from a large sepsis study looking at the effect of secondary infections on mortality. Their data only looked at a small array of mostly proinflammatory cytokine genes but did look at IL-10 expression. They found no correlation between gene expression and outcomes other than some differences in genes associated with glucose metabolism.

SUMMARY

Reviewing the recent literature on the role immunosuppression plays in the course of the illness, it is clear that a more tailored precision treatment strategy is not far away. Despite some conflicting data from the last 20 years it is more likely than not that immunosuppression occurs in a significant fraction of patients and that this immunosuppression can affect outcomes. The lack of a clear signal likely reflects a combination of factors, such as technical challenges and lack of standardization with the different assays and the timing of their measurement. Additionally, the naturally occurring heterogeneity of patients with sepsis and their medications adds further confounders to this problem.

Recently, several agents have been shown to reverse some aspects of sepsis immunosuppression. Two studies showed that administration of γ-interferon to alveolar macrophages could stimulate them to a more proinflammatory state[44,46] and IL-7 has been shown to reverse some aspects of T-cell dysfunction. The key to therapies like these going forward is real-time identification of patients who have these specific defects. Both researchers and clinicians must hope that from these initial biomarker studies identifying immunosuppression in sepsis there will eventually emerge more effective immunostimulatory therapies that are timed and individualized for each patient. Perhaps then additional reductions in the mortality of this disease can be seen through a better understanding of the complex immune response.

REFERENCES

1. Bone RC. Sir Isaac Newton, sepsis, SIRS, and CARS. Crit Care Med 1996;24(7): 1125–8.
2. Ward NS, Casserly B, Ayala A. The compensatory anti-inflammatory response syndrome (CARS) in critically ill patients. Clin Chest Med 2008;29(4):617–25, viii.
3. Ward PA. Immunosuppression in sepsis. JAMA 2011;306(23):2618–9.
4. Stephan RN, Kupper TS, Geha AS, et al. Hemorrhage without tissue trauma produces immunosuppression and enhances susceptibility to sepsis. Arch Surg 1987;122(1):62–8.
5. Denzel C, Riese J, Hohenberger W, et al. Monitoring of immunotherapy by measuring monocyte HLA-DR expression and stimulated TNFalpha production during sepsis after liver transplantation. Intensive Care Med 1998;24(12):1343–4.
6. Voll RE, Herrmann M, Roth EA, et al. Immunosuppressive effects of apoptotic cells. Nature 1997;390(6658):350–1.
7. Hotchkiss RS, Swanson PE, Freeman BD, et al. Apoptotic cell death in patients with sepsis, shock, and multiple organ dysfunction. Crit Care Med 1999;27(7): 1230–51.
8. Hotchkiss RS, Tinsley KW, Swanson PE, et al. Sepsis-induced apoptosis causes progressive profound depletion of B and CD4+ T lymphocytes in humans. J Immunol 2001;166(11):6952–63.
9. Le Tulzo Y, Pangault C, Gacouin A, et al. Early circulating lymphocyte apoptosis in human septic shock is associated with poor outcome. Shock 2002;18(6): 487–94.
10. Roger PM, Hyvernat H, Ticchioni M, et al. The early phase of human sepsis is characterized by a combination of apoptosis and proliferation of T cells. J Crit Care 2012;27(4):384–93.
11. Chung KP, Chang HT, Lo SC, et al. Severe lymphopenia is associated with elevated plasma interleukin-15 levels and increased mortality during severe sepsis. Shock 2015;43(6):569–75.

12. Drewry AM, Samra N, Skrupky LP, et al. Persistent lymphopenia after diagnosis of sepsis predicts mortality. Shock 2014;42(5):383–91.
13. Venet F, Lukaszewicz AC, Payen D, et al. Monitoring the immune response in sepsis: a rational approach to administration of immunoadjuvant therapies. Curr Opin Immunol 2013;25(4):477–83.
14. Christou NV, Meakins JL, Gordon J, et al. The delayed hypersensitivity response and host resistance in surgical patients. 20 years later. Ann Surg 1995;222(4): 534–46 [discussion: 46–8].
15. MacLean LD, Meakins JL, Taguchi K, et al. Host resistance in sepsis and trauma. Ann Surg 1975;182(3):207–17.
16. Kung CT, Su CM, Chang HW, et al. The prognostic value of leukocyte apoptosis in patients with severe sepsis at the emergency department. Clin Chim Acta 2015; 438:364–9.
17. Inoue S, Sato T, Suzuki-Utsunomiya K, et al. Sepsis-induced hypercytokinemia and lymphocyte apoptosis in aging-accelerated Klotho knockout mice. Shock 2013;39(3):311–6.
18. Albertsmeier M, Quaiser D, von Dossow-Hanfstingl V, et al. Major surgical trauma differentially affects T-cells and APC. Innate Immun 2015;21(1):55–64.
19. Otto GP, Sossdorf M, Claus RA, et al. The late phase of sepsis is characterized by an increased microbiological burden and death rate. Crit Care 2011;15(4):R183.
20. Wherry EJ, Kurachi M. Molecular and cellular insights into T cell exhaustion. Nat Rev Immunol 2015;15(8):486–99.
21. Boomer JS, Shuherk-Shaffer J, Hotchkiss RS, et al. A prospective analysis of lymphocyte phenotype and function over the course of acute sepsis. Crit Care 2012;16(3):R112.
22. Hofmeister R, Khaled AR, Benbernou N, et al. Interleukin-7: physiological roles and mechanisms of action. Cytokine Growth Factor Rev 1999;10(1):41–60.
23. Mazzucchelli R, Durum SK. Interleukin-7 receptor expression: intelligent design. Nat Rev Immunol 2007;7(2):144–54.
24. Mackall CL, Fry TJ, Gress RE. Harnessing the biology of IL-7 for therapeutic application. Nat Rev Immunol 2011;11(5):330–42.
25. Unsinger J, McGlynn M, Kasten KR, et al. IL-7 promotes T cell viability, trafficking, and functionality and improves survival in sepsis. J Immunol 2010;184(7): 3768–79.
26. Sportes C, Hakim FT, Memon SA, et al. Administration of rhIL-7 in humans increases in vivo TCR repertoire diversity by preferential expansion of naive T cell subsets. J Exp Med 2008;205(7):1701–14.
27. Morre M, Beq S. Interleukin-7 and immune reconstitution in cancer patients: a new paradigm for dramatically increasing overall survival. Target Oncol 2012; 7(1):55–68.
28. Rosenberg SA, Sportes C, Ahmadzadeh M, et al. IL-7 administration to humans leads to expansion of CD8+ and CD4+ cells but a relative decrease of CD4+ T-regulatory cells. J Immunother 2006;29(3):313–9.
29. Francois B, Jeannet R, Daix T, et al. Interleukin-7 restores lymphocytes in septic shock: the IRIS-7 randomized clinical trial. JCI Insight 2018;3(5) [pii:98960].
30. Roche PA, Furuta K. The ins and outs of MHC class II-mediated antigen processing and presentation. Nat Rev Immunol 2015;15(4):203–16.
31. Asadullah K, Woiciechowsky C, Docke WD, et al. Very low monocytic HLA-DR expression indicates high risk of infection: immunomonitoring for patients after neurosurgery and patients during high dose steroid therapy. Eur J Emerg Med 1995;2(4):184–90.

32. Fumeaux T, Pugin J. Role of interleukin-10 in the intracellular sequestration of human leukocyte antigen-DR in monocytes during septic shock. Am J Respir Crit Care Med 2002;166(11):1475–82.

33. Haveman JW, van den Berg AP, van den Berk JM, et al. Low HLA-DR expression on peripheral blood monocytes predicts bacterial sepsis after liver transplantation: relation with prednisolone intake. Transpl Infect Dis 1999;1(3):146–52.

34. van den Berk JM, Oldenburger RH, van den Berg AP, et al. Low HLA-DR expression on monocytes as a prognostic marker for bacterial sepsis after liver transplantation. Transplantation 1997;63(12):1846–8.

35. Volk HD, Reinke P, Docke WD. Immunological monitoring of the inflammatory process: which variables? When to assess? Eur J Surg Suppl 1999;(584):70–2.

36. Volk HD, Reinke P, Krausch D, et al. Monocyte deactivation: rationale for a new therapeutic strategy in sepsis. Intensive Care Med 1996;22(Suppl 4):S474–81.

37. Allen ML, Peters MJ, Goldman A, et al. Early postoperative monocyte deactivation predicts systemic inflammation and prolonged stay in pediatric cardiac intensive care. Crit Care Med 2002;30(5):1140–5.

38. Su L, Zhou DY, Tang YQ, et al. Clinical value of monitoring CD14+ monocyte human leukocyte antigen (locus) DR levels in the early stage of sepsis. Zhongguo Wei Zhong Bing Ji Jiu Yi Xue 2006;18(11):677–9 [in Chinese].

39. Hynninen M, Pettila V, Takkunen O, et al. Predictive value of monocyte histocompatibility leukocyte antigen-DR expression and plasma interleukin-4 and -10 levels in critically ill patients with sepsis. Shock 2003;20(1):1–4.

40. Perry SE, Mostafa SM, Wenstone R, et al. Is low monocyte HLA-DR expression helpful to predict outcome in severe sepsis? Intensive Care Med 2003;29(8):1245–52.

41. Oczenski W, Krenn H, Jilch R, et al. HLA-DR as a marker for increased risk for systemic inflammation and septic complications after cardiac surgery. Intensive Care Med 2003;29(8):1253–7.

42. Gomez HG, Gonzalez SM, Londono JM, et al. Immunological characterization of compensatory anti-inflammatory response syndrome in patients with severe sepsis: a longitudinal study*. Crit Care Med 2014;42(4):771–80.

43. Bundschuh DS, Barsig J, Hartung T, et al. Granulocyte-macrophage colony-stimulating factor and IFN-gamma restore the systemic TNF-alpha response to endotoxin in lipopolysaccharide-desensitized mice. J Immunol 1997;158(6):2862–71.

44. Docke WD, Randow F, Syrbe U, et al. Monocyte deactivation in septic patients: restoration by IFN-gamma treatment. Nat Med 1997;3(6):678–81.

45. Hershman MJ, Appel SH, Wellhausen SR, et al. Inter'-gamma treatment increases HLA-DR expression on monocytes in severely injured patients. Clin Exp Immunol 1989;77(1):67–70.

46. Nakos G, Malamou-Mitsi VD, Lachana A, et al. Immunoparalysis in patients with severe trauma and the effect of inhaled interferon-gamma. Crit Care Med 2002;30(7):1488–94.

47. Pfortmueller CA, Meisel C, Fux M, et al. Assessment of immune organ dysfunction in critical illness: utility of innate immune response markers. Intensive Care Med Exp 2017;5(1):49.

48. O'Garra A, Stapleton G, Dhar V, et al. Production of cytokines by mouse B cells: B lymphomas and normal B cells produce interleukin 10. Int Immunol 1990;2(9):821–32.

49. Oberholzer A, Oberholzer C, Moldawer LL. Interleukin-10: a complex role in the pathogenesis of sepsis syndromes and its potential as an anti-inflammatory drug. Crit Care Med 2002;30(1 Supp):S58–63.
50. Berg DJ, Kuhn R, Rajewsky K, et al. Interleukin-10 is a central regulator of the response to LPS in murine models of endotoxic shock and the Shwartzman reaction but not endotoxin tolerance. J Clin Invest 1995;96(5):2339–47.
51. Howard M, Muchamuel T, Andrade S, et al. Interleukin 10 protects mice from lethal endotoxemia. J Exp Med 1993;177(4):1205–8.
52. van der Poll T, Jansen PM, Montegut WJ, et al. Effects of IL-10 on systemic inflammatory responses during sublethal primate endotoxemia. J Immunol 1997;158(4):1971–5.
53. Remick DG, Garg SJ, Newcomb DE, et al. Exogenous interleukin-10 fails to decrease the mortality or morbidity of sepsis. Crit Care Med 1998;26(5):895–904.
54. Steinhauser ML, Hogaboam CM, Kunkel SL, et al. IL-10 is a major mediator of sepsis-induced impairment in lung antibacterial host defense. J Immunol 1999;162(1):392–9.
55. Ashare A, Powers LS, Butler NS, et al. Anti-inflammatory response is associated with mortality and severity of infection in sepsis. Am J Physiol Lung Cell Mol Physiol 2005;288(4):L633–40.
56. Song GY, Chung CS, Chaudry IH, et al. What is the role of interleukin 10 in polymicrobial sepsis: anti-inflammatory agent or immunosuppressant? Surgery 1999;126(2):378–83.
57. Doughty L, Carcillo JA, Kaplan S, et al. The compensatory anti-inflammatory cytokine interleukin 10 response in pediatric sepsis-induced multiple organ failure. Chest 1998;113(6):1625–31.
58. Ahlstrom A, Hynninen M, Tallgren M, et al. Predictive value of interleukins 6, 8 and 10, and low HLA-DR expression in acute renal failure. Clin Nephrol 2004;61(2):103–10.
59. Simmons EM, Himmelfarb J, Sezer MT, et al. Plasma cytokine levels predict mortality in patients with acute renal failure. Kidney Int 2004;65(4):1357–65.
60. van Dissel JT, van Langevelde P, Westendorp RG, et al. Anti-inflammatory cytokine profile and mortality in febrile patients. Lancet 1998;351(9107):950–3.
61. Gogos CA, Drosou E, Bassaris HP, et al. Pro- versus anti-inflammatory cytokine profile in patients with severe sepsis: a marker for prognosis and future therapeutic options. J Infect Dis 2000;181(1):176–80.
62. Frencken JF, van Vught LA, Peelen LM, et al. An unbalanced inflammatory cytokine response is not associated with mortality following sepsis: a prospective cohort study. Crit Care Med 2017;45(5):e493–9.
63. van Vught LA, Klein Klouwenberg PM, Spitoni C, et al. Incidence, risk factors, and attributable mortality of secondary infections in the intensive care unit after admission for sepsis. JAMA 2016;315(14):1469–79.
64. Fairfax BP, Humburg P, Makino S, et al. Innate immune activity conditions the effect of regulatory variants upon monocyte gene expression. Science 2014;343(6175):1246949.
65. Davenport EE, Burnham KL, Radhakrishnan J, et al. Genomic landscape of the individual host response and outcomes in sepsis: a prospective cohort study. Lancet Respir Med 2016;4(4):259–71.

The Future of Biomarkers

Jean-Louis Vincent, MD, PhD*, Elisa Bogossian, MD,
Marco Menozzi, MD

KEYWORDS

• Precision medicine • Phenotypes • Biomarker panels • Sensitivity • Specificity

KEY POINTS

• New biomarkers are being developed that will facilitate the move toward personalized medicine.
• Combinations of biomarkers are more likely to be of use than single biomarkers.
• Developments in omics will add new biomarkers to the traditional protein and cytokine markers.

CASE PRESENTATION IN THE INTENSIVE CARE UNIT IN 2040

Mr X, a postoperative patient on the general surgical floor, develops a temperature of more than 38°C. In just 2 minutes, his bedside sepsis panel alerts that he has an infection. In just 7 minutes, the presence of *Klebsiella* is identified from a blood sample and its antibiotic sensitivities provided. Appropriate antibiotics are started according to a computerized algorithm. The antibiotic doses given are higher than usual because tests suggest he has increased renal clearance of drugs. Nevertheless, his bedside renal panel indicates he is at high risk of developing renal failure likely to require renal replacement therapy (RRT) in the next few days, so immediate transfer to the intensive care unit (ICU) is organized. His urine output then starts to fall, and his blood volume biomarker level indicates a risk of fluid overload showing that he needs close monitoring, especially because his acute respiratory destress syndrome (ARDS) risk panel is also in the red zone. These results suggest RRT should be started, even before his creatinine levels increase significantly (in any case, creatinine levels are no longer trusted very much; there are better markers now). The new lung protective agent will also be prescribed, even though this drug is costly.

Disclosure Statement: The authors have no conflicts of interest to declare.
Department of Intensive Care, Erasme Hospital, Université libre de Bruxelles, Route de Lennik 808, Brussels 1070, Belgium
* Corresponding author.
E-mail address: jlvincent@intensive.org

Crit Care Clin 36 (2020) 177–187
https://doi.org/10.1016/j.ccc.2019.08.014
0749-0704/20/© 2019 Elsevier Inc. All rights reserved.

INTRODUCTION

Markers of disease have been used for centuries, but it was only really in the 1980s that the term, *biomarker*, came into widespread use. Biomarkers can range from simple physiologic measurements of, for example, pulse and blood pressure, to highly complex and expensive molecular or imaging variables. Since the early 1980s, biomarker research across all fields of medicine has increased dramatically and this expansion shows no sign of slowing down as new technology assists in facilitating the development of new biomarkers and assessing their place in modern medicine. In some fields, for example, oncology, biomarkers have played a key role in defining distinct disease entities that respond to specific treatments, enabling precision medicine to be applied to individual patients. In the critical care arena, progress has been much slower, partly because much critical illness, for example, ARDS and sepsis, is syndromic and heterogeneous rather than consisting of clearly defined, homogeneous disease states.[1,2] With increasing availability of data from large patient databases and improved technology to analyze and identify potential biomarkers, huge advances will be seen in this field in the future.

GENERAL BIOMARKER APPLICATIONS

Importantly, biomarkers can have multiple applications. The US Food and Drug Administration (FDA) and the National Institutes of Health have recently listed 7 categories of biomarker: susceptibility/risk, diagnostic, monitoring, prognostic, predictive, pharmacodynamic/response, and safety[3] (**Table 1**). There may be some overlap between categories and any 1 biomarker may meet the criteria for several different categories. The fictional case history at the beginning of this article demonstrates some of these uses, with biomarkers for diagnosis, prediction, therapeutic response, and prognosis. This article explores 2 of the key applications for biomarkers in the ICU, focusing on how each will likely evolve in the future.

Table 1
Categories of biomarker with some possible examples from critical care medicine

Category[a]	Example of Use…	…To Guide/Assess in This Context
Susceptibility/risk	ARDS, risk of respiratory arrest	Early endotracheal intubation
Diagnostic	Infection	Early and adequate antibiotic therapy
Monitoring	Fluid status	Fluid management
Prognostic	Risk of multiple organ failure /death	ICU admission
Predictive	Good outcome	ICU discharge
Pharmacodynamic/response	Serial sepsis biomarkers	Duration of antibiotic therapy
Safety	Chloride levels	Stop saline infusions

[a] Categories as proposed by the US Food and Drug Administration and the National Institutes of Health Biomarker Working Group.
Data from FDA-NIH Biomarker Working Group. BEST (Biomarkers, EndpointS, and other Tools) Resource: Glossary. Available at: https://www.ncbi.nlm.nih.gov/books/NBK338448/pdf/Bookshelf_NBK338448.pdf. Accessed 9/7/19.

Diagnostic Biomarkers

A diagnostic biomarker is used to identify or confirm the presence of a disease or condition.[4] The number of available diagnostic markers is vast, enabling identification of diseases ranging from myocardial infarction to prostate cancer to lactose intolerance. Some of these tests are highly sensitive for the condition in question, others much less so. The same applies to specificity. New diagnostic biomarkers are being developed on a daily basis as understanding of disease pathogenesis improves and ability to reliably detect and measure even very low concentrations of substances increases. The challenge is to ensure that such biomarkers are correctly validated and relevant. Moreover, diagnostic biomarkers are of limited interest if the information they provide is not associated with the ability to offer appropriate treatment of the condition in question or to influence clinical decision making so that patient outcomes can be improved. This is particularly true in critical care medicine.

Diagnostic markers also can be used to assess disease severity, which can be helpful when evaluating the need for aggressive therapies, such as a surgical intervention or a costly medication. Assessing severity also can help in deciding whether a patient in an emergency department should be oriented toward the ICU or the general floor. This type of biomarker use may be especially important in the middle of the night, when doctors are often less experienced or may not be fully awake. Increasingly, artificial intelligence and machine-learning systems will combine biomarker information with other elements, for example, patient age and medical history, to provide accurate patient triage based on known outcomes.[5]

Given the high morbidity and mortality associated with sepsis and the recognized importance of early appropriate management, availability of a biomarker able to accurately diagnose sepsis would be a major breakthrough. Over the years, many candidate markers of sepsis have been identified, proposed, and studied[6]; however, none is perfect and can unequivocally and reliably differentiate all patients with sepsis from those without. Even procalcitonin (PCT) and C-reactive protein, the 2 most widely studied sepsis biomarkers, have many limitations.[7] A major problem is the lack of a gold standard against which biomarkers can be tested: there is and will always be a gray zone between demonstrated, suspected, possible, and unlikely infections.[8]

Will there be better sepsis markers in the future? Unfortunately, given the highly complex nature of the sepsis response and the heterogeneity of the patients sepsis can affect, it is unlikely that 1 biomarker will be found that can definitively separate septic from nonseptic patients. Rather than relying on single biomarkers, combinations or panels of biomarkers probably will be used in the future. As an example, SeptiCyte (Immunexpress, Seattle, WA) is a test based on the expression of 4 key genes involved in the host response to infection: *CEACAM4*, *LAMP1*, *PLAC8*, and *PLA2G7*. Septicyte is the first host response gene expression assay authorized by the FDA for the diagnosis of sepsis in ICU patients. In a clinical trial,[9] the assay was able to differentiate sepsis from sepsis-like states on the first day of ICU admission with good sensitivity and specificity, combined in an area under the receiver operating characteristic curve of approximately 0.85. It performed better than other markers of sepsis, including PCT.[9] Nevertheless, the test results currently take an average of 6 hours to become available, limiting its usefulness to guide initiation of treatment. Clearly these time delays will be much shorter in the future.

In another approach, Langelier and colleagues[10] used metagenomics next-generation sequencing to develop pathogen, microbiome diversity, and host gene expression metrics to differentiate critically ill patients with lower tract respiratory infections from those without. Combining the 3 metrics together resulted in a negative predictive value of 100%. Combining bacterial and host characteristics will be a key feature of future biomarkers.

Importantly, markers of sepsis should be distinguished from tests to identify the presence of microorganisms. There is no doubt that rapidly identifying the presence of microorganisms will be possible in the near future,[11–13] without having to rely on time-consuming microbiological cultures. As these tests are refined and they are more widely used, the time needed to obtain a result will decrease from several hours to minutes, and the price, which remains a strong limitation to their use today, will go down. Nevertheless, the distinction between colonization and infection may never be entirely clear. Hence, it is likely that combinations of sepsis markers, to assess the presence of sepsis and its severity, with microbiological tests, to choose the correct antibiotic, will always be needed.

Response Biomarkers

Therapeutic response biomarkers are vitally important because they can help guide treatment decisions to optimize patient outcomes. Monitoring of biomarker levels over time after treatment start can help determine whether the treatment is effective or needs to be reviewed and altered. This approach is widely used in many medical conditions, including chronic hypertension and diabetes. In critical illness, response biomarkers will be increasingly used to guide antibiotic duration in sepsis, to decide when to start and stop RRT or to determine ongoing fluid needs.

Antibiotic doses and durations in patients with sepsis are largely determined from data in noncritically ill populations. Yet critically ill patients frequently have acute hepatic and renal dysfunction, which can influence drug metabolism and clearance; capillary leak and fluid resuscitation, which can alter volumes of distribution; and comorbid conditions that can also alter antibiotic response. Moreover, the rapid and multiple changes in physiologic alterations during critical illness make it difficult to predict how a patient will respond to a particular dose. Antibiotic doses, therefore, need to be individualized much more than is currently the case. This will be facilitated in the future by more rapid and widely available drug-level monitoring.

The duration of therapy is also important. Giving antibiotics for an arbitrary planned duration of 4 days, 7 days, or 10 days exposes patients to risk of inadequate or excessive treatment as well as increased risks of adverse events when treatment is prolonged and promotion of the development of resistance. Again, durations should be personalized based on identified pathogens and individual clinical response. Some patients will recover quickly even from bad infections, whereas others remain febrile and acutely ill for longer periods of time. Changes in levels of biomarkers over time may help adjust the duration of antibiotic therapy in individual patients. This approach has already been studied with several biomarkers, notably PCT and C-reactive protein. In a multicenter randomized controlled trial in the Netherlands, patients who received antibiotics for presumed infection were randomized to PCT-guided (advice to discontinue antibiotics if PCT decreased by 80% or more of its peak value or to less than or equal to 0.5 μg/L) or standard-of-care antibiotic discontinuation.[14] Antibiotic duration was lower in the PCT-guided group (absolute difference 1.22; 95% CI, 0.65–1.78; $P<.0001$) and mortality rates also were lower in this group. Importantly, however, although use of PCT to guide initiation of antibiotics in stable patients with respiratory tract infections was associated with reduced antibiotic durations with no increase in mortality,[15,16] in critically ill patients, use of PCT for initiation or escalation of antibiotics had no impact on antibiotic durations and was associated with worse outcomes.[17] In a meta-analysis of 15 studies in critically ill patients, Lam and colleagues[18] reported no difference in short-term mortality for studies using PCT to guide antibiotic initiation but lower mortality in studies using PCT to guide antibiotic discontinuation. Current recommendations for patients with sepsis suggest use of PCT only to guide antibiotic discontinuation.[19] PCT has now been approved by the FDA for use by clinicians to help guide antibiotic management decisions in patients with sepsis or lower respiratory tract infections. This strategy will be increasingly used in the future and should help decrease the emergence of multidrug resistant organisms, a major concern worldwide.

The use of biomarkers can also help identify the need to re-explore a source of sepsis. Hence, the evaluation of the time course of a biomarker will help assess patient course. Persistence of high levels of sepsis markers suggests that treatment is not effective and should trigger further reevaluation of the patient and repeated exploration for a possible source.[20]

THE FUTURE OF ORGAN-SPECIFIC BIOMARKERS

Biomarkers can provide important information related to organ function in critically ill patients in terms of diagnosis, prediction, prognosis, and treatment guidance and response (**Table 2**). As for sepsis, when considering organ function, the ability to diagnose organ dysfunction early is paramount so that treatments, if available, can be started promptly. Current markers are often limited by delay in appearance as well

Table 2
Examples of future applications of biomarkers per organ system

Organ System	Signal	Potential Therapeutic Implications
Cerebral	Encephalopathy Cell alterations	Cerebral/metabolic support Adapted monitoring Therapeutic limitation
Pulmonary	Overdistension/parenchymal alterations Respiratory muscle and diaphragmatic dysfunction	Decrease tidal volume Adjust PEEP level Start ECMO/ECCO2R Start corticosteroids Need for lung transplantation
Cardiovascular	Risk of myocardial ischemia Altered cell oxygen supply	Need for PTCA Antiplatelet agent Myocardial protective substance Need for LVAD/transplant
Renal	Altered perfusion Impending injury	Fluids (albumin?) Renal protective agents Specific vasoactive agent Start RRT Expect long-term failure
Coagulation	Subtle coagulopathy Endothelial activation	Adjust (anti)hemostatic agents Give an anticoagulant/endothelial protective agent (thrombomodulin?)
Gastrointestinal	Dysfunction	Withhold enteral nutrition Give a specific nutrient
Hepatic	Dysfunction	Liver protective agent Need for liver transplantation
Metabolic, cellular	Deficiencies	Add proteins, amino acids Add vitamins and other trace elements

Abbreviations: ECCO2R, extracorporeal CO_2 removal; LVAD, left ventricular assist device; PTCA, percutaneous transluminal coronary angioplasty.

as problems with sensitivity and specificity. Combinations of multiple markers in the future are likely to be more accurate than single markers.

Cerebral Function

Brain injury can be the result of direct and indirect brain injury, but, whatever the cause, cerebral biomarkers will increasingly be used to predict which patients will survive with a good as opposed to a bad neurologic outcome.[21,22] Accurate prediction of prognosis will help provide appropriate treatment, limit premature withdrawal of life-sustaining therapy in patients who may go on to survive with good outcomes, help inform discussions with relatives, and potentially reduce the economic burden on society.[23]

Several biomarkers have already been studied for this purpose, including neuron-specific enolase and S-100B protein, but many can be produced by extracerebral sources so are not specific to cerebral injury or can be influenced by other factors. MicroRNAs are so-called functional biomarkers that play an important role in the pathophysiology of organ dysfunction. Importantly, some microRNAs are tissue-specific, potentially making them valuable biomarkers of injury to the tissue in question.[23,24] Recently, Tissier and colleagues[25] analyzed gene expression profiles in comatose survivors of out-of-hospital cardiac arrest and, using functional enrichment analysis, identified differential expression of more than 300 genes, involved in innate and adaptative immunity, in patients with unfavorable compared with those with favorable outcomes. The transcriptomic signature was able to predict outcome already at hospital admission. Although single tests will never alone be sufficient to lead to a decision to withhold/withdraw life-sustaining therapy in these patients, as part of the total information available, they can help inform these difficult decisions.

Respiratory Function

Important future roles for biomarkers in patients with acute respiratory failure will be to accurately determine whether or when to start mechanical ventilation or extracorporeal membrane oxygenation (ECMO), how to adjust ventilatory conditions for an individual patient, and when and how to wean the patient from mechanical ventilation. Recently, latent class analysis has identified patients with ARDS who have different subphenotypes, based in part on differences in concentrations of the inflammatory biomarkers interleukin (IL)-6, IL-8, soluble tumor necrosis factor receptor 1 and plasminogen activator inhibitor 1. The 2 groups were found to respond differently to different fluid management strategies[26] and to different positive end-expiratory pressure (PEEP) settings[27] and had different responses to simvastatin treatment.[28]

Cardiovascular Function

Biomarkers will help evaluate more rapidly the presence myocardial function and the need for intervention, including some myocardial protection. Acute aortic syndromes, which are particularly challenging to diagnose, also will be more easily recognized, probably by combinations of several biomarkers.[29]

In circulatory shock, biomarkers will increasingly be used to evaluate the need for fluid therapy. For example, natriuretic peptides can reflect the degree of myocardial fiber distension and, therefore, potentially indicate adequate fluid status or fluid overload. Use of natriuretic peptides is already widespread in the diagnosis of heart failure,[30] but their usefulness in critically ill patients is unclear.[31] The combination of biomarkers with the colloid osmotic pressure and bioimpedance techniques could help identify and quantitate fluid overload.[32]

In addition to what some people call macrohemodynamic alterations, the role of the microcirculation in critical illness has gained interest in recent years as techniques have been developed that enable its assessment. Importantly, in patients with shock, microcirculatory changes persist even when global hemodynamic parameters seem to have normalized, making normalization of the microcirculation a potentially important resuscitation target. Markers of endothelial damage, such as endothelial progenitor cells and endothelial microparticles, have been associated with outcomes[33,34] and may help determine the best therapeutic support for the microcirculation and to monitor treatment success in the future.[33]

Renal Function

Evaluation of renal hemodynamics will help select the right drug, for example, angiotensin II in certain patients to increase postglomerular perfusion. Although not yet possible with sufficient accuracy,[35] renal biomarkers will be developed to decide when to start and when to stop RRT, thus avoiding unnecessary treatments in some and providing maximum benefit in others. They also can help predict long-term renal outcomes, which is important for organizational and sometimes ethical decisions. Several new biomarkers, urinary-based or blood-based, of renal dysfunction have been proposed in recent years and been shown to have various degrees of accuracy in prediction and prognosis, including insulin-like growth factor binding protein 7 and tissue inhibitor of metalloproteinase 2, neutrophil gelatinase–associated lipocalin, and kidney injury molecule-1. Combinations of these biomarkers are likely to be most useful[36] but some work remains to determine which panels are most effective for each purpose and to develop rapid point-of-care assays that can be used at the bedside.

Hemostatic Function

Biomarkers of coagulopathy can include markers of platelet activation and function, for example, platelet-derived microparticles.[37] Markers of endothelial cell dysfunction can also indicate development and prognosis of coagulopathy. Panels of different biomarkers will enable the underlying cause of the coagulopathy to be identified enabling appropriate treatment.

Gastrointestinal Function

The importance of adequate nutrition in ICU patients is well recognized but the ability to provide correct nutrition to individual patients is currently limited. Biomarkers of gastrointestinal function will enable in evaluating the potential benefits but also the likely risks of enteral feeding more accurately. Instead of the vague current recommendation that enteral nutrition should be withheld in the presence of profound shock,[38] quantifying the precise degree of gut impairment and its evolution over time will be possible, enabling feeding to be started in a timely manner.

Biomarkers will also enable the diagnosis of certain conditions, for example, acute mesenteric ischemia, to be made noninvasively instead of surgically,[39] thus reducing risks associated with surgery and anesthesia and making diagnosis, and therefore treatment initiation, more rapid.

Hepatic Support

Few interventions are currently available that can improve liver function, but new liver support systems and drugs for hepatic protection are being developed. Current markers of liver dysfunction or injury, including bilirubin and liver enzymes, are elevated late in the disease course, and biomarkers that can identify liver dysfunction early are needed.

THERANOSTICS

The term, *theranostics*, refers to the use of techniques, including biomarkers and phenotypes, to guide therapeutic interventions. This approach is widely used in cancer therapy and in rheumatoid arthritis.[40] In the field of sepsis, it is highly unlikely that sepsis drugs that are effective in all patients will be developed, because of the complexity of the condition, with an immune response that changes over time and varies among individuals. Rather, a theranostic approach will increasingly be used. For example, corticosteroids in septic shock will be guided by genetic expression signatures or metabolic response.[41,42] Corticosteroids in patients with ARDS may be guided by a mediator in the bronchoalveolar fluid. In a multicenter study by Steinberg and colleagues,[43] mortality rates were lower in patients with ARDS treated with methylprednisolone who had high bronchoalveolar procollagen type III levels compared with those who had lower levels. A randomized controlled trial is currently ongoing to assess whether procollagen II can indeed be used to guide corticosteroid use in persistent ARDS (Procollagen-3 Driven Corticosteroids for Persistent Acute Respiratory Distress Syndrome; ClinicalTrials.gov Identifier: NCT03371498).

In a retrospective analysis, Seymour and colleagues[44] identified 4 clinical phenotypes of sepsis based on clinical characteristics and organ dysfunction patterns. The different phenotypes were associated with different outcomes and different measures of host-response measured using biomarkers of coagulation, inflammation, and endothelial and renal injury. Importantly, in simulation models, estimated treatment effects of early goal-directed therapy, activated protein C, and eritoran varied according to the relative frequencies of the 4 phenotypes, suggesting these phenotypes could potentially identify groups of patients more likely to respond to these interventions. As discussed previously, latent class analysis has identified subphenotypes of ARDS that respond differently to different management strategies.[26–28]

SUMMARY

The numbers of biomarkers in critical care medicine is increasing rapidly, but there is a real need to improve analysis and validation. Groups, such as the Operation Brain Trauma Therapy,[45] a multicenter preclinical therapy and biomarker screening consortium, will help speed progress in this field, and big data analytics and machine learning will facilitate translation of research to clinical application.[46]

Although it is not impossible that a biomarker will be 100% sensitive and 100% specific for a certain condition or application, it is clear that the vast majority of biomarkers will not attain this ideal. Combined panels of biomarkers, therefore, will increasingly be used[9,36] rather than focusing on single compounds, especially as technology enables multiple markers to be assessed simultaneously from 1 blood sample or sensor at point of care and costs begin to decrease (**Table 3**). Importantly, biomarkers should not be used alone to make diagnostic, prognostic, or treatment decisions but rather to guide them, combined with physician expertise and clinical judgment.[47] The focus on traditional markers, for example, proteins and cytokines, has begun to move toward newer omics markers,[48] using transcriptomics, metabolomics, and genomics. The potential for use of biomarkers to advance the move toward personalized medicine is exciting. As new biomarkers appear and are validated, panels with have to be altered accordingly and increasingly it will be possible to accurately predict and diagnose conditions and complications, target treatments for individual patients and monitor doses and treatment durations, and prognosticate short-term and long-term outcomes. The future of biomarkers will be one of constant evolution.

Table 3
General evolution of biomarker characteristics over time

Characteristic	Present	Future
Sensitivity	Very good	Very good (even better)
Specificity	Very good	Very good (even better)
Reproducibility	Very good	Very good (even better)
Cost	High	Low
Practicality	Complex methods	Simplified test
Delay in obtaining the results	Long	Short

REFERENCES

1. Ware LB. Biomarkers in critical illness: new insights and challenges for the future. Am J Respir Crit Care Med 2017;196:944–5.
2. Sweeney TE, Khatri P. Generalizable biomarkers in critical care: toward precision medicine. Crit Care Med 2017;45:934–9.
3. FDA-NIH Biomarker Working Group. BEST (biomarkers, EndpointS, and other tools) resource: glossary. Available at: https://www.ncbi.nlm.nih.gov/books/NBK338448/pdf/Bookshelf_NBK338448.pdf. Accessed July 7, 2019.
4. Califf RM. Biomarker definitions and their applications. Exp Biol Med (Maywood) 2018;243:213–21.
5. Raita Y, Goto T, Faridi MK, et al. Emergency department triage prediction of clinical outcomes using machine learning models. Crit Care 2019;23:64.
6. Pierrakos C, Vincent JL. Sepsis biomarkers: a review. Crit Care 2010;14:R15.
7. Vincent JL, Van NM, Lelubre C. Host response biomarkers in sepsis: the role of procalcitonin. Methods Mol Biol 2015;1237:213–24.
8. European Society of Intensive Care Medicine. The problem of sepsis. An expert report of the European Society of Intensive Care Medicine. Intensive Care Med 1994;20:300–4.
9. Miller RR III, Lopansri BK, Burke JP, et al. Validation of a host response assay, SeptiCyte LAB, for discriminating sepsis from systemic inflammatory response syndrome in the ICU. Am J Respir Crit Care Med 2018;198:903–13.
10. Langelier C, Kalantar KL, Moazed F, et al. Integrating host response and unbiased microbe detection for lower respiratory tract infection diagnosis in critically ill adults. Proc Natl Acad Sci U S A 2018;115:E12353–62.
11. Vincent JL, Brealey D, Libert N, et al. Rapid Diagnosis of Infection in the Critically III (RADICAL), a multicenter study of molecular detection in bloodstream infections, pneumonia and sterile site infections. Crit Care Med 2015;43:2283–91.
12. Jagtap P, Singh R, Deepika K, et al. A flowthrough assay for rapid bedside stratification of bloodstream bacterial infection in critically ill patients: a pilot study. J Clin Microbiol 2018;56 [pii:e00408-18].
13. Zhang C, Zheng X, Zhao C, et al. Detection of pathogenic microorganisms from bloodstream infection specimens using TaqMan array card technology. Sci Rep 2018;8:12828.
14. de Jong E, van Oers JA, Beishuizen A, et al. Efficacy and safety of procalcitonin guidance in reducing the duration of antibiotic treatment in critically ill patients: a randomised, controlled, open-label trial. Lancet Infect Dis 2016;16:819–27.

15. Christ-Crain M, Stolz D, Bingisser R, et al. Procalcitonin guidance of antibiotic therapy in community-acquired pneumonia: a randomized trial. Am J Respir Crit Care Med 2006;174:84–93.

16. Schuetz P, Christ-Crain M, Thomann R, et al. Effect of procalcitonin-based guidelines vs standard guidelines on antibiotic use in lower respiratory tract infections: the ProHOSP randomized controlled trial. JAMA 2009;302:1059–66.

17. Jensen JU, Hein L, Lundgren B, et al. Procalcitonin-guided interventions against infections to increase early appropriate antibiotics and improve survival in the intensive care unit: a randomized trial. Crit Care Med 2011;39:2048–58.

18. Lam SW, Bauer SR, Fowler R, et al. Systematic review and meta-analysis of procalcitonin-guidance versus usual care for antimicrobial management in critically ill patients: focus on subgroups based on antibiotic initiation, cessation, or mixed strategies. Crit Care Med 2018;46:684–90.

19. Rhodes A, Evans LE, Alhazzani W, et al. Surviving sepsis campaign: international guidelines for management of sepsis and septic shock: 2016. Crit Care Med 2017;45:486–552.

20. Schmit X, Vincent JL. The time course of blood C-reactive protein concentrations in relation to the response to initial antimicrobial therapy in patients with sepsis. Infection 2008;36:213–9.

21. Annborn M, Nilsson F, Dankiewicz J, et al. The combination of biomarkers for prognostication of long-term outcome in patients treated with mild hypothermia after out-of-hospital cardiac arrest-A pilot study. Ther Hypothermia Temp Manag 2016;6:85–90.

22. Isenschmid C, Kalt J, Gamp M, et al. Routine blood markers from different biological pathways improve early risk stratification in cardiac arrest patients: results from the prospective, observational COMMUNICATE study. Resuscitation 2018; 130:138–45.

23. Devaux Y, Stammet P. What's new in prognostication after cardiac arrest: micro-RNAs? Intensive Care Med 2018;44:897–9.

24. Devaux Y, Dankiewicz J, Salgado-Somoza A, et al. Association of circulating microRNA-124-3p levels with outcomes after out-of-hospital cardiac arrest: a substudy of a randomized clinical trial. JAMA Cardiol 2016;1:305–13.

25. Tissier R, Hocini H, Tchitchek N, et al. Early blood transcriptomic signature predicts patients' outcome after out-of-hospital cardiac arrest. Resuscitation 2019; 138:222–32.

26. Famous KR, Delucchi K, Ware LB, et al. Acute respiratory distress syndrome subphenotypes respond differently to randomized fluid management strategy. Am J Respir Crit Care Med 2017;195:331–8.

27. Calfee CS, Delucchi K, Parsons PE, et al. Subphenotypes in acute respiratory distress syndrome: latent class analysis of data from two randomised controlled trials. Lancet Respir Med 2014;2:611–20.

28. Calfee CS, Delucchi KL, Sinha P, et al. Acute respiratory distress syndrome subphenotypes and differential response to simvastatin: secondary analysis of a randomised controlled trial. Lancet Respir Med 2018;6:691–8.

29. Yildiz M, Oksen D, Behnes M, et al. Contribution and value of biomarkers in acute aortic syndromes. Curr Pharm Biotechnol 2017;18:495–8.

30. Chow SL, Maisel AS, Anand I, et al. Role of biomarkers for the prevention, assessment, and management of heart failure: a Scientific Statement from the American Heart Association. Circulation 2017;135:e1054–91.

31. Matsuo A, Nagai-Okatani C, Nishigori M, et al. Natriuretic peptides in human heart: novel insight into their molecular forms, functions, and diagnostic use. Peptides 2019;111:3–17.
32. Massari F, Scicchitano P, Iacoviello M, et al. Serum biochemical determinants of peripheral congestion assessed by bioimpedance vector analysis in acute heart failure. Heart Lung 2019;48(5):395–9.
33. Tapia P, Gatica S, Cortes-Rivera C, et al. Circulating endothelial cells from septic shock patients convert to fibroblasts are associated with the resuscitation fluid dose and are biomarkers for survival prediction. Crit Care Med 2019;47:942–50.
34. van Ierssel SH, Jorens PG, Van Craenenbroeck EM, et al. The endothelium, a protagonist in the pathophysiology of critical illness: focus on cellular markers. Biomed Res Int 2014;2014:985813.
35. Klein SJ, Brandtner AK, Lehner GF, et al. Biomarkers for prediction of renal replacement therapy in acute kidney injury: a systematic review and meta-analysis. Intensive Care Med 2018;44:323–36.
36. Kashani K, Al-Khafaji A, Ardiles T, et al. Discovery and validation of cell cycle arrest biomarkers in human acute kidney injury. Crit Care 2013;17:R25.
37. Melki I, Tessandier N, Zufferey A, et al. Platelet microvesicles in health and disease. Platelets 2017;28:214–21.
38. Singer P, Blaser AR, Berger MM, et al. ESPEN guideline on clinical nutrition in the intensive care unit. Clin Nutr 2019;38:48–79.
39. Treskes N, Persoon AM, van Zanten ARH. Diagnostic accuracy of novel serological biomarkers to detect acute mesenteric ischemia: a systematic review and meta-analysis. Intern Emerg Med 2017;12:821–36.
40. Kaneko Y, Takeuchi T. Targeted antibody therapy and relevant novel biomarkers for precision medicine for rheumatoid arthritis. Int Immunol 2017;29:511–7.
41. Wong HR, Atkinson SJ, Cvijanovich NZ, et al. Combining prognostic and predictive enrichment strategies to identify children with septic shock responsive to corticosteroids. Crit Care Med 2016;44:e1000–3.
42. Antcliffe DB, Burnham KL, Al-Beidh F, et al. Transcriptomic signatures in sepsis and a differential response to steroids. From the VANISH randomized trial. Am J Respir Crit Care Med 2019;199:980–6.
43. Steinberg KP, Hudson LD, Goodman RB, et al. Efficacy and safety of corticosteroids for persistent acute respiratory distress syndrome. N Engl J Med 2006;354:1671–84.
44. Seymour CW, Kennedy JN, Wang S, et al. Derivation, validation, and potential treatment implications of novel clinical phenotypes for sepsis. JAMA 2019;321:2003–17.
45. Kochanek PM, Dixon CE, Mondello S, et al. Multi-center pre-clinical consortia to enhance translation of therapies and biomarkers for traumatic brain injury: Operation Brain Trauma Therapy and beyond. Front Neurol 2018;9:640.
46. Vincent JL, Creteur J. Big data are here to stay. Anaesth Crit Care Pain Med 2019;38:339–40.
47. Vincent JL, Teixeira L. Sepsis biomarkers. Value and limitations. Am J Respir Crit Care Med 2014;190:1081–2.
48. Rello J, van Engelen TSR, Alp E, et al. Towards precision medicine in sepsis: a position paper from the European Society of Clinical Microbiology and Infectious Diseases. Clin Microbiol Infect 2018;24:1264–72.

Moving?

Make sure your subscription moves with you!

To notify us of your new address, find your **Clinics Account Number** (located on your mailing label above your name), and contact customer service at:

Email: journalscustomerservice-usa@elsevier.com

800-654-2452 (subscribers in the U.S. & Canada)
314-447-8871 (subscribers outside of the U.S. & Canada)

Fax number: 314-447-8029

Elsevier Health Sciences Division
Subscription Customer Service
3251 Riverport Lane
Maryland Heights, MO 63043

*To ensure uninterrupted delivery of your subscription, please notify us at least 4 weeks in advance of move.

ELSEVIER